The Pathophysiology
of Psyche

The Pathophysiology of Psyche

La Maladie de Psychisme

Darko Pozder

To order additional copies of this book, contact:
Xlibris
AU TFN: 1 800 844 927 (Toll Free inside Australia)
AU Local: 0283 108 187 (+61 2 8310 8187 from outside Australia)
www.Xlibris.com.au
Orders@Xlibris.com.au
824015

CONTENTS

I dedicate this book to my beloved parents Djuro and Jadranka.
Ante familia nihil venit (Before my family comes nothing).

PREFACE

Depression is as rare as the individual who has not experienced its touch and as old as the `human race. At times with no obvious reason, a person experiences too much sadness where the world becomes grey. For some people, this experience is momentary, or something one can dismiss with good sense or practical actions. Nevertheless, for some people, this experience is like a prison whose wall is impenetrable or a ghost whose presence ruins every happy occasion. In the twenty-first century, depression has been referred to as a disease and treated with various therapies and pills. For some people, this treatment has beneficial, and the depression issue is permanently solved. Nonetheless, for some individuals, therapy and medicines bring temporary relief only, and they have to seek for natural methods for relief.

Mental health is ever-changing and vibrant; this book looks at various aspects of depression, borderline personality disorder, narcissism, post-traumatic stress disorder, and schizophrenia. Chapter 1 begins by defining depression and looking at the different types of depression. The relationship between depression and brain anatomy is an issue that cannot be ignored; therefore, this chapter addresses this issue in depth. Does depression cause inflammation or is the opposite true? This has been discussed in chapter 2. There exists a correlation between the immune system, depression, and neurological disorders; chapter 3 looks at this correlation. At times depression can be resistant to conventional treatment; chapter 4 discusses how buprenorphine can be used to treat this kind of depression and how buprenorphine's chemical structure should be used in order to develop a new more effective mu opioid receptor and antagonist at the kappa receptors.

People's way of life (lifestyle) has significantly contributed to depression. Many people nowadays are eating junk foods, are living sedentary lifestyles, have become addicted to illegal substances, nicotine, and alcohol. This kind of lifestyle has increased the risk of depression among many people. Chapter 5 addresses the impact this lifestyle has on depression and measures those engaged in such destructive habits can adopt to reduce their risk of depression or learn how to manage their depressive symptoms. Possible causes, neurological roots, brain anatomy, comorbid diagnosis, and common misdiagnosis of borderline personality disorder, as well as self-harm and narcissism, is pinpointed in chapters 6 and 7. Chapter 8 is stressing about current unsuccessful treatments for borderline personality disorder; therefore, new promising treatments are proposed in chapter 9. What is a hidden relationship between a silence stroke and PTDS symptoms is discussed in chapter 10. The last chapter is looking deep into the direct correlation between structural damages of gastrointestinal tract and antibodies as well as their impact on brain-derived neurotropic factor or BDNF and neuroplasticity in people diagnosed with schizophrenia spectrum disorders. In addition, new treatments are proposed such as faecal transplant and anti-inflammatory diet to improved symptoms and quality of life of people diagnosed with schizophrenia.

It is more important to know what sort of person has a disease than to know what sort of disease a person has.

—Hippocrates

CHAPTER 1

Introduction

Depression as a mental illness fills both the print and mass media news regularly; it can be described as an illness that adversely affects how a person feels, acts, and thinks. It is normal to feel depressed or sad when faced with life's stressors; nevertheless, when these feelings of hopelessness and sadness become intense, and last for extended periods, this could be an indication of depression. Depression can make an individual lose interest in things which they once enjoyed. Depression can be described as a mood disorder which leads to constant feelings of unhappiness (Moragne, 2011).

Based on the *Diagnostic and Statistical Manual of Mental Disorders* (*DSM*-5) diagnostic criteria, a mental health practitioner can diagnose depression when several symptoms are present. These symptoms include experiencing depressed mood throughout the day, and particularly in the morning (no author found, 2013). Also, the constant lack of energy daily can be a symptom of depression according to the *DSM*-5 criteria. Other symptoms of depression might entail feelings of guilt and worthlessness, lack of sleep, or sleeping extensively, and feeling suicidal (Moragne, 2011).

An individual can also be said to be experiencing depression if they portray no interest in things which previously they enjoyed. Additionally, according to *DSM*-5, the inability to make decisions, remember details, and restlessness could be an indication of depression. Five of these symptoms should be present for more than two weeks, for an individual to be diagnosed as being affected by depression, according to *DSM*-5 (Roberts and Louie, 2015).

During the diagnosis, the mental health professional should rule out that the symptoms named above are not a result of other medical conditions or a direct result of some medications the person could be using. Depression can impede an individual's capacity to enjoy life, sleep, study, and work. At times, the person that is affected by depression may experience intense feelings of hopelessness without any relief (Roberts and Louie, 2015). People that have experienced depression describe it differently; some say that they feel empty and lifeless, while others describe what they feel, as having a fear of looming doom (Roberts and Louie, 2015). Whichever way an individual experiences depression; if the condition is not treated it can develop into a severe health condition.

Depression affects people of all ages, races, and genders and social, economic status; this means that men, women, and adolescents are all at risk of developing depression. The symptoms of depression seem to vary based on gender and age. For instance, among men, depression often manifests in the form of fatigue, changes in sleep patterns, becoming easily irritable, and losing interest in hobbies and work (Lynch and Kilmartin, 2013). On the other hand, women experiencing depression often talk of experiencing intense emotions of guilt, sleeping excessively, and gaining weight due to overeating (Lynch and Kilmartin, 2013).

Among teenagers and adolescents, depression may be expressed through anger, becoming short-tempered, and experiencing physical pains such as stomach aches and headaches (Springer, Rubin, and Beevers, 2011). For the older adults affected by depression, they tend to talk more concerning their physical and not emotional symptoms. Some of them complain of loss of memory, fatigue, and physical pains that cannot be explained (Serani, 2016). The older adults might also become negligent regarding their physical appearance and may even cease from taking medicines that are critical for their health.

Other long-term illnesses such as schizophrenia, obsessive

compulsive disorder, and anxiety can come as a result of depression. According to the World Health Organization 2015 statistics, over three hundred million individuals were affected by depression by 2015. The study also stated that men are less likely to experience depression than women. Depression has also been shown to be a significant cause of death through suicide among young people aged between fifteen to twenty-nine years.

Anxiety

Anxiety can be described as a person's natural reaction to stressful situations. It is a term that is often used to describe various disorders that lead to worry, fear, nervousness, and dread (Freeman and Freeman, 2012). Anxiety refers to feelings of apprehension and fear regarding the future. If the anxious feelings last for extended periods, are intense, and impede a person's life, then this can be termed as an anxiety disorder life (Hyman and Pedrick, 2012). The various disorders associated with anxiety influence how an individual acts and feels.

Anxiety and anxiety disorders are different in that anxiety that is normal though unpleasant may encourage an individual to work more. Also, normal anxiety does not last for long and does not obstruct an individual's life. On the contrary, a person that is experiencing an anxiety disorder is always anxious, and the anxiety tends to interfere with their life (Hyman and Pedrick, 2012).

Any person, regardless of their age, race, gender, or socioeconomic class, can be affected by anxiety disorders. Some of the symptoms of anxiety include restlessness, breathing rapidly, difficulty in concentrating and falling asleep (Hyman and Pedrick, 2012).

Various factors can lead to anxiety, and they include, among others genetics, where the condition is inherited (Daitch, 2011). Additionally, environmental factors, for example, traumatic events in a person's life, financial challenges, and stresses that come from work or relationships, can cause anxiety (Daitch, 2011). Medical factors like stress arising from specific medical conditions, or the adverse side effects of particular medications and individual could be using, can also lead to anxiety.

According to the *Diagnostic and Statistical Manual of Mental Disorders* (*DSM*-5), general anxiety can be diagnosed by checking if the individual is experiencing symptoms that indicate the presence of the disorder (ISHIBASHI, 2015). For instance, for the generalised anxiety disorder, the mental health professionals check to see if the person has difficulty in managing their worry.

The other symptom which is used to determine the presence of generalised anxiety is ascertaining if the person has experienced the worry for more than six months (ISHIBASHI, 2015). The professional also checks if the fear is accompanied by symptoms of restlessness, fatigue, disturbances in sleep, challenges in concentrating, muscle stiffness, and irritability.

There are various types of anxiety disorders, namely generalised anxiety disorder, panic disorders, social anxiety disorder, separation anxiety disorders, among others. Based on *DSM*-5, the panic disorder is characterised by sweating, shaking or trembling, palpitations, fear of death, the fear of losing one's mind, and smothering, among others. During diagnosis, the mental health practitioner should rule out the existence of other likely causes of the attack, such as substance abuse or other health conditions (Roberts and Louie, 2015).

Regarding social anxiety, *DSM*-5 defines the condition as the fear that is constant concerning social situations, where the individual is afraid that they might act in embarrassing ways. For a person to be diagnosed with social anxiety disorder, they should have experienced constant fear for more than six months (First, 2014). When the individual that is experiencing social fear is exposed to the situation that they are afraid of, they immediately become afraid. Often, the individual realises that the fear they are experiencing is unreasonable. Furthermore, the person tends to avoid the feared social situations, or they might endure them with extreme anxiety (First, 2014).

Another anxiety disorder is the social separation disorder which *DSM*-5 states that it is a condition that starts during one's childhood and seldom during adolescence. Some of the symptoms of the disorder include excessive fear when expecting separation (Nussbaum, 2013). Additionally, as a response to the fear of being separated from others, the person might demonstrate extreme worry concerning experiencing an adverse event such as illness or becoming lost (Silove *et al.*, 2010).

Often, anxiety is left untreated, and only when an individual experiences complications from the condition do they seek treatment. Anxiety disorders can be treated in various ways, namely therapies such as psychotherapy and cognitive behavioural therapy (Starcevic, 2010). Moreover, medications such as antidepressants, selective serotonin reuptake inhibitor, or sedatives can be used to alleviate the symptoms of the anxiety (Kramer, 2015). Self-care, which involves physical exercises, management of stress, and relaxation techniques have also proven to be a great way of controlling the symptoms of anxiety.

Homeostasis, Depression, and Anxiety

Homeostasis can be defined as an attempt by the body to sustain an internal environment that is both continuous and stable; this necessitates constant observation and adjustment to the changes in the conditions. The regulation of the physiological systems in the body is referred to as homeostatic regulation, which involves the receptor, the effector, and the control centre.

The receptor gets the message that there is something within the environment that is changing. The control centre receives the message from the receptor and processes it; the effector as a response can either oppose or boost the stimulus. This process is continuous and works at sustaining homeostasis. For instance, when the body is regulating temperature, the skin receptors communicate to the brain which is the control centre, and this information is relayed to the effectors (sweat glands and blood vessels) in the skin. The objective of homeostasis is to maintain equilibrium in the body.

Extended periods of depression, if not treated, can significantly affect an individual's body and emotions. Depression can have a significant impact on homeostasis, continuous feelings of worthlessness, hopelessness, and low moods can significantly disturb the body's metabolism. If these symptoms related to depression are not treated, it can lead to other disorders such as major depressive disorder, fibromyalgia, generalised anxiety disorder, and depression, among others. These conditions can also adversely impact the physical body of a person through lethargy, headaches, and weight issues.

Anxiety tends to activate the brain's limbic system by putting on the flight or fight survival reaction, which in turn controls an individual's feelings, perceptions, and body reactions. After the activation of the limbic system, the person tends to feel threatened even though the situation they are in might not be threatening. Being in a *limbic state,* it disrupts the physiological reaction or homeostasis, where the adrenaline levels are increased, the heart rate and blood pressure also rises. The person might also experience, digestion that is inhibited, some tension in their muscles and shortness in their breath.

It is necessary to bring back to normal the internal environment which has been disrupted by anxiety to avoid an adverse impact on a person's well-being and health. The person that is experiencing anxiety can bring back to normal their internal environment through therapy, mindfulness, or various medications.

Types of Depression

There are various types of depression namely melancholia, major depressive disorder, psychotic depression, manic depression/ bipolar I, II, mixed, antenatal and postnatal depression, cyclothymic disorder, and seasonal affective disorder.

Melancholia

This is a major depressive disorder where the affected person exhibits melancholic traits. Melancholia is a type of depression where the affected person loses interest in nearly everything (Andrews, 2010). Those affected by the melancholic depression tend to feel hopeless and sad; their sleep patterns and appetite are also adversely affected. A particular event rarely triggers the melancholic episodes; the person's mood rarely improves even for short periods.

For an individual to be diagnosed with melancholic depression, several symptoms have to be present. These symptoms include the presence of an intense emptiness, where the person is not sad due to the events that might have occurred in their life such as the diagnosis of an incurable disease or the death of a loved one (Andrews, 2010). Another symptom that indicates melancholia is the depression seems to be worse in the morning. Weight loss and guilt that is inappropriate could be other symptoms of melancholia.

Melancholic depression can also lead to feelings of anxiety and irritability, difficulties in concentration, and changes in appetite where the person either eats too little or too much (Andrews, 2010). Some of the causes of melancholic depression are believed to be biological, where the individual may have inherited it from their parents. Environmental factors such as life stressors can also cause this kind of depression. Melancholia is often experienced during old age and can be mistaken for dementia.

The severity and type of melancholic depression vary from one person to another, where most of these symptoms are manageable and treatable.

The Treatment of Melancholia

After an individual has been diagnosed with melancholic depression treatment should ensue immediately. Some of how this kind of depression is treated and managed includes

➢ *medication*—this is mostly recommended since the primary cause of the depression is biological as no other causes have so far been established. Various antidepressants can be used to treat melancholia; some of those employed are selective serotonin reuptake inhibitors (SSRIs) (Acton, 2012).

The selective serotonin reuptake inhibitors antidepressant works by altering the way through which the neurotransmitter serotonin works in an individual's brain thereby improving their mood, some of the medications under this class include Lexapro, Paxil, and Zoloft.

Another antidepressant that is used to treat melancholia is the serotonin-norepinephrine reuptake inhibitors (SNRIs), which affect the work of norepinephrine and serotonin in the brain. Atypical antidepressants such as Oleptro, Viibryd, and Brintellix, can also be used to improve the affected individual's mood.

➢ *therapy*—at times melancholic depression can become resistant to medications or antidepressants (Taylor and Fink, 2006). In such circumstances, psychotherapy such as cognitive behavioural therapy, group, and interpersonal therapy is recommended. Through cognitive behavioural therapy, the affected individual learns ways to change their negative pattern of thinking and develop a positive mindset (Taylor and Fink, 2006).

Interpersonal therapy is also useful as it focuses on interpersonal relationships and looks into areas that could be aggravating the symptoms of melancholia. This therapy is aimed at assisting the affected person in enhancing their interpersonal relationships and changing their expectancy level regarding them (Taylor and Fink, 2006).

The process of learning how to cope with melancholic depression is long, but the person should not lose hope. Though the journey to recovery might be extended, combining therapy, medication, and a strong support system might ease the melancholic symptoms and enable the individual to live a healthier and happier life.

Major Depression/Major Depressive Disorder

Major depression is often characterised by a lack of interest in external stimuli and feeling sad (Pierce, 2018). The major depressive disorder is a mental disorder that is often characterised by low moods for more than two weeks. The *Diagnostic Statistical Manual of Mental Disorder (DSM)* has laid down the criteria to be followed in diagnosing an individual with a major depressive disorder. The person should at least have more than five of the symptom which *DSM* has laid down as being an indication of the presence of a major depressive disorder.

Some of the symptoms *DSM* has laid down as criteria for diagnosing major depression entail constant feelings of irritability and sadness (McIntyre and Nathanson, 2010). Also, the loss of interest in activities which previously the person might have enjoyed and the feelings of restlessness could be an indication of major depression. Other symptoms of major depression, according to *DSM*, include lack of sleep or sleeping excessively and gaining or losing weight and changes in the individual's appetite. Lack of energy, feelings of guilt or worthlessness, trouble in concentrating, and thoughts of suicide can also be an indication of a major depressive disorder (McIntyre and Nathanson, 2010).

The actual cause of the major depressive disorder remains unknown, but stress and biological factors can affect the chemistry of the brain, thereby decreasing an individual's ability to sustain the stability of their mood (Kim, 2017). Additionally, hormonal imbalances could also trigger major depressive disorder. Alcohol, substance and drug abuse, some types of medical conditions, for instance, cancer, and some kinds of medications such as steroids can all trigger major depression.

Treating Major Depression

After an individual has been diagnosed with a major depressive disorder, there is a need to commence treatment immediately, some of the ways of treating this condition include

> ➢ *medication*—antidepressants such as selective serotonin reuptake inhibitors (SSRIs) are often prescribed to treat major depression. SSRIs help in preventing the serotonin breakdown in the brain, which leads to higher levels of this neurotransmitter, which might increase the individual's mood and sleeping pattern (Acton, 2012). Atypical depressants can also be used in case other drugs have failed.

> ➢ *psychotherapy*—individuals affected by major depression can benefit from talk therapy, where the therapist and the person meet regularly to talk concerning the condition and other associated issues. Psychotherapy might help the individual to adjust to events that are stressful in their life. Additionally, it might assist them in replacing their negative thoughts and beliefs with those that are healthy (Taylor and Fink, 2006).

> Psychotherapy is also beneficial in assisting an individual in developing high self-esteem and in discovering better ways of coping with difficulties and solving problems. An individual is also through psychotherapy able to regain control over their life.

> ➢ *changes in one's lifestyle*—a person can learn how to manage the symptoms of major depression through lifestyle changes. Some of the lifestyle changes entail having a healthy

diet, avoiding alcohol, substance abuse, and foods that are processed (Thanavaro and Moore, 2017).

Alcohol tends to worsen the symptoms of the major depression as it is a nervous system depressant.

Although some of the symptoms of a major depressive disorder can make the affected individual feel extremely tired, it is essential for them to become physically active to enhance their mood. Also, having adequate sleep can be crucial in managing major depressive disorder (Thanavaro and Moore, 2017). In circumstances that the affected person is having trouble sleeping, they should talk to their doctor.

Psychotic Depression

Psychotic depression is one that occurs mostly in people that are affected by a major depressive disorder or bipolar disorder. This kind of depression involves some psychosis such as hallucinations where the individual hears voices or delusions where they experience intense feelings of failure or worthlessness. Psychotic depression can make the affected person not to be in touch with reality (Swartz and Shorter, 2007). For instance, the person might believe that those around have plans of harming them or that evil spirits possess them.

Psychotic depression can lead to unwarranted anger, or the affected individual might spend their time alone or sleeping during daytime and being awake at night. The person could also become negligent concerning their physical appearance by not changing their clothes or even bathing. At times, the person's speech can also become incoherent; also the delusions or hallucination which these people experience are often linked with depressive thoughts and feelings such as hopelessness and helplessness (Swartz and Shorter, 2007).

Some of the symptoms that could be indications of psychotic

depression are anxiety, becoming easily agitated, hallucinations or delusions, insomnia, becoming physically immobile, and experiencing intellectual impairment (Swartz and Shorter, 2007). More than half of the individuals that are affected by the psychosis depression experience various delusions that are not accompanied by hallucinations. Moreover, most of the individuals affected by this kind of depression cannot experience pleasure (anhedonia).

Psychotic depression is often genetic, but other factors make an individual prone to the disorder. Some of these factors are gender—women are more prone to psychotic depression than men, also a difficult childhood can make one predisposed, thus developing this condition.

The Treatment of Psychotic Depression

Generally, psychotic depression is done in a hospital set-up for the mental health professionals to monitor the patient closely. The treatment of this condition can be done through ways such as

> ➢ *medication*—there are various medications which can be used in stabilising the mood of the affected individual; they include antipsychotic drugs and antidepressants. The antipsychotic drugs tend to impact the neurotransmitter which permits the communication amongst the nerve cells in regions of the brain which controls a person's capacity to recognise and manage information around them (Rothschild, 2010).

> Some of the antipsychotic medications commonly used are cariprazine, risperidone, and olanzapine, among others. The medicines are usually effective in treating the psychotic depression, where those affected tend to recover within a few months.

> ***electroconvulsive therapy (ECT)***—when the psychotic depression does not respond to medication, electroconvulsive therapy can be used (Ottosson and Fink, 2012). ECT entails passing electric current that is cautiously controlled through a person's brain. Electroconvulsive therapy is used when the condition seems to be life-threatening or when other treatments have failed. This therapy can decrease symptoms of depression that are severe more than other forms of treatment (Ottosson and Fink, 2012).

Some of the side effects of electroconvulsive therapy include loss of memory a condition that resolves after several weeks but can extend for more extended periods. Owing to this side effect, electroconvulsive therapy should only be provided with the individual's full consent that is if they can provide their consent. In situations where the person is incapable of providing their consent, their caregivers and family can do so with the approval of the necessary mental health authorities.

Antenatal and Postnatal Depression

Antenatal or prenatal depression refers to a clinical depression, which affects a pregnant woman during the duration of the pregnancy. Antenatal depression can adversely impact foetal development, later causing harm to both the child and the mother. Some of the symptoms associated with antenatal depression include having feelings of numbness, worthlessness, and worthlessness. The affected woman might also feel emotional, irritable, angry, and resentful of others (Curham, 2012). Other symptoms of antenatal depression can be experiencing changes in sleeping patterns, where the person either wants to sleep always or is unable to sleep.

Weight gain or loss due to changes in appetite might also be an indication of antenatal depression. Feelings of isolation, thoughts of harming the child and oneself, and the inability to cope with daily responsibilities can also be symptoms of antenatal depression (Curham, 2012). Some of the causes of antenatal depression can be hormonal imbalance during pregnancy. Sickness during pregnancy, the anxieties of how to cope as a mother, financial, and relationship challenges can also lead to antenatal depression.

Postnatal depression, on the other hand, means the kind of depression which most parents experience after the birth of the baby. Some of the symptoms of postnatal depression include experiencing low moods, hopelessness, exhaustion, guilt, sadness, anxiety, and failure as a parent (Curham, 2012). Postnatal depression can also lead to excessively worry regarding the baby by the parents. Excessive sleeping or trouble sleeping and fear of being alone could be other symptoms of postnatal depression.

Treatment of Antenatal and Postnatal Depression

It is necessary to receive treatment one's an individual has been diagnosed with either antenatal or postnatal depression. Some of the treatment methods can include

> ➤ ***therapy and counselling***—these are talking therapies where the affected individual is provided with a chance to look at the hidden factors that could have led to the depression. Therapy and counselling also assist in changing how the individual feels (Milgrom and Gemmill, 2015).

> ➤ ***medication***—in some circumstances the healthcare provider may prescribe antidepressants. Some of the commonly prescribed antidepressants are the selective serotonin reuptake inhibitors (SSRIs) which are considered safe both for the women that are pregnant and the mothers that are nursing. The affected individual should discuss with

their physician on whether the antidepressants are safe for them and the baby during pregnancy or breastfeeding.

➤ **support groups**—those affected by either the antenatal or postnatal depression can significantly benefit by interacting with someone that has gone through a similar experience (Milgrom and Gemmill, 2015). It is necessary to ensure that the peer support group has volunteers and staff that have adequate training and can quickly gain access to clinical supervision.

➤ **lifestyle changes**—parents that are affected by either antenatal or postnatal depression can overcome their condition by applying various changes in their lifestyle (Maizes and Dog, 2010). Some of the changes might entail taking care of their hygiene.

When an individual is experiencing depression, this might be the last thing they want to do, but little things like a change of clothes, taking a shower can impact significantly on how a person feels. Another lifestyle change can include becoming kind to oneself; the individual might have had expectations for themselves as a parent, and they should not be hard on themselves when these expectations are not always met.

Manic Depression/Bipolar I, II, III

Bipolar disorder can also be referred to as manic depression or main depressive condition. This disorder is a type of mood disorder that is often characterised by hypomanic or manic episodes (Leonard and Jovinelly, 2012). This disorder usually is caused by factors that are either genetic or non-genetic. The affected individual tends to experience either clinical depression or excessive energy and elation, which are referred to as mania. These mood episodes can either be mild or extreme and may occur unexpectedly or progressively.

Some of the common symptoms that are associated with bipolar disorder include experiencing shifts in one's moods (Leonard and Jovinelly, 2012). Also, changes might occur in an individual's level of energy, sleeping patterns, and behaviours. Suicide ideation and attempt, difficulties in concentrating, and restlessness can also be indications of the disorder. Some individuals affected by bipolar disorder may also experience both the manic and depressive symptoms together. Bipolar disorder can lead to poor performance in a person's job and might damage an individual's relationship.

There are three classifications of bipolar disorder namely:

Bipolar I

BipolarI1, this is a type of mental illness where the affected individual has experienced a manic episode that lasted for more than a week. A manic episode can be described as unusual high energy and mood going along with strange behaviour that interrupts the individual's life. Most individuals affected by bipolar I disorder also experience periods of depression. Frequently, the person might experience cycles of depression and mania, which gave rise to the term manic depression. Any person is at risk of developing bipolar I disorder 1.

Bipolar II

Bipolar I and II are similar except that an individual that is affected by bipolar II, the high moods never become mania that is full-blown (Roberts, Sylvia, and Harrington, 2014). For a person to be diagnosed with bipolar II, they must have had more than one hypomanic experience in their life. Individuals affected by bipolar II disorder tend to experience depression frequently, and they are more prone to experience psychotic symptoms while deeply depressed.

Some of the symptoms of bipolar disorder include enhanced self-confidence, a reduced need for sleep, talking more than the person typically does, olfactory and visual hallucinations, and inability to make decisions.

Bipolar III

Bipolar III is a mild kind of bipolar disorder which usually begins during teen years or early adulthood and affects men and women in equal measure. At times, this condition is misdiagnosed as those affected may be diagnosed as experiencing other mental illnesses such as depression. Most people with bipolar III disorders rarely seek treatment since they only experience mild symptoms. The actual causes of bipolar III disorders remain unknown, but some factors such as life stressors and genes can trigger the condition.

Some of the symptoms of the disorder include restlessness, irritability, excessive talking, euphoria, and becoming physically overactive.

Treatment of Bipolar Disorder

The treatment of bipolar disorder is aimed at assisting the affected individual in learning how to manage their symptoms. Some of the treatment methods used entail

> ➤ **medication**—after the diagnosis with any bipolar disorder, it is imperative to start medication immediately to balance the individual's moods. Some of the medicines that are commonly prescribed include antipsychotic and selective serotonin reuptake inhibitor (Hunt, 2011).

> ➤ **hospitalisation**—if the affected individual's behaviour is dangerous to themselves and those around them, the mental healthcare provider can endorse their hospitalisation (Court

and Nelson, 2013). Receiving treatment from a psychiatric hospital can help the individual to remain calm.

> ***therapies***—various therapies such as psychotherapy, psychoeducation, and cognitive behavioural therapy have proved beneficial in the treatment of bipolar disorders.

Cyclothymic Disorder

Cyclothymic disorder is an uncommon mood disorder that has similar features to the bipolar disorder. The people affected tend to have cyclic lows and highs that persist for more than two years (Sadock and Sadock, 2008). The lows tend to be characterised by mild depressions while the highs comprise of mania that is not severe. In between the highs and the lows, the person tends to feel normal. The cyclothymic disorder can enhance the chance of an individual developing bipolar disorder. Women and men tend to be affected by the disorder in equal measures.

Some of the depressive symptoms of the cyclothymic disorder are irritability, hopelessness, restlessness, experiencing a disturbance in one's sleep, feelings of guilt, and worthlessness. Others include fatigue, suicidal thoughts, difficulties in concentrating, and developing an impaired judgement (Sadock and Sadock, 2008). On the other hand, the hypomanic symptoms may include having self-esteem that is inflated, euphoria, a reduced need for sleep, excessive talking and physical activity, impulsivity, irresponsibility, and becoming easily distracted.

The real cause of the cyclothymic disorder remains unknown, but genes or family history can lead to the development of the disorder. Environmental factors such as sexual or physical abuse and traumatic events in an individual's life can also lead to the development of the disorder. It is crucial for an individual that exhibits the symptoms listed above to seek mental healthcare services for a proper diagnosis.

Cyclothymic Disorder Treatment

Once the various diagnosis forms of treatment can be recommended by the mental healthcare professional such as

> ➤ **psychotherap**y—the kind of therapies used in the treatment of bipolar disorder can also be used to treat the cyclothymic disorder. One of them is the cognitive behavioural therapy which aims at changing the negative thought pattern of an individual and helps them to develop positive thoughts (Starcevic, 2010). Dialectical behavioural therapy can also be used to teach the affected individual how to regulate their emotions and learn how to tolerate distress.

> ➤ **medication**—presently medications that can treat cyclothymic disorder efficiently remain unknown. Nevertheless, medicines used to treat bipolar disorder can also be used in the treatment of the cyclothymic disorder (Sadock and Sadock, 2008). Some of the drugs that are usually prescribed include atypical antipsychotics and anticonvulsants such as quetiapine and lithium. Antidepressants are rarely used in the treatment of the cyclothymic disorder as they have not been seen to be efficient.

Dysthymic Disorder

Dysthymic disorder is a mild depression that is chronic and lasts for an extended period. The disorder often begins in early adulthood, and a person may experience it for a long time (Sadock and Sadock, 2008). The late onset of the dysthymic disorder is often related to stress or the loss of a loved one. Studies show that women are more likely to be affected by the disorder than men. The causes of the disorder remain mostly unknown, but a family history of people affected by the disorder can lead to the development of the condition in a person. Furthermore, neurotransmitters change in a person's brain can lead to dysthymia disorder.

Stress, becoming socially isolated, and health conditions can also lead to the development of the dysthymic disorder. Mental illnesses such as borderline personality disorder can also increase an individual's risk of developing the disorder. Some of the symptoms of the dysthymic disorder include low self-esteem, changes in sleep patterns, feelings of hopelessness, difficulties in concentrating, and changes in the person's appetite (Sadock and Sadock, 2008). The diagnosis is often made when a person has been chronically depressed for more than two years.

Individuals affected by the dysthymia disorder might not view themselves as being depressed and often seek medical health services for physical conditions rather than psychological issues. When this condition is not diagnosed and treated at the right time, it can lead to suicide or substance and drug abuse.

Treatment of Dysthymia Disorder

In most cases, depression and dysthymia are treated using a similar approach, which is through psychotherapy and medication.

> *Medication*—antidepressants such as selective serotonin reuptake inhibitors (SSRIs) such as citalopram, fluoxetine, and paroxetine are used in the treatment of the dysthymic disorder (Sadock and Sadock, 2008).

> *Therapy*—cognitive behavioural therapy is often applied in the treatment of dysthymia as it helps the person affected to understand how their emotions and thoughts impact on their behaviour (Starcevic, 2010). Interpersonal therapy can also help the affected individual to focus on the problems they might be experiencing in their relationship with others (Taylor and Fink, 2006). Group therapy can also be used

in the management of the disorder through the support the person receives from others experiencing a similar condition.

> ***Peer support***—the support groups help an individual that is affected by the dysthymia disorder to share with others who are going through a similar experience or have learned to manage their condition. In the support groups, the patients are encouraged to develop new ways of coping with their condition and also cognitive restructuring (Sadock and Sadock, 2008).

Seasonal Affective Disorder (SAD)

The seasonal affective disorder is a kind of depression that is linked to seasonal changes; this disorder starts and ends almost at a particular time of each year. This disorder is often experienced during the beginning of winter or late fall and ceases during summer and spring (Oginska and Bruchal, 2014). The seasonal affective disorder is more common among young people and women and individuals that reside far away from the equator. Furthermore, an individual that has a family history of people affected by the seasonal affective disorder is at higher risk of developing the disorder.

The actual causes of the disorder remain mostly unknown, but studies have shown that people affected by the disorder often have a serotonin imbalance, which is a chemical in the brain that influences one's moods. Additionally, those affected seem to produce much melatonin, which is the hormone that controls an individual's sleep, and they also tend to produce inadequate vitamin D (Partonen and Perumal, 2010). The occurrence of the seasonal affective disorder has been connected to the imbalance of biochemical in the brain, which is stimulated by less sunlight and fewer daylight hours and occurs during winter.

Some of the symptoms of the seasonal affective disorder include sadness, little energy, lack of sleep or excessive sleep, having suicidal thoughts, feelings of worthlessness, hopelessness, irritability, and loss of interest in activities which previously the individual enjoyed (Partonen and Perumal, 2010). The disorder can occur at any age but often happens when an individual is between eighteen and thirty years of age.

Treatment of Seasonal Affective Disorder

After the diagnosis of the seasonal affective disorder, treatment is imperative. Some of the commonly used methods of treating the disorder include

> ➤ *light therapy*—in this therapy, the affected individual, is expected to sit before a light therapy box which radiates a very bright light. The sessions often last for around twenty minutes every day during the winter season and are usually conducted in the morning (Partonen and Perumal, 2010). To avoid relapse, light therapy treatment is continuously provided throughout the winter period. Due to the expected reoccurrence of the symptoms, those affected by the disorder tend to start the light therapy treatment at the beginning of the fall as a measure of preventing the symptoms.

> ➤ *talk therapy*—an example of a talk therapy that is used in the treatment of the seasonal affective disorder is the cognitive behavioural therapy which helps the affected person to recognise and change negative thought patterns which makes worse how they feel (Starcevic, 2010). This therapy is also useful in learning better ways of coping with the symptoms of the disorder and the management of stress.

> ➤ *medications*—some individuals, affected by the seasonal affective disorder, tend to benefit only from medications such as antidepressants. One of the antidepressants commonly

used in the treatment of the disorder is bupropion. At times, the mental health professional might recommend that the individual begins the treatment before the occurrence of the symptoms. It is necessary to note that one may need to try various medications before they find one that is suitable for them (Partonen and Perumal, 2010).

Depression and the Brain Anatomy

When a person has been affected by depression, various parts of the brain tend to be affected; these parts will be discussed below.

Insular Cortex

The insular cortex is a part of the cerebral cortex situated within the lateral sulcus, which is the fissure that separates the temporal lobe from the frontal and parietal lobes. The insular cortex has various functions regarding a person's emotions or in the regulation of the homeostasis. Some of these functions are self-awareness, perception, interpersonal experience, motor control. The insular cortex helps in the perception of pain and the formation of taste memory (Smith and Verberne, 2011).

The insular cortex consists of two parts, namely the large anterior insula and the small posterior insula. When an individual is experiencing depression for the first time, studies demonstrate that the volume of the insular cortex seems to reduce (Takahashi *et al.*, 2010).

Hippocampus and Depression

Hippocampus is a vital part of the brain, which plays a significant role in the limbic system. The hippocampus helps in the creation of new memories and is also linked with emotions and learning (Byrne,

2009). The hippocampus is responsible for the storage of long-term memories; it would not be possible to remember the location of one's house without the hippocampus.

Studies have shown that individuals that are affected by depression continuously tend to have a smaller hippocampus, which is the part of the brain that forms new memories and findings. Furthermore, people that became affected with major depressive disorders before they were twenty-one years of age also tend to have a smaller hippocampus (Campbell *et al.*, 2004). Hippocampus tends to regulate the prefrontal cortical function, and when it is disrupted, it may lead to a lowered level of concentration, which is one of the symptoms of people affected by the major depressive disorder.

Further studies have demonstrated that adverse circumstances early in an individual's life put them at a higher risk of developing a major depressive disorder. Adults and young people exposed to harmful or traumatic events early in their lives tend to have a smaller volume of the hippocampus (Woon and Hedges, 2008).

The shrinkage of the hippocampus tends to weaken an individual's capacity to experience various emotions usually. For instance, individuals that are affected by psychotic depression tend to experience little or no feelings, which could be attributed to the decrease in the size of the hippocampus. Also, the shrinkage of the hippocampus makes an individual have less control of their impulses and become susceptible to a negative thought pattern which proves difficult to escape.

The decrease of the hippocampus tends to harm a person's cognitive functions and interrupts the process of developing memories which profoundly impacts the capacity to create a stable sense of self (Rubin *et al.*, 2014). People that are affected by various types of depression tend to find it challenging to create and maintain interpersonal relationships or even make decisions that are acceptable socially. The reason for this can be attributed to the changes in the hippocampus.

A study done in 2014 showed that when the hippocampus is damaged, the capacity for social and cognitive behaviour is hindered

(Rubin *et al.*, 2014). When flexible social and cognitive behaviours are hindered, the person cannot interpret or respond to information accurately. The person's capacity to bond socially also becomes impaired, which is evident amongst most people that are affected by various types of depression (Rubin *et al.*, 2014).

Amygdala and Depression

Amygdala is that part of the brain that is used to detect fear and helps an individual to prepare for emergencies. Fear is necessary for self-preservation, where a person protects him/herself from danger. Humans have two amygdalae with one on each side of the brain. The amygdala assists a person to perceive various emotions such as sadness, fear, and sadness (Whalen and Phelps, 2009). The amygdala stores memories and feelings of multiple events that assist a person in identifying similar situations in the future. For instance, if a person has ever fallen on a slippery floor, the amygdalae help in enhancing the individual's alertness when near wet floors (Whalen and Phelps, 2009).

When an individual is affected by depression, the activity in their amygdala tends to increase. People affected by major depressive disorder tend to have an enlarged amygdala, which is more active due to the continual exposure to cortisol levels that are high (Beck and Alford, 2014). A hyperactive and enlarged amygdala together with other unusual activities in different regions of the brain can lead to sleep disturbance, which is common among people affected by various types of depression.

Furthermore, an enlarged amygdala can cause a person's body to produce irregular levels of hormones and chemicals in one's body, causing more complications (Beck and Alford, 2014). When an individual is experiencing depression, the amygdala becomes highly active, which can lead to interrupted physical activity. Therefore, the size of the amygdala can be used by scientists to predict if an individual will become depressed in the future or not.

Studies have shown that individuals that affect depression regularly tend to have a smaller hippocampus, which is the part of the brain that forms new memories and findings. Furthermore, people that became affected with major depressive disorders before they were twenty-one years of age also tend to have a smaller hippocampus (Campbell *et al.*, 2004). Hippocampus tends to regulate the prefrontal cortical function, and when it is disrupted, it may lead to a lowered level of concentration, which is one of the symptoms of people affected by major depressive disorder.

Further studies have demonstrated that adverse circumstances early in an individual's life put them at a higher risk of developing a major depressive disorder. Adults and young people exposed to harmful or traumatic circumstances early in their lives tend to have a smaller volume of the hippocampus (Woon and Hedges, 2008).

The shrinkage of the hippocampus tends to weaken an individual's capacity to experience various emotions normally. For instance, individuals that are affected by psychotic depression tend to experience little or no feelings, which could be attributed to the decrease in size of the hippocampus. Also, the shrinkage of the hippocampus makes an individual to have less control of their impulses and become susceptible to a negative thought pattern which proves difficult to escape.

The decrease of the hippocampus tends to harm a person's cognitive functions and interrupts the process of developing memories which deeply impacts the capacity to create a stable sense of self (Rubin *et al.*, 2014). People that are affected by various types of depression tend to find it difficult to create and maintain interpersonal relationships or even make decisions that are acceptable socially. The reason for this can be attributed to the changes in the hippocampus.

A study done in 2014 showed that when the hippocampus has damaged the capacity for social and cognitive behaviour is hindered (Rubin *et al.*, 2014). When flexible social and cognitive behaviours are hindered, the person cannot interpret or respond to information accurately. The person's capacity to bond socially also becomes impaired, which is evident amongst most people that are affected by various types of depression (Rubin *et al.*, 2014).

Nucleus Accumbens and Depression

Nucleus accumbens is a portion of the brain that is involved in various functions like reward and motivation (Reeve, 2015). The nucleus accumbens, which is located in the basal region of the brain, is contained in all cerebral hemispheres. The nucleus accumbens has the functions of receiving brain connections that are related to the emotions such as the hypothalamus and amygdala, and also, it connects to motor areas and memory.

Nucleus accumbens is considered as the brain's centre of pleasure; when a person performs activities that are pleasurable, dopamine neurons tend to be activated. The dopamine neurons further increase the levels of nucleus accumbens dopamine levels to be enhanced, leading to a pleasurable sensation. Anhedonia, which is the incapacity to experience pleasure and is one of the symptoms of people affected by psychotic depression and other types of depression, is attributed to changes in the nucleus accumbens dopamine level (Ritsner, 2014).

Studies have demonstrated that the nucleus accumbens of people that are affected by depression is not as active as for those that are not experiencing depression. Additionally, among people having depression, there are changes on the way through which nucleus accumbens releases and processes dopamine. The nucleus accumbens helps an individual to form attachment in their relationships. Among individuals that are affected by depression, this becomes difficult as there is an imbalance in nucleus accumbens, which explains why these individuals opt to stay alone most of the times.

The critical function, as stated earlier of the nucleus accumbens, involves intervening on the reward system, and when it malfunctions, it leads to various psychological disorders such as depression (Reeve, 2015). The dopamine activity in the nucleus accumbens is often controlled by multiple substances such as CART and dynorphin among others. Therefore, in most circumstances when dopamine reuptake inhibitors have been used in the treatment of patients affected by major depressive disorders, they have proven successful.

Anterior Cingulate Cortex and Depression

The anterior cingulate cortex is a part of the brain that is situated at the centre of the frontal lobe. It is positioned at the front part of the corpus callosum which links and the right and left brain hemispheres. The anterior cingulate cortex may be divided based on emotional and cognitive components. The dorsal or cognitive part is connected to the parietal and prefrontal cortex and the motor system. The ventral part, on the other hand, is connected to the anterior insula, amygdala, hypothalamus, and the nucleus accumbens. The dorsal anterior cingulate cortex of individuals affected by depression and panic disorders tends to be smaller (Asami *et al.*, 2008).

Research has shown that individuals affected by major depressive disorders tend to have high levels of activity in the dorsal anterior cingulate cortex in various areas (Graham *et al.*, 2013). For instance, people affected by major depression tend to have a hyperactive the dorsal anterior cingulate cortex reaction in processing information that is negative (Hamilton *et al.*, 2011).

The anterior cingulate cortex is accountable for various psychological functions and physiological such as the ability to make decisions, regulation of emotions, executive functions, and regulation of emotions. Individuals that are affected by major depressive disorders tend to have reduced levels of the anterior cingulate cortex (Asami *et al.*, 2008). Moreover, abnormal activation of the subgenual anterior cingulate cortex has been associated with significant depression.

Cerebellum and Depression

The cerebellum is an easily identifiable region of the brain due to its distinct position and shape. It is exceptionally significant in helping an individual to perform their daily activities such as writing and walking. The cerebellum, which is situated at the back of a person's brain also helps a person to stay upright and balanced (Thomson, Hahn, and Johnson, 2012). The cerebellum comprises two hemispheres that are linked together between the slim midline regions. The cerebellum consists of white matter and the grey matter.

The cerebellum has various functions which include the coordination of the voluntary movements of the body. Movement is a process which involves multiple groups of muscles that work together. Though the cerebellum does not start the movement, it assists in coordinating the actions of the group of muscles involved in the specific movement. Another function of the cerebellum is the maintenance of posture and balance, the intake of alcohol tends to have an immediate impact on the cerebellum leading to disruption in the coordination of the body (Thomson, Hahn, and Johnson, 2012).

The cerebellum also assists in motor learning, where a person learns to carry out new skills like riding or learning and play a particular game. Patients that have been diagnosed with the major depressive disorder tend to have a decreased size of the cerebellum and a heightened level of activities in the cerebellum.

Studies have emerged showing that the cerebellum has other roles such as the regulation of emotions, hindering impulsive decision making and working memory (Schmahmann, Weilburg, and Sherman, 2007). Studies have also suggested that emotional and cognitive abnormalities can arise from damages to some regions of the cerebellum which projects to the limbic system, prefrontal cortex, and motor areas. The cerebellum thus is involved in emotional behaviours that are fear-related.

Cingulate Gyrus and Depression

The cingulate gyrus is a curved fold which envelops the corpus callosum. The cingulate gyrus is a part of the limbic system; it takes part in the regulation of behaviour and the processing of information.

The cingulate gyrus comprises of two sections, namely the posterior and anterior sections. When the cingulate gyrus is damaged, it can lead to behavioural, emotional, and cognitive disorders. Some of the functions of the cingulate gyrus include regulation of hostile behaviours, communication, the making of decisions, emotional reaction to pain, and maternal bonding (Vogt, 2009).

In circumstances that the cingulate gyrus becomes damaged, it can lead to various behavioural and emotional disorders such as obsessive compulsive disorder, anxiety disorders, schizophrenia, attention deficit disorders, and depression. Furthermore, this could lead to the individual engaging in addictive behaviours such as substance and alcohol abuse and eating disorders. People whose cingulate gyrus is not functioning correctly might have challenges handling changing circumstances or may experience problems in their communication (Vogt, 2009). Due to this, these individuals can become easily upset and angry or might experience aggressive and emotional flare-ups. An increase in the microglial quinolinic acid in some parts of the anterior cingulate gyrus has been linked to depression.

Hypothalamus and Depression

The hypothalamus is a small part of the brain which is situated at the bottom of the brain close to the pituitary gland. The hypothalamus has three main parts namely the anterior, middle, and posterior regions (FitzGerald, Gruener, and Mtui, 2012). The anterior region has the role of the body's thermoregulation and also regulates a person's sleep. Some of the hormones that are produced by the anterior region comprise of corticotrophin-releasing hormone which controls the body's reaction to emotional and physical stress. Oxytocin is another hormone produced by the anterior region of the hypothalamus, whose primary role is the control of various emotions and behaviours such as recognition, trust, and sexual arousal.

The middle section of the hypothalamus has a role in the body's development and growth through the arcuate and ventromedial nuclei which control appetite. The posterior or the mammillary section, on the other hand, is involved in memory function (FitzGerald, Gruener, and Mtui, 2012). The hypothalamus can be viewed as the brain's manager where the body's signals go through it to the cerebral cortex where all thinking takes place before affecting other body parts.

The hypothalamus controls the homeostasis of the body and can be considered as the brain's emotional seat. Depression can be linked to an overactive hypothalamus (Goldberg, 2010). When a person has an overactive hypothalamus, it often leads to irritability and moodiness, hopelessness, negative view of situations, and negative thoughts. Additionally, an overactive hypothalamus can also lead to social isolation, changes in sleep pattern, all of which are symptoms of depression.

An individual that is affected by depression can heal their hypothalamus in various ways. One of the ways is by eating a balanced diet to reduce inflammation of the hypothalamus and other parts of the body (Dalvi et al., 2017). Physical exercise is another way through which the inflammation of the hypothalamus can be lessened (Yi et al., 2012).

Meditation can also heal the hypothalamus as it decreases the production of the norepinephrine leading to a reduction in the corticotrophin-releasing hormone level. The reduced levels of cortisol lead to less stress, and it also ensures that the hypothalamus is not over-activated. Meditation also impacts positively on serotonin, GABA, dopamine, among other neurotransmitters that work together with the hypothalamus.

Sleep is necessary for both the physical and mental health of an individual and assists in the reduction of stress and inflammation, which often leads to depression (Kim et al., 2014). Reducing the levels of stress which an individual is exposing themselves to can be another way of healing the hypothalamus and thereby depression. A study done showed that some stress levels interrupt the downstream and luteinizing hormones' secretion. The outcome can be the role of cortisol in the negative feedback loop affecting the hypothalamic pathways (Ciechanowska *et al.*, 2016).

Pituitary Gland and Depression

The pituitary gland is a gland that is small in size, and its primary responsibility is to regulate the body functions that are vital to the general health of an individual. The hormones produced by the pituitary gland controls most of the processes that happen in the body. The pituitary gland senses the needs which the body has and transmits signals to various glands and organs in the body to control their function and ensure that a suitable environment is maintained.

When the pituitary gland becomes enlarged, studies have shown that it can lead to major depressive disorders (Soares and Young, 2007). Additionally, when the levels of blood in the cortisol hormone are not suppressed, it can also lead to major depression. The pituitary gland is prone to disorders which can lead to imbalances in an individual's hormone. Some of the symptoms of hormonal imbalance due to pituitary/master gland disorder include depression, mood swings, inability to sleep, eating disorders, and anger among others.

The pituitary gland regularly checks the hormones' blood levels, including the thyroid's blood level. When the level of blood of thyroid hormones reduces, the pituitary gland utilizes the thyroid-stimulating hormone to assist the thyroid to thrust production. As a reaction, the thyroid tends to use the iodine that comes from food to produce T3 and T4 hormones (Philip *et al.*, 2010).

When the thyroid and the pituitary gland are working usually, T3 and T4 are secreted into the bloodstream steadily. In circumstances that the thyroid hormones have reduced, the body's internal systems and other organs tend to work more slowly, leading to various conditions such as depression. Hypothyroidism a condition where the thyroid gland produces low levels of the hormone is often linked to depression. More women are affected by hypothyroidism than men, and the condition is more prevalent among older adults.

In some situations during the treatment of depression, antidepressants and thyroid drugs are combined to enhance the mood of the affected individual even though the thyroid could generally be functioning (Philip *et al.*, 2010). The theory behind this is that thyroid drugs improve the brain's chemical activity, thus enhancing the concentration and mood of the affected individual. Most individuals affected by hypothyroidism realise that depression and other negative symptoms abate through hypothyroidism treatment.

Rostral Raphe and Caudal Raphe Nuclei and Depression

The word raphe means a line that divides two symmetrical regions of the body and is used in identifying the raphe nuclei since they are a compilation of nuclei gathered together around the centre of the brainstem. The raphe nuclei comprise of various nuclei found on the centre of the brain to the spinal cord. The serotonin neurotransmitter is located in the raphe nuclei, where it is synthesised and sent to the central nervous system.

Often the raphe nuclei are divided into a rostral cluster which is near the peak of the brainstem and caudal cluster which is near the base of the brainstem. Eighty-five per cent (85%) of the brain's serotonin neurons are contained in the rostral group nuclei (Hornung, 2003). Serotonin tends to influence one's sleep when a person is asleep, and when they have a dream, it increases their serotonin level.

Serotonin is also believed to influence an individual's mood, and this can be linked to depression as a reduction of serotonin level in the brain can lead to mood swings which are one of the symptoms of depression (Iler and Jacobs, 2010). When there is a reduction in the serotonin level in an individual's brain, often it leads to various conditions such as suicidal thoughts, depression, insomnia, aggressive behaviour, and addiction among others.

The transmission of serotonin from the rostral and caudal raphe nuclei tends to be reduced in individuals affected by depression in comparison to those that do not have the disorder. Increasing the serotonin in the pathways and decreasing the reuptake of serotonin, thereby enhancing its function is one of the therapies used in the treatment of depression (Iler and Jacobs, 2010).

Neurotransmitters and Depression

Neurotransmitters can be described as the chemical messengers of the body; they are used to send messages from neurons to muscles or between neurons. Neurons communicate in the synaptic cleft, which is the little gap linking the neurons' synapses. Neurotransmitters influence neurons in one of the three ways, namely modulatory, inhibitory, or excitatory. A neurotransmitter is regarded as either inhibitory or excitatory depending on the receptor it attaches itself. Depression is often associated with brain imbalances particularly with the neurotransmitters acetylcholine, dopamine, norepinephrine, glutamate, and GABA (Gotlib and Hammen, 2014).

Acetylcholine and Depression

Acetylcholine is a neurotransmitter mostly found in the peripheral nervous system and the central nervous system (Picciotto, Higley, and Mineur, 2012). This chemical is comprised of acetic acid and choline, which make up the name acetylcholine. In the central nervous system, acetylcholine balances the different neurons in parts of the brain, which manage attention, motivation, and arousal. When the signalling of acetylcholine in the hippocampus is interrupted, it tends to enhance anxiety and depression.

The impact of acetylcholine is dependent on the location, timescale, and pattern of its release. The release of acetylcholine is provoked by stressors that are environmental in various parts of the brain which includes the hippocampus and the prefrontal cortex, the two regions involved in mood regulation and depression (Drever, Riedel, and Platt, 2011). The acetylcholine signalling may harmonise the neuronal network's response to the neuronal network's response concerning the stress-sensitive brain parts which are appropriate for behaviours linked to depression and anxiety.

Stress-induced acetylcholine might lead to responses that are adaptive to environmental stimuli. On the other hand, a constant increase of the acetylcholine signalling might cause mood disorders, conceivably by stimulating synaptic plasticity in various neuronal subtypes within the hippocampus and leading to encoding stimuli memories linked with events that are stressful (Drever, Riedel, and Platt, 2011)

Serotonin and Depression

Serotonin is a transmitter that assists in transmitting signals between different parts of the brain. Even though the brain manufactures serotonin, its principal functions are in the blood platelets and the digestive tract. There is a belief that serotonin influences various body and psychological functions due to its extensive cell distribution. A large number of brain cells such as those associated with sleep, mood, and sleep tend to be influenced by serotonin (Monti, 2008). Serotonin may also affect an individual's muscles and cardiovascular system.

Various studies have demonstrated that an imbalance in the levels of serotonin can adversely impact a person's mood in a way that could cause depression (Miller, 2008). The imbalance of the serotonin levels could be as a result of the brain cells producing low levels of serotonin. Another factor that might cause the imbalance is lacking receiving sites or a shortfall in tryptophan, the chemical that forms serotonin. Researchers believe that when there are problems with the serotonin; it can lead to panic, depression, and anxiety (Miller, 2008).

Furthermore, it is believed that new brain cells are regenerated by serotonin, and when this process is suppressed, it leads to stress and eventually to depression. The commonly used antidepressants such as the selective serotonin reuptake inhibitors (SSRIs) are intended to enhance the serotonin levels through the production of new brain cells, a process that helps in the management of depression. Studies have shown that administering selective serotonin reuptake inhibitors often leads to positive changes in the manner in which evaluates the information that is emotionally balanced (Harmer, Goodwin, and Cowen, 2009).

The selective serotonin reuptake inhibitors alleviate depression by boosting the serotonin levels in the brain (Acton, 2012). The selective serotonin reuptake inhibitors hinder the reabsorption of serotonin in the brain, causing the availability of more serotonin. In comparison to moods, emotions tend to be a brief unintentional response to external and internal stimuli, and in individuals affected by depression, emotional reactions tend to be negatively biased. Owing to this, boosting the serotonin activity among individuals affected by depression helps in positively changing their unconscious emotional reactions (Acton, 2012).

Norepinephrine and Depression

Norepinephrine is a chemical that occurs naturally in one's body and acts as a neurotransmitter and a stress hormone. In circumstances where the brain discerns that there is the occurrence of an event that is stressful, norepinephrine is released into the blood, causing leading to more heart contractions. Norepinephrine is a stress hormone that is linked with the flight or fight reaction; it also increases the flow of blood to one's muscles and helps in boosting energy (Wolfe, 2010). Norepinephrine influence the approach through which the brain reacts and gives attention to circumstances.

Studies have shown that norepinephrine influences an individual's capacity to concentrate and also their mood. Additionally, low levels of norepinephrine might lead to depressive feelings while high norepinephrine levels might lead to anxiety Miller, 2008). Low levels of norepinephrine can leave an individual with feelings of fatigue, mental cloudiness, and lack of interest in day-to-day activities.

An individual can boost their norepinephrine levels in various ways such as exercise which assists in alleviating feelings of mental fogginess and sluggishness, which are signs of low norepinephrine (Arden, 2012). Eating a balanced diet can also boost the level of norepinephrine in the minds further helping a person to overcome depressive symptoms associated with low norepinephrine levels.

Dopamine and Depression

Dopamine refers to a neurotransmitter that assists in controlling the pleasure and reward centres of the brain. Dopamine is also useful in regulating emotional responses and movements of the body; it also helps an individual to see rewards and engage in action to assist them in attaining the rewards (Estren and Potter, 2013). Dopamine secretions assist in boosting a person's memory, thereby affecting their learning process and how information is retained. The presence of dopamine during a particular event helps a person to remember it; nevertheless, when dopamine is absent, the person might not remember anything regarding the event.

Dopamine is linked to the reward centre; therefore, if a person has no interest regarding a particular activity, then the levels of dopamine in the prefrontal cortex tend to reduce. When this occurs, the individual does not feel motivated to recall the information presented to them (Estren and Potter, 2013). Dopamine also assists a person to pay attention and to keep focus; when the dopamine level is very low, it leads to a lack of concentration. Since dopamine is a chemical that enhances pleasurable feelings, it makes an individual anticipate enjoying various activities. When there is a dopamine imbalance, the person might experience anhedonia, which is a symptom of depression.

Dopamine also plays a significant role in sleep; often more dopamine is secreted by the brain in the daytime to help in wakefulness. Nonetheless, the levels of dopamine are reduced at night, and melatonin is produced to enhance the feeling of sleepiness.

When the dopamine levels are too low, a person tends to become unmotivated, depressed, or bored (Estren and Potter, 2013). There are no definite ways of determining the dopamine levels in a person's brain. When we talk of low levels of dopamine, it means that there is little production of dopamine being made, the breaking down of dopamine is happening too fast or that the dopamine receptors are too little.

People are often motivated to take actions towards their objectives and goals by dopamine. Therefore, low levels of dopamine make it unlikely that people will work towards attaining their desires, objectives, and goals (Estren and Potter, 2013). Individuals that have been diagnosed with clinical depression tend to have high levels of monoamine oxidase, an enzyme that helps in breaking down various transmitters such as norepinephrine, serotonin, and dopamine.

An individual can have a deficiency in their dopamine level due to various factors, one of which is poor diet. Diets that are high in saturated fats and sugar tend to restrain dopamine; also insufficient protein in one's diet can lead to little l-tyrosine, which is an amino acid that helps in the dopamine production. Some of the symptoms of low dopamine level include fatigue, insomnia, loss of memory, mood swings, incapacity to experience pleasure (anhedonia), and forgetfulness among others (American Psychiatric Association, 2013).

A person can enhance their dopamine level in various ways. One of the methods is by engaging in physical exercises regularly (Burchard, 2017). Exercise helps in increasing new brain cells production, which reduces the ageing process of the brain cells, thereby increasing the dopamine levels. Getting adequate sleep is another way of increasing the level of dopamine in the brain since lack of sleep tends to decrease neurotransmitters concentration, which includes dopamine. Meditation can also be useful in enhancing an individual's dopamine level as it increases the concentration capacity of the person.

Glutamate and Depression

Glutamate refers to the neurotransmitter that transmits messages in the brain and the body nerves. Glutamate is an excitatory neurotransmitter; this means that it raises the possibility that a nerve cell will fire an action potential. Among other brain neurotransmitters, glutamate is the most vital for the normal functioning of the brain (Chayat and Yedidya, 2012). Besides its excitatory role, glutamate also helps in memory and learning. One of the crucial functions of this neurotransmitter is to convey instructions that control the development of the brain and establishes the survival of cells.

Glutamate also has a significant role in the production of cell energy and synthesis of protein. The gamma-aminobutyric acid (GABA), which helps in the reduction of anxiety, is produced by the body through glutamate. Too little or too much glutamate can prove dangerous; therefore, there must be the correct concentration in the right position of the brain in the appropriate time for processes to be executed without causing any damage to cells.

Excessive glutamate can overexcite the nerve cells that are accepting their signals. Glutamate could also facilitate the reinforcement of signals linking two neurons that happen with constant use. When the glutamate levels in the brain are elevated, it can lead to depression. Studies have demonstrated that people affected by depression tend to have high levels of glutamate in their brains (Sancora *et al.*, 2008). Glial cells tend to have significant responsibility for regulating glutamate signalling and might have a role in depression (Sancora and Banasr, 2013).

Glial cells have the role of clearing glutamate through the excitatory amino acids from the synaptic cleft, producing and releasing trophic factors. When there is a glia loss, in the prefrontal cortex, research shows that it leads to various mood disorders (Sancora and Banasr, 2013).

Stress can contribute to changes in the glutamate synapses which often lead to cellular signalling disruption and a decrease in the resilience of the cells in the brain circuits that are necessary for the regulation of mood (Manji*et al.*, 2003). These molecular changes are often associated with the deformities that are commonly found among people that are affected by major depressive disorders, which include changes in the volume and levels of glutamate (Yüksel and Öngür, 2010).

Ketamine is more efficient than other antidepressants in the treatment of depression as it adjusts the glutamate system, which is connected in an individual's emotional response, reaction to stress, and neuroplasticity. Nevertheless, ketamine has other side effects, such as causing impairment in a person's judgement, hallucinations, and developing false beliefs (Matthew and Zarate, 2016).

Gamma-Aminobutyric Acid (GABA) and Depression

GABA is a significant neurotransmitter in the central nervous system (Erdö., 2012). Glutamate is responsible for the production of gamma-aminobutyric acid in the brain. The production of GABA is dependent on the capacity of the brain to create and degenerate glutamate through the use of glutamic acid decarboxylase. GABA receptors are widely distributed in different parts of the brain like the cortex and basal ganglia. The cortex is the brain layer linked to seizures, and this is the reason most anti-seizure drugs work to enhance the proportion of the GABA inhibitory action over the glutamate excitatory response.

The cortex, in conjunction with other brain parts, also controls how a person feels, thinks, perceives, moves, and behaves. GABA has the responsibility of transmitting signals to the cortex and other regions of the brain initiate and restrain muscle groups' movements in the body. GABA also plays a vital role in the neurons (central nervous system cells) development. GABA permits the cells to differentiate into suitable numbers of neurons throughout the formation of the brain and afterwards.

GABA is that component of the brain system which allows people to control their actions, moods, and thoughts with an astonishing level of detail. Studies have shown that a shortage of GABA can lead to depression. As a way of compensation, the body tends to increase glutamate production. During the initial stages, the increase in glutamate leads to excitation of neurons. However, ultimately, the glutamate receptors withdraw, hindering the firing of the brain cells. The outcome is that a person tends to feel numb and disengaged from the world around them, rarely become excited, which are signs of depression.

It is necessary to note that most brain functions tend to be controlled by GABA and its receptors. Individuals that are affected by major depressive disorder tend to have distorted GABA functions. Therefore, drugs that can correct the GABA imbalance might assist in treating major depressive disorders. Anaesthetic ketamine can be used to provide temporary relief to symptoms of depression. Ketamine tends to stimulate glutamate receptors and the function of GABA, thereby reinstating the stability between glutamate and GABA (Mathew and Zarate, 2016).

CHAPTER 2

Inflammation and Depression

Various studies have linked inflammation to depression and held the view that the two are related and tend to affect each other (Dowlati *et al.*, 2010). The relationship between the two shows that depression can lead to inflammation and vice versa. It is widely believed that the immune system and particularly increased inflammation levels play a significant role in a person developing depression (Bufalino *et al.*, 2013). The majority of the facts that link depression to inflammation is based on the fact that most people with the disorder tend to portray high levels of inflammatory markers in their blood even when they do not have any other medical illness.

Inflammatory markers tend to change the signalling sequence of the brain, which can lead to symptoms that are related to depression (Krishnadas and Cavanagh, 2012). The degree to which inflammation can lead to depression is mostly unknown (Raison and Miller, 2011). Illnesses such as asthma, cardiovascular diseases, asthma, rheumatoid arthritis, and diabetes among others raise the risk of depression, but this is not the only cause for depression as they are other factors involved (Slavich and Irwin, 2014).

Nevertheless, not every person that has an increased inflammation ends up developing symptoms of depression. This shows that inflammation does not always lead to depression; it is just only one of the factors that can lead to depression (Dantzer and Capuron,

2017). It is necessary to note that even though inflammation can lead to mental illness in a particular person, mental disorders are not inflammatory conditions.

Inflammation creates changes in the functioning of a person's brain or body, and it can lead to the development of various psychiatric disorders such as depression. However, inflammation is one of the many factors that predispose a person to mental illnesses. The other risk factors that could lead to depression besides inflammation are life stressors or genetic factors (Dantzer and Capuron, 2017).

There are risk factors that can make a person vulnerable to depression as a result of inflammation. One of the risk factors can be the time when an individual is exposed to inflammation. Furthermore, the age in which a person becomes exposed to inflammation can be a contributing factor to the development of depression (Kalmakis and Chandler, 2015).

When a child experiences hardships early in life, studies have shown that this can increase the risk of them developing depression either during adolescence or later in their adulthood (Colman et al., 2014). Therefore, it appears that harsh conditions early on in life can lead to depression later in life. Undoubtedly, there are times early in life when a person is most vulnerable when exposed to trauma or hard conditions. For instance, when a child's immune system is still developing, it is more sensitive to toxins that are induced through the environment in comparison to an individual whose immune system is fully matured (Dietert, 2013).

An inflammation early in an individual's life can lead to impairment of various biological systems, and this can become a significant cause of depression in a person's life (Rivest, 2010). Few studies have been done showing the relationship between maternal infection and depression (Knuesel et al., 2014). One of the studies done in this area has demonstrated that prenatal infection rarely increases the risk of developing depression later in life for the unborn child (Pang et al., 2009). For instance, prenatal exposure to the human immunodeficiency virus, according to various studies, has not led to depression later in the child's life.

A study done on the impact of chronic illness among children on depression in Britain showed that there existed little connection between psychiatric illnesses, including depression and chronic illness. Nonetheless, children that were ill in their childhood and later when they were twenty-one years of age were more likely to develop psychiatric disorders. This shows that the age a person is exposed to medical inflammation- linked, can lead to mental disorders such as depression in some individuals.

On the contrary, a study done in the United States demonstrated that exposure to chronic illness in childhood could increase the risk of developing depression later in life for some individuals (Ferro and Boyle, 2015). Additionally, obesity during childhood does not necessarily lead to depression later in life. There are contradictory results regarding the relationship between depression and obesity during adolescence.

Some of the studies indicate that depression and obesity during adolescence have a positive relationship while others state that there exists no association between depression and obesity in adolescence (Marmorstein *et al.*, 2014). Another health condition which is of interest in this discussion regarding its relationship to depression is diabetes mellitus. Studies have demonstrated that individuals diagnosed with diabetes rarely develop depression (Lašaite *et al.*, 2015).

The above examples demonstrate that depression, among other psychiatric disorders, is not inflammation or infection and that infection does not always cause depression (Dantzer and Capuron, 2017). Scientists assume that the immune response of the body to a particular inflammation can lead to a psychiatric disorder in some people.

Some people may experience a similar kind of immune system response when experiencing psychological trauma while other individuals might be struggling with an overactive immune system. In these different cases, the immune response of the body tends to interrupt the normal functioning of the brain leading to severe psychological symptoms.

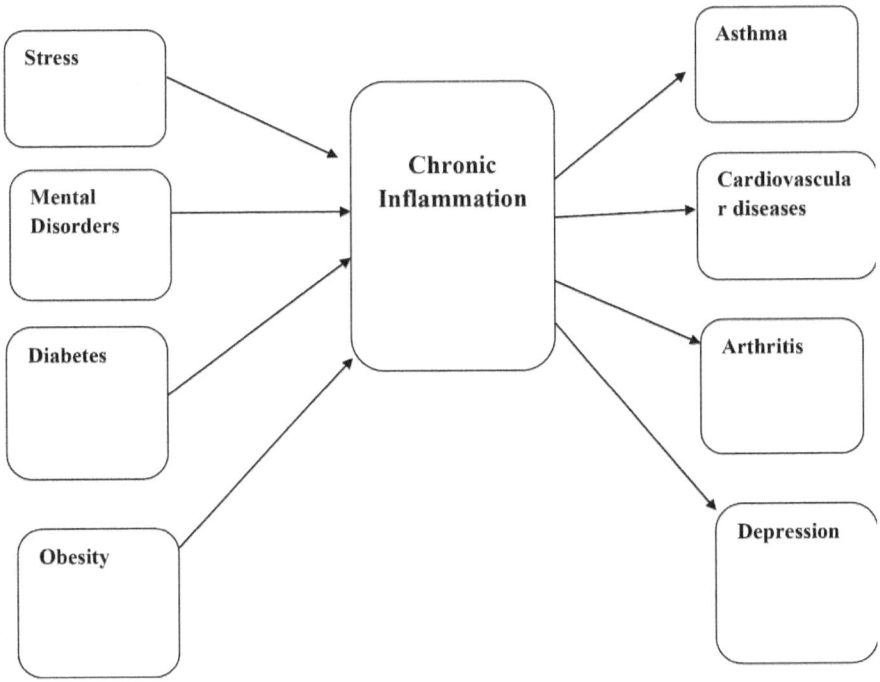

The Impact of Chronic Inflammation on Hyperactive and Irritable Behaviour

Inflammation is a critical part of the body's immune response. It can be described as the response of the immune system to infection, environmental toxins, and irritants (Stewart, 2013). Often it is the attempt the body makes in healing itself after it has been injured or protect itself from foreign intruders like bacteria, parasites, or viruses. When intruders activate the immune system, there are signals sent to the white blood cells to go to the infected tissue and clean it. After the intruders have been subdued, the healing process by the anti-inflammatory agents begins (Stewart, 2013).

The absence of inflammation could lead to deadly infections (Stewart, 2013). Redness, pain, warmth, or swelling can be some of the indications of inflammation. For instance, when a person hurt a part of their body, cytokines are released by biochemical processes. The cytokines bring hormones and the body's immune cells to manage the condition. The flow of blood increases and capillaries become more porous to enable the hormones and white blood cells to go into the spaces in the cells. The white blood cells go to the injured part and ingest the invaders as a way of assisting the body in healing.

There are two types of inflammation, namely, chronic and acute (Miyasaka and Takatsu, 2016). Acute inflammation is often a result of a scrape or a cut in a person's skin, a sprained ankle, an ingrown nail that is infected, appendicitis, or a sore throat. This means that acute inflammation diminishes after a short period. On the contrary, chronic inflammation occurs due to the body's wear and tear and lasts for an extended period (Miyasaka and Takatsu, 2016). Some of the conditions that might cause wear and tear include autoimmune diseases like rheumatoid arthritis, allergies, lupus, and asthma among others.

Environmental factors such as exposure to toxins in the environment repeated infections, and chronic stress, lack of sleep and exercise can lead to inflammation (Jain, Pandley, and Shukla, 2014). Behavioural factors which include a poor diet, smoking, excess weight, stress, lack of exercise, and excess intake of alcohol can lead to chronic inflammation.

Chronic inflammation occurs when an individual's body makes an inflammatory response to a supposed internal danger, which does not need the response (Miyasaka and Takatsu, 2016). Owing to this, the white blood cells flock, but since they have no place to go and nothing to do, they begin ambushing internal organs and other vital cells and tissues. There are various risks associated with chronic/ persistent inflammation, and they include, among others, anger and stress.

Individuals with psychological stress are often vulnerable to viruses that cause common colds. The viruses are usually not the cause of the cold but rather adverse effects of the inflammatory reaction as a means through which the body heals itself of the infection. When a person is stressed, the cells in the immune system are not able to respond to the hormonal balance (Mertsalove, 2017).

As a result, inflammation occurs, which leads to other illnesses and diseases.

Depression can lead to increased levels of inflammation. Individuals that are affected by major depressive disorder tend to have higher amounts of pro-inflammatory cytokines, which are accountable for causing inflammation in a person's body (Dowlati *et al.*, 2010).

Research has demonstrated that individuals with an intermittent explosive disorder (IED) often struggle with inflammation. IED is a mental disorder which is characterised by repeated aggressive outbursts, hostility, and impulsivity. Recent studies have shown that the inflammation blood markers in people who have the intermittent explosive disorder are often too. This study has shown a direct connection between aggression, impulsivity, and anger with inflammatory markers (Liveley and Larstone, 2018).

The two markers time and again draw a parallel with impulsivity and aggressive behaviour and not with other mental disorders. Individuals with the disorder tend to overreact to stressful situations, often with rage and uncontrollable anger. An intermittent explosive disorder can make a person susceptible to various mental illnesses such as anxiety disorders and depression. The two markers of inflammation include interleukin- 6(IL-6) and C-reactive protein (CRP) (Liveley and Larstone, 2018). Both of these markers are linked to aggressive behaviour.

The liver produces the C-reactive protein in response to an injury or infection; it assists the immune system to focus on cells that are either damaged or dead (Karst, 2006). On the other hand, the white blood cells secrete the interleukin-6 to help in stimulating the responses of the immune system. Individuals with intermittent explosive disorder tend to have high levels of C-reactive protein, and the interleukin- 6 (Lochman and Matthys, 2018).

When the body is experiencing inflammation, the immune system hastens to protect it (DeFranco, Locksley, and Robertson, 2007). Nevertheless, when the inflammation is chronic and intense, the immune can become worn out, reducing its capacity to repair itself.

Since the mind and the body are devised to operate in good health, inflammation can make the body to turn against itself, resulting in emotional and cognitive self-attack.

Ways in which Depression and
Anxiety Lead to Inflammation

Depression is a mental disorder that can cause much emotional distress. The changes that occur in the brain can have a significant impact on the body, which explains why people affected by depression experience various physical health conditions. Depression can adversely affect the immune system, which makes it difficult for the body to confront or challenge infections. Various physical changes that occur due to depression like insomnia are believed to weaken the immune system (Beck, 2011).

Research has demonstrated that anxiety, stress, or depression can increase the body's inflammation, which is the response of the body to injury, which can be physical, emotional, or mental. When inflammation occurs in the body, the first thing to become affected is the microbiome and gut. Stress or anxiety tends to create inflammatory cytokines which can change the way an individual's nervous system, brain, and gut responds; this can lead to anxiety, a leaky gut, and depression (Bosch and Bird, 2018).

Depression and anxiety might be mental conditions, but prolonged adverse physical effects are bound to occur as a result. Anxiety tends to stress the body with such magnitude that cortisol, which is a stress hormone, is released in all parts of the body. Anxiety and depression affect the immune system by causing chronic inflammation that is damaging to the tissues, which makes one susceptible to various diseases. Additionally, anxiety and depression tend to suppress the immune cells which are required in fighting infection (Beck, 2011).

Anxiety makes an individual vulnerable to autoimmune and infectious diseases. It seems that chronic stress or anxiety decreases the ability of the immune system to fight against intruders and antigens that cause disease, which makes a person prone to disease and infections.

The Fight-or-Flight Response and Cortisol

The fight-or-flight response is triggered by the sympathetic nervous system when a person perceives danger (Berne, Koeppen, and Stanton, 2010). During this period, epinephrine (adrenaline) and norepinephrine (noradrenaline) get released in the body. This leads to a rise in the blood pressure, more alertness, and senses become more enhanced (Berne, Koeppen and Stanton, 2010). Furthermore, digestion and other systems are slowed down since, at that time, all the energy is required to live. When a person is experiencing stress or anxiety, and they are in a flight or fight mode, the body starts to produce more cortisol, which is the stress hormone that is produced by the adrenal gland.

Most of the cells have cortisol receptors; thus, cortisol has various actions which depend on the type of cell they are acting upon. Some of the actions involve regulating the levels of blood sugar, which assists in controlling a person's metabolism. Additionally, cortisol influences the formation of memory acts as an anti-inflammatory and influences blood pressure (Bergström and Söderström, 2015). Cortisol is primarily managed by three parts of the body, which include the hypothalamus, adrenal and pituitary glands.

When the level of cortisol in the blood is low, the hypothalamus part of the brain releases the corticotrophin hormone, which makes the pituitary gland to secrete into the bloodstream the adrenocorticotropic hormone. When the adrenocorticotropic hormone level is high, it leads to elevated cortisol level. The rising level of cortisol tends to obstruct the hypothalamus from releasing the corticotrophin hormone. Owing to this, the level of the adrenocorticotropic hormone begins to go down, leading to a reduction on the cortisol levels.

When high levels of cortisol are maintained for an extended period by the body, it can cause Cushing's syndrome. Additionally, this can lead to an immune system that is suppressed; increasing the vulnerability a person has to various illnesses.

High Levels of Cortisol and the Immune System

The primary purpose of cortisol is to reinstate homeostasis after a person the experience of stress by an individual (Nelson and Collins, 2008). The highest level of cortisol occurs in the morning when a person wakes up and falls during the day. For people that work at night, the reverse is true. When a person is experiencing stress, their immune response tends to become compromised. When the immune system is suppressed by cortisol, the body becomes more vulnerable to diseases. Anxiety, which can result from stress, tends to impact the body adversely in various ways (Beck, 2011). For instance, it takes a prolonged period for the body to recover from infection. Also, the susceptibility to infection tends to increase.

Cortisol assists the body in fleeing from the danger it might be facing. Cortisol accomplishes this by subduing the immune whereby the quantity protein needed for messaging other immune cells is reduced. As a result, lymphocytes (B and T cells), which are immune cells, tend to be reduced. T cells assist in the production of cytokines, which direct and magnify the other part of the immune system. The T cells tend to lock on intruders who have gained access to a cell and destroy them (Brannon, Feist, and Updegraff, 2018). B cells, on the other hand, create antibodies that assist in deactivating bacterial toxins in hindering their access to cells.

B lymphocytes can also be described as the military intelligence system of the body which look for targets and send defences against them. T cells, on the other hand, can be defined as soldiers that B lymphocytes (intelligence system) have recognised. When unknown substances attack a person's body, various cells come together to identify them and respond. As a response, the B lymphocytes are activated to create antibodies that lock onto particular antigens. When produced, the antibodies tend to stay in an individual's body such that if they come across the antigen again, the antibodies are there to counter them.

Even though antibodies can identify a particular antigen and hold onto it, they have no capacity of destroying it, devoid of assistance. T cells help in destroying antigens which the antibodies have tagged or infected or altered them (Brannon, Feist, and Updegraff, 2018). Furthermore, T cells send messages to other cells to perform their role. An immune system works by differentiating itself from non-self; it achieves this by identifying proteins that exist on all cells' surface. The immune system learns how to overlook its proteins early.

Cortisol is only useful at low levels, but when a person experiences extended stress, the T cells are suppressed, thereby weakening the immune system. Due to this, a person might become ill, and their recovery process tends to become longer due to their lowered immunity (Dalal and Misra, 2012). The body requires T cells to fight invaders, but when the immune system is being suppressed by depression or anxiety, this becomes difficult.

With fewer lymphocytes, the body's risk to diseases and infections is increased, thus becoming more vulnerable to contracting various illnesses. Furthermore, the body takes longer to recover from illnesses and wounds. Eventually, the immune system becomes weak, leading to other infections such as diabetes, cardiovascular disease, and asthma among others. Chronic anxiety and stress make the levels of cortisol to continue increasing, but with time, this becomes ineffective in the management of inflammation (Cohen *et al.*, 2012). The inefficiency is caused by the immune cells becoming less sensitive to cortisol, which leads to the dysregulation of the immune system, causing inflammation.

Cortisol partially regulates inflammation, and when it is inhibited in its function, inflammation can get out of hand. When the cortisol levels are too high, the immune response is suppressed, making an individual prone to infection and inflammation (Blum and Bender, 2013). Stress hormones are intended to provide chemical reactions to the body that is brief and intense. Extended anxiety and stress change the ability of cortisol in regulating the inflammatory response since it reduces the tissue responsiveness to itself. This puts the body at risk of developing high blood pressure, digestive health conditions, and heart diseases among others.

When the stress level steadily increases over an extended period, the body's internal organs deplete the materials required in the production of neurotransmitters and primary hormones, which leads to adrenal fatigue. Constant activation of the flight or fight mode leads to the production of large quantities of cortisol, which is a stress hormone. The immune cells thus become incapable of a normal response, which can lead to inflammation and infections (Blum and Bender, 2013).

The fight-or-flight reaction (sympathetic nervous system), which is a part of the autonomic nervous system makes the body ready for action (Berne, Koeppen, and Stanton, 2010). The organs concerned prepare to either challenge or retreat from the situation. On the other hand, the parasympathetic nervous system, which is also a part of the autonomic nervous system, assists in the maintenance of the body's equilibrium.

The sympathetic nervous system tends to trigger the adrenal gland, which further releases hormones into an individual's bloodstream. The hormones also trigger the target glands and muscles, making the body become uptight, more vigilant. Other functions that are not instantly necessary, such as the digestive and immune system are closed to some extent. When the sympathetic nervous activation is maintained for a long time, the tissues that are affected experience a phase change and become flexible for adaptation to occur. The adverse effect of this is that the tissues tend to become prone to inflammation and infections.

The release of too much cortisol can lead to a decline in the body's immune system since in times of extreme stress or anxiety, the role of cortisol is to decrease inflammation by making weak, several antibodies that could increase inflammation (Talbott, 2007). Additionally, cortisol turns on the body's natural immunity and takes away particular immunities leading to vulnerability to infections and inflammation.

The immune system can be described as the body's protection against infections and diseases. For an immune system to function correctly, it needs to identify various agents which are known as pathogens. Additionally, the immune system should have the capacity to distinguish the pathogens from parasites and viruses. On coming into contact with bacterium, parasite, or viruses, the immune system mounts the immune response (Chiras, 2013). For an immune system to distinguish between itself and invaders, it detects proteins that are usually on the exterior of cells.

The immune cells tend to become less responsive to the regulatory impact of cortisol. Due to this, runaway inflammation is believed to enhance the growth of other diseases. The persistent inflammation reduces the body's resistance, increasing its vulnerability to various diseases. Since most of the immune system is in the gut, the gastrointestinal system's health suffers, and as a result, different autoimmune system conditions such as Celiac disease may occur (Blumer and Crowe, 2010).

Other issues that might arise when the body maintains an elevated level of cortisol includes

> ➢ ***diabetes and imbalances in the blood sugar***—when a person is faced with stressful situations, cortisol gives the body glucose by accessing the protein storage in the liver. The energy derived can assist an individual to flee or fight the danger they are facing. Nevertheless, a constant increase of cortisol, which continuously generates glucose can lead to a rise in the levels of the blood sugars (Stephenson, Hicks, and Hicks, 2011). There is a belief that this mechanism may raise the risk of a person developing diabetes type 11.

> ➢ ***obesity or weight gain***—a constant increase of cortisol may lead to weight gain. Having elevated levels in the blood glucose combined with the suppression of insulin can lead to cells which have insufficient glucose since these cells require more energy, and the way to achieve this is by sending to

the brain hunger signals, which can lead to overeating and ultimately weight gain. Moreover, cortisol can also influence a person's appetite directly by changing other factors related to stress response and hormones to activate appetite (Geissler and Powers, 2011).

➢ *suppression of the immune system*—cortisol helps in reducing inflammation and infection in the body. Nevertheless, by reducing inflammation, cortisol might also repress the immune system. A weakened immune system tends to increase the vulnerability of the body to various physical health conditions such as cancer and food allergies among others.

➢ *cardiovascular diseases*—cortisol tends to narrow the blood vessels which raise the blood pressure to boost the release of oxygenated blood. This process is beneficial in the fight and flight response but can be harmful when it occurs consistently. The constriction of the blood vessels and a constant increase in the blood pressure may place an individual at risk of developing cardiovascular diseases (Olpin and Hesson, 2015).

Having discussed how anxiety and depression lead to the body's inflammation, thereby weakening the have on the immune system, we will look at the various ways in which inflammation can be reduced.

Natural Ways of Reducing Inflammation as a Means of Managing Depression

The Impact of Stress Levels, Inflammation, and Depression

Research has demonstrated that chronic stress may make worse inflammation, which might lead to damaging mental and physical effect. It is necessary to find ways of taking care of oneself to lessen stress; some of the ways this can be achieved is through

> ➢ **gratitude**—this can assist in relieving stress as the person tends to focus on positive things in their life. Even though people have different temperaments, every person can develop a positive outlook on life since the brain is a muscle. Writing down what one is grateful for can be one way of establishing a positive mindset through gratitude (Burke and Page, 2017). At times, stress can arise when a person wrongfully compares him/herself to others. A person might always be comparing themselves with people that seem to be better than them, rather than being grateful for who they are and what they have. The habit of comparison can lead to stress, thus should be avoided at all costs.

> ➢ **spending time with family**—life has many stressors; family members can come in handy during such times (Rosenberg and Pehler, 2011). Most people spend most of their time working and away from their loved ones and family, which can make life stressors to overwhelm them. Spending time with family should be planned as it is one of the ways through which one can reduce their stress levels. A study done in this area has shown that when women spend time with their family and friends, oxytocin which relieves stress naturally is released. The effect of the release of oxytocin acts in contrast to the flight or fight reaction.

Spending quality time with family should be planned; it does not occur automatically. To avoid stress, a person should talk regarding their day at work with their family. It is by spending time with family that one learns how to manage conflict, which can be useful in avoiding and reducing stress (Rosenberg and Pehler, 2011).

➤ **laughter**—laughing is another way through which a person can reduce their stress level and as a result, decrease inflammation in their body (King, 2016). It is challenging to be stressful while laughing; thus, this practice is useful as a means of stress reduction. Happy chemicals which boost the immune response are released during laughter; they include among others serotonin, NK cells, and endorphins. Furthermore, laughter reduces cortisol secretion and simultaneously enhances the reaction of the immune system.

Stress hormones such as cortisol tend can be reduced through laughter. Laughter can also help in removing the body emotions that could be increasing the stress level (King, 2016). Laughter is also useful in activating circulation and aids in the relaxation of muscles, and both are useful in relieving the physical signs of stress. When a person is laughing, their focus tends to stay away from negative emotions such as anger and guilt; this is useful in reducing the level of stress a person could be experiencing.

Research demonstrates that the response a person has to stressful circumstances determines how they view the situation (King, 2016). In such cases, laughter can provide a more light-hearted perspective, making the issue to seem less challenging.

➤ **learning to say no**—for some people it is not easy to say no, nevertheless, agreeing to every demand can lead to anxiety and stress as one might not be able to fulfil all their obligations (Tucker, 2014). It is necessary to know that saying no does not mean that one is selfish; instead, the person may want to devote their time in their existing obligations.

Over-commitment can lead to stress and eventually to inflammations and infections. Some stressors are beyond a person's control; therefore, one should take charge over the parts of their life which they can adjust and which could be causing them stress. For instance, an individual could be assuming more responsibilities than they can handle since they do not want to disappoint those around them (Tucker, 2014). For such an individual to reduce their level of stress, they would have to accept only responsibilities which they can handle.

When a person says no, others can step in to offer their help, or the individual may pass on some of their responsibilities to other people, which can help in reducing their stress level. Learning to say no at the beginning can be challenging; hence, a person should stand by their decision despite the pressure to give in (Tucker, 2014).

➢ ***steer clear of procrastination***—stress can arise from procrastination; therefore, it is crucial for a person to avoid it. Procrastination, whether viewed as a trait or a state, tends to harm an individual's psychological health. Often procrastination is linked to negative emotions such as guilt, shame, and stress (Stead, Shanahan, and Neufeld, 2010). Procrastination might lead to reactive behaviour and actions where a person is rushing to meet deadlines and this can lead to stress (Sirois, 2014).

Research has shown that stress is the link that exists between poor health, which involves infection and inflammation and procrastination (Sirois, 2007). To reduce stress levels, a person can develop the practice of developing a to-do schedule which they arrange by priority. Also, establishing realistic deadlines can help in avoiding procrastination. Things that need to be attended to today should be given an uninterrupted time, and one should avoid multitasking as at times it can lead to stress.

The Impact of Diet on Inflammation and Depression

A balanced diet is suitable for both mental and physical health. Various studies have demonstrated that there is a link between what a person eats and how their brain functions (Moon, 2016). Many people that are affected by depression try to manage their condition through medication; however, a balanced and healthy diet can also lessen the symptoms that are associated with the condition. Having a diet change can be useful in the treatment of depression and various inflammations in the body.

More studies are revealing that an unhealthy diet increases the risk of developing depression. On the other hand, a healthy diet works as a defence mechanism against depression and other emotional and disorders. A healthy diet helps in increasing one's energy level and also helps the body to function at its best (Moon, 2016). The serotonin levels in the brain can be affected by the nutrients a person gets. The food an individual eats can either sustain or hamper a healthy gut.

At times, when a person is depressed, he/she may yearn for foods that have high sugar and fats as a means of comfort (Otto, Smits, and Smits, 2011). Though temporarily, the person may feel better, in the long run, the effect is adverse. The consumption of too much processed foods and refined sugar exposes the brain to inflammation and free radicals, and this can be linked to depression.

There are foods which a person that is experiencing depression should avoid, and they include among others:

> ➢ **Fast foods**—most of these food items have little or no nutrient since they are highly processed (Otto, Smits, and Smits, 2011). Fast foods tend to raise inflammation, perhaps by influencing gut health. Junk food may weaken the lining of the gut barrier, which hinders the leaking of food particles into the bloodstream. Since the food particles by being in the bloodstream are not in their proper place, the inflammatory response becomes low, which is believed to increase the risk

of developing depression. The preservatives and chemicals in fast foods can cause moodiness (Otto, Smits, and Smits, 2011).

> ***Refined sugars and artificial sweeteners***—these sugars often lead to a drop in the levels of blood glucose; this leaves the person feeling irritable and tired. Research done in London found out that people that consumed foods that were processed had a higher likelihood of being diagnosed with depression than those who consumed whole foods (Akbaraly *et al.*, 2009).

A diet that is high in sugar increase the risk of inflammation. The reason being when a person consumes artificial sugar, there is a rapid increase in their blood sugar, which tends affects insult. As a result, insulin takes away blood sugar, causing a crash in the blood sugar and cortisol comes in to try and get out the sugar from storage into the bloodstream. This process referred to as hypoglycaemia can lead to irritability, anxiety, and eventually depression (Chow and Chow, 2011).

Sugar tends to spike insulin and harms the gut microbiome leading to inflammation, which is a critical factor that causes depression. The sweeteners tend to obstruct the production of serotonin, and this can lead to headaches, insomnia, and mood swings.

Weight gain is another issue that can be linked to the intake of refined sugars; inflammation has been linked to excess body fat due to the body's resistance to insulin (Watts and Magee, 2012). Refined sugar alone cannot cause inflammation, but other factors such as smoking, medication, excessive body fats, and stress can be contributing factors.

> ***Alcohol***—since it is an antidepressant, it increases the feelings and symptoms that accompany depression. Excess dopamine

and **GABA** tends to be released when one consumes alcohol (Nairne, 2014). When these neurotransmitters are released excessively, it may lead to delusions, high blood pressure, and increase symptoms related to depression. Additionally, consumption of alcohol may cause the release of excess endorphins, which can lead to depression.

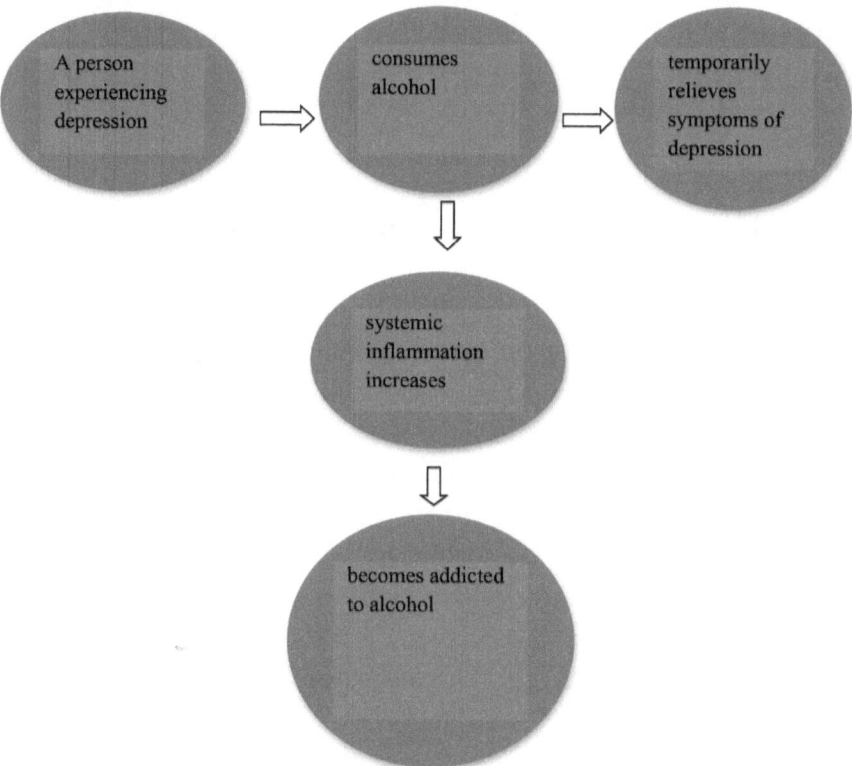

> ➤ **Caffeine**—the production of serotonin tends to be inhibited by caffeine, and this makes it difficult for the person to sleep.

Having looked at the foods that increase inflammation and depression, the next part will be dedicated to foods that can reduce both depression and inflammation. These foods include among others:

➤ *Leafy greens*—they include green vegetables such as spinach and kale, which contain vitamin K, folate, magnesium, and calcium (Preston and Kirk, 2010). Folate is necessary for reducing alleviating the symptoms of depression. Low folate has been associated with symptoms of depression and lack of response to antidepressants. Foods such as vegetables which are rich in folate also increase the serotonin level, and this helps in alleviating the symptoms linked to depression. Leafy greens or vegetables contain vitamin B, which tends to have an impact on chemicals in the brain that is linked to a person's mood (Preston and Kirk, 2010). The leafy greens play a significant part in protecting a person's body from inflammation.

➤ *Berries*—besides being sweet, berries have nutritional value. Berries have many antioxidants such as anthocyanins and flavonoids, which help in maintaining the health of cells and protect them from oxidative stress and environmental toxins. Anthocyanins assist in reducing inflammation in the body (Energy, 2017).

Furthermore, research has demonstrated that often people affected by depression tend to have in their blood low antioxidant levels. Therefore, the consumption of berries can enhance the antioxidant levels in the blood of those affected by depression. Antioxidants are essential in repairing cells and protecting them from various inflammations.

Blueberries have also been shown as being useful in promoting a positive mindset, alertness, and resilience (Energy, 2017). Studies have shown that compounds found in grapes are anti-depressive. The compounds work through the modulation of inflammation.

The fibre that comes from vegetables or plants tends to

ferment in the gut and produces fatty acids which help in regulating the immune system and influence the expression of the gene in the brain and other parts of the body. Food that is rich in fibre is useful in getting various bacteria that affect a person's mood (Li *et al.*, 2017).

> ➤ **Walnuts**—they are a rich source of Omega-3 fatty acids, which are essential for the functioning of the brain and also alleviate the symptoms linked to depression (Hallahan and Garaland, 2005). Walnuts based on some studies are also a rich source of magnesium, which plays a significant role in decreasing the risk of developing depression in a person.

> ➤ **Fruits**—various fruits such as Apple have iron, fibre and are full of antioxidants which provide healing to the body on a cellular level (Greener, 2015). Most fruits contain natural sugars, minerals, and vitamins which help in supporting other body organs, thereby reducing inflammation.

> ➤ **Onions**—they have antioxidant properties which are useful in providing healing to cells that have been damaged. Some of the symptoms of depression, which include the feeling of sadness can be improved by taking onions which tend to act as mood enhancers (Barton, 2017). Onions also have healthy nutrients that help in fighting various inflammations such as heart diseases and rheumatoid arthritis. Onions can be eaten as part of salads, put in sandwiches, or added to vegetables.

> ➤ **Turkey**—it contains tryptophan a chemical that activates serotonin. Also, turkey has selenium mineral, which acts as an anti-inflammatory and is useful in fighting depression (Barton, 2017).

> ➤ **Fermented foods**—these foods tend to contain bacteria that are healthy and which help in soothing the inflammation

in the gut. Studies have demonstrated that there exists a relationship between the brain and digestive health, which is referred to as *gut-brain axis*. Some critical chemicals in the brain include serotonin, which acts as mood booster, is manufactured in the gut. Therefore, there is a belief that an unhealthy gut harms a person's mood. By taking these foods, a person can fight depression (Barton, 2017).

The Impact of Physical Exercise on Inflammation and Depression

Besides a healthy diet, exercise is another way of reducing both depression and inflammation levels. Being physically inactive has been linked to both depression and inflammation (Roshanaei-Moghaddam, Katon, and Russo, 2009). Studies have shown that exercise, whether aerobic or non-aerobic can lower the C-reactive protein level, which the inflammation marker by the body. When the C-reactive proteins (CRP) are low, inflammation also tends to reduce. Physical exercise that is both planned and regular tends to have the same effects as antidepressants (Schuch *et al.*, 2016).

Furthermore, exercise stimulates the anti-inflammatory outcome primarily by releasing anti-inflammatory cytokines like IL-10, which is helpful for inflammations (Schuch *et al.*, 2016). Physical activity has numerous benefits such as weight management, decreasing the risk of developing heart diseases and strengthening the bones, muscles, and heart.

Exercises enhance the anti-inflammatory response by triggering the sympathetic nervous system (Schuch *et al.*, 2016). As a result, norepinephrine and epinephrine hormones are released by the body, which furthers activates the immune cell receptors. The release of norepinephrine enhances alertness, arousal, vigilance, and attention, which decreases the symptoms linked to depression.

Exercise can be placed at the same level as cognitive behavioural therapy and antidepressants in the treatment of depression, whether moderate or mild (Carek, Laibstain, and Carek, 2011). Though the actual mechanisms through which exercise lessens inflammation might not be fully understood, some studies have pointed out various factors that might contribute. One of the factors includes exercise can reduce the proportion of an individual's body fat, which could be a contributing factor to inflammation.

Another factor proposed by scientists regarding the way exercise reduces inflammation that exercise induces the body into producing a large number of antioxidants which search for and wipe out radicals that might be linked to inflammation (Lamprecht, 2015). In fighting depression, exercise is beneficial since it brings several changes to the brains, which comprise neural growth and new patterns of activity that can enhance feelings of well-being and calmness. When a person is engaged in exercise or physical activity, the brain releases endorphins, which are essential chemicals in energizing the mind.

Engaging in exercise is also beneficial as it provides distraction enabling the person that is affected by depression to break from the negative thought pattern that increases depression (Horowitz, 2017). Additionally, the growth of new cells in the brain can also be stimulated through exercise. When a person engages in regular exercise, their self-esteem tends to be enhanced; the person may begin to feel good regarding him/herself and his/her achievements. All these are essential factors in reducing depression.

Exercise enhances synaptic plasticity; this occurs when the systems that maintain plasticity are strengthened. Furthermore, physical exercise decreases other risk factors such as hypertension, cardiovascular disease, and diabetes, which can lead to depression (Hillegass and Sadowsky, 2010). Therefore, by reducing risk factors assists in ensuring the brain functions efficiently.

Engaging in physical exercise tends to bring a calming effect on the amygdala, thereby controlling the fight-or-flight response. Also, the process of cellular healing is activated through exercise by enhancing the competence of the production of intercellular energy. Exercise activates the making of more insulin receptor, which translates to the efficient use of blood glucose and cells that are strong. When a person engages in physical exercises, this brings relaxation to their muscles, which sends a message to the brain, just like the body; it ought to relax (Horowitz, 2017).

At times, people that are affected by depression may experience insomnia or changes in their sleep pattern; exercise can prove useful as it assists in regulating an individual's sleep pattern (Horowitz, 2017). Depression can lead to destructive behaviours such as drug and substance abuse, alcohol abuse, among other practices. Exercise helps a person that is affected by depression to cope with the symptoms that are healthily linked to depression. Also, when one makes exercise a regular habit, this can boost their immune system.

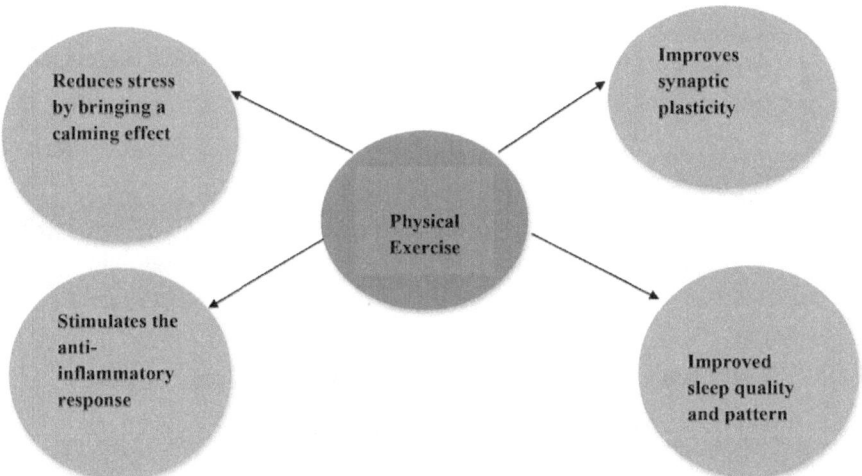

To benefit from the anti-inflammatory effect of exercise a person should

> ➢ ***make exercise a habit***—a person that wants to fight both inflammation and depression through physical exercise should make it a habit (Meadows, 2018). It is wise to start exercising for short periods and engage in activities such as swimming, walking, or running.

➢ ***engage in various activities***—to lower the levels of C-reactive proteins (CRP), a person should participate in multiple exercises such as walking, riding a bike, running, or lifting weights among others (Meadows, 2018). These exercises can be done in a gym or the comfort of one's home.

➢ ***avoid overdoing the exercises***—being overzealous can hurt both the joints and muscles and can be detrimental to a person's health, which can increase rather than reduce inflammation. Therefore, a person should engage in a few exercises and for a short period when starting on making exercise a habit (Meadows, 2018).

To get the anti-inflammatory benefits of physical exercise, a person does not have to engage in it for an extended period. Studies have shown that half an hour a day of physical exercise is enough to experience the anti-inflammatory benefits. This amount of physical exercise can decrease the inflammation markers in a person's body.

The Impact of Slow Breathing in Reducing Stress and Improving the Immune System

The brain's respiratory centre controls breathing when a person is feeling stressed, the pattern and rate of breathing changes. As luck would have it, human beings have the power to control their breathing. Scientific studies have demonstrated that controlling one's breath may assist in the management of stress and thereby, depression (Matzo and Sherman, 2010). The primary function of breathing is to inhale oxygen and exhale carbon dioxide. When a person is stressed, the pattern of breathing tends to change. Usually, a person when anxious tends to take shallow breaths through the use of their muscles rather their diaphragm. This kind of breathing interrupts the stability of gases in an individual's body.

Stress can cause hinder the glutamate surplus to the hippocampus, thus causing damage; this can cause the death of cells leading to memory loss. Over time, the release of excess cortisol tends to destroy the pathways that exist between the amygdala and the hippocampus, and this leads to a dangerous spiral. This forms a brain that is inclined to be in a continuous condition of fight-or-flight. Stress also can reduce the size of dendrites, in so doing hinders the hippocampus from forming new cells; this causes the amygdala to work itself to exhaustion (Andersen, 2007).

Moreover, stress makes the amygdala to form additional connections which continue firing and causes the release of more cortisol than required. As the amygdala continues to fire, it becomes stronger and ultimately subdues the hippocampus. Eventually, a constant feeling of fear, stress, and anxiety gains control over the brain in spite of the prevailing circumstances due to the control of the brain by the amygdala.

Breathing can be done through either the abdomen or the chest. Abdominal breathing begins by relaxing the abdomen and taking deep and slow breaths. As a result, for the lungs to be filled with air, the diaphragm tends to move downward, and this causes an expansion in the belly. Breathing through the abdomen brings the feeling of a balloon that is expanding gently as one inhales and exhales (Hamilton and McClellan, 2014).

On the other hand, chest breathing is often shallow where expansion occurs only in the chest (Pearlman et al., 2014). This kind of breathing makes just a small amount of oxygen to get into the blood, which increases the heart rate and leads to muscle tension. Chest breathing often occurs when an individual is experiencing stress, are in pain, or anxious.

Practising shallow breathing for an extended period can have a disastrous effect on a person's health. Studies have shown that shallow breathing can be linked to chronic stress and less quantity of lymphocyte (Pearlman et al., 2014). When a person has low quantity lymphocyte, which is a kind of white cells that are useful in protecting the body from intruders, it can raise the risk of contracting various illnesses and extending the healing period.

When chest breathing is practised, it may lead to various physical health issues such as the chest, neck, and shoulder muscles are sued to enlarge the lungs. It can lead to headaches and neck pain (Pearlman *et al.*, 2014). The shoulders tend to bend forward, and this can change the posture of a person. On the contrary, breathing by the use of the diaphragm can decrease the heart rate, blood pressure, and reduce stress.

When relaxed, a person's breathing tends to be both gentle and slow. Controlling one's breath may lead to physiological changes such as having low blood pressure and fewer stress hormones in the blood (Hamilton and McClellan, 2014). Additionally, slow breathing may assist in balancing the carbon dioxide and oxygen levels in the blood, enhance feelings of well-being and calmness, experience more physical energy, and improving the functioning of the immune system.

According to some studies, the pattern of breathing produces in the brain electrical activity, which influences what a person can remember; this means that hat it has an impact on the memory. Controlled or slow breathing can enhance the immune system and raise the energy metabolism (Hamilton and McClellan, 2014). Slow breathing activates a parasympathetic response which can improve the resilience of the immune system. Some theories hold the view that controlled or slow breathing can alter the autonomic nervous system's response.

Changing the way a person breathes tends to convey to the brain the need to regulate the parasympathetic region of the nervous system. By doing this, the heart rate slows down, and the feelings of calmness and well-being are enhanced. The sympathetic system which manages the release of cortisol, which is a stress hormone, also improves through controlled breathing. Stress has the potential to exacerbate conditions such as depression and anxiety. By breathing slowly, the message is sent to the brain that everything is alright, and this activates the parasympathetic response (Hamilton and

McClellan, 2014). Additionally, by breathing slowly, the sympathetic reaction is triggered, and this tends to calm down the brain.

Through slow breathing, a person can decrease their blood pressure by managing stress, which is the primary factor that causes high blood pressure and other cardiovascular diseases (Ahem, 2009). When a person has stress, their mind, emotions, and physical bodies are affected. The heart rates increases and blood pressure rises simultaneously, which is referred to as the fight-or-flight mode. The fight-or-flight response is useful when one is in danger but unhelpful when the situation is not life-threatening.

The immune system can be suppressed by stress; for instance, a person might become vulnerable to various infections. Suppressing the immune system can be dangerous since a person may be at risk of getting into physical and mental health conditions. Breathing slowly often leads to calmness and may alleviate anxiety; fast breathing can lead to panic. The calmness that comes from slow breathing activates the nervous system, which calms the nerves (Ahem, 2009). Slow breathing stimulates the region of the nervous system, which enhances relaxation. The result becomes a reduction of inflammation in the body, which improves the efficiency of the immune system.

The levels of stress in the body are controlled by the autonomic nervous system, which comprises two mechanisms which counterbalance one another. The two mechanisms are the sympathetic and parasympathetic nervous systems. The sympathetic nervous system assists during periods of infection or stress and helps a person to manage the danger they may be perceived by triggering the fight-or-flight response (Bennett *et al.*, 2015). The activation of the sympathetic nervous system increases the heart rate, blood pressure, and one begins to breathe more rapidly.

The parasympathetic nervous system brings relaxation and calmness to the body, which counterbalances the impact of the sympathetic nervous system (Arden, 2009). Due to this, the breathing and heart rate becomes slower, which decrease inflammation and hinders the over-responsiveness of the immune system. The incorrect working of the parasympathetic nervous can lead to fast breathing causing constant inflammation.

Stress can adversely affect the various aspect of an individual's physical and mental health. Therefore, it is necessary to note early enough when one is becoming stressed and avoid going that route. By exercising deep or slow breathing, research has shown that brain size can increase. Slow breathing stimulates relaxation, which can alter the expression of the genes, particularly the ones that are involved in the secretion of insulin, energy metabolism, and the immune system (Westra, 2012). Having control over one's breathing can prevent stress, which often affects the brain adversely.

The Impact of Mind and Body Exercises on Stress

The mind-body exercise is one that merges the movement of the body, mental focus, and slow breathing to assist in enhancing balance, strength, and general health (Iknoian, 2011). The mind influences how the body works, therefore understanding the link between the body and the mind is vital in reducing stress. By learning how to use one's thoughts to influence the physical body responses, a person can control their stress level. Mind and body exercises bring a calming effect, which helps in changing the way a person perceives and responds to a situation (Iknoian, 2011).

One of the mind-body exercises commonly applied in the reduction of stress is yoga. A primary concept which yoga applies is becoming non-judgemental towards oneself and others. By not judging oneself, a person can reduce their stress levels since most of the stress experienced comes from self-judgement (Iknoian, 2011). One of the primary rules in yoga is that the mind and body are linked, and stress tends to affect both.

Most people live either through their mind or body, which produces a lack of balance or awareness. For instance, individuals whose careers involve much analysis tend to spend most of their time using their mind. These people might not comprehend the amount of tension their body keeps as a result of spending most of their times in their mind. Another example involves people that use their bodies most of the time like the athletes who might be more aware of their bodies than their mind. In both cases, yoga aids in balancing the relationship between the mind and the body (Iknoian, 2011).

Yoga helps in training the parasympathetic nervous system, which is involved in stress response. When a person engages in the practice of yoga regularly, the level of their stress hormone tends to drop (Iknoian, 2011).

Other Symptoms of Depression and Anxiety besides Inflammation

There has been a long-held belief that depression and anxiety disorders are primarily caused by the imbalances of chemicals such as serotonin in the brain. This current school of thought also views the presence of inflammation in the inflammatory markers in the blood indicate depression. This current school of thought that has attributed depression to inflammation is inaccurate since other factors can be connected to the development of the condition.

This school of thought attributes depression to inflammation holds the view that if a diagnosis of a patient does not show any inflammatory agents, then the patient has no depression is erroneous. The reason being at times a patient might portray no signs of inflammation, yet they are affected by depression. The treatment that is most offered to patients affected by depression based in this school of thought is aimed at enhancing the serotonin levels (Cook, 2016). Advertisements by pharmaceutical companies have popularised this school of thought by showing that medications alone can restore the serotonin levels, thereby alleviating depression.

Research has demonstrated that people affected by depression and other mental disorders, such as schizophrenia and anxiety disorders, have high levels of inflammatory markers (Raison *et al.*, 2013). Also as discussed earlier, people that are affected by depression can have a suppressed immune system (Bufalino *et al.*, 2013). However, inflammation or a suppressed immune system does not always lead to depression, but it is one of the factors which may cause depression.

Although inflammation may lead to mental illness such as depression in a particular individual, mental disorders are not inflammatory conditions. The notion that chemical imbalances in the brain are the primary cause of depression is deeply rooted in our brain though this is not always true (Dantzer and Capuron, 2017). Most advertisements regarding depression portray antidepressants as the ultimate cure for depression as it corrects serotonin, which, according to popular belief, its deficiency is the primary cause of depression.

Nevertheless, no research has shown the existence of a relationship between mental disorders such as depression and chemical imbalances in the brain (Dantzer and Capuron, 2017). Hence, an individual might be affected by depression, yet the results show no inflammation or chemical imbalances in their brain. The belief that chemical imbalances in the brain always lead to depression can be misleading since no evidence indicates that when dopamine, norepinephrine, and when dopamine levels are low, the patient is affected by depression. Furthermore, studies have shown that only a small percentage of people affected by depression have reduced serotonin and norepinephrine levels.

The view that reduced serotonin levels lead to depression is so prevalent that people often talk about enhancing their serotonin levels in various ways, such as exercise and medications (Acton, 2012). This theory is erroneous since cocaine and amphetamine are drugs that improve the norepinephrine and serotonin levels but do not alleviate the symptoms of depression. Also, some people affected by depression tend to have high norepinephrine and serotonin levels, and other people with no depression have low levels of these chemicals. Therefore, inflammation cannot be viewed as the only factor that causes depression.

Measuring norepinephrine and serotonin in the brain is also difficult since only small amounts of these agents in cerebrospinal fluid and urine are from the brain. Most of the serotonin and norepinephrine come from other parts of the body. Hence, the results from inflammatory markers in a patient's blood cannot be relied on to ascertain whether a person is affected by depression or not since chemical imbalances do not just cause the disorder in the brain.

The absence of inflammation cannot make a mental health practitioner conclude that the patient has no depression. Instead, in such cases other symptoms that can indicate the presence of depression should be looked into, they include among others:

> ➤ **Feelings of hopelessness**—people that are affected by depression tend to feel hopeless regarding their circumstances (Yapko, 2013). The person might feel there is no point in living; therefore, they can become suicidal. Thus, even though in the blood there might be no inflammatory markers indicating inflammation, hopelessness can be a sign that the person is affected by depression.

> ➤ **Lack of interest in things previously enjoyed**—when a person is affected by depression, this can take away the pleasure of enjoying things they earlier loved (Edlin and Golanty, 2016). When a person loses interest in participating in activities that they enjoyed before, such as music, baking, or sports, this can be indicating that they could be experiencing depression.

> ➤ **Changes in sleep patterns and fatigue**—depression can occur with feelings of an overwhelming lack of energy, which can lead to too much sleeping (Edlin and Golanty, 2016). Depression can also lead to a lack of sleep or insomnia, leading to immense feelings of fatigue.

> ➤ **Anxiety**—though depression does not lead to anxiety, the two can co-occur. Symptoms of anxiety, such as restlessness, fast breathing, increased heart rate, fear, or panic can also

be linked to depression (Edlin and Golanty, 2016). Therefore, if the patient is exhibiting such symptoms even though no inflammation can be detected, these symptoms can be signs of depression.

➢ ***Lack of control regarding one's emotions***—individuals experiencing depression can experience mood swings. These people tend to switch from happiness to sadness regularly even though their external circumstances may be unchanged (Edlin and Golanty, 2016).

➢ ***Becoming suicidal***—if a person is always talking about death or self-harm, this can be an indication that they are affected by depression (Edlin and Golanty, 2016). The person can also develop an unusual desire for death; he/she might even begin to act recklessly in a manner that shows the desire to die. For instance, the individual might start driving carelessly as if they want to cause an accident. Also, calling people and bidding them goodbye can be a sign of the desire to commit suicide.

Additionally, statements such as 'people are better off when I am not around' should not be ignored as the person could be planning on how to end their lives. Even though the blood test might show no inflammation, suicidal thought and talks can be taken as an indication of depression.

➢ ***Changes in appetite***—some individuals when anxious or depressed tend to overeat while others eat very little or have to be forced to eat (Edlin and Golanty, 2016). Changes in a person's appetite should not be ignored, but the person should be observed keenly to ascertain whether they are affected by depression or not.

➢ **Self-hate or low self-esteem**—a person with low self-esteem or self-hate is vulnerable to developing depression (Edlin and Golanty, 2016). When a physician comes into contact with an individual whose self-esteem is low, even though the inflammatory markers in their blood may indicate no inflammation, they should be viewed as being affected by depression.

➢ **Psychomotor impairment**—a person that is affected by depression might feel as if things have slowed down. For instance, the person might start experiencing slowed speech, lethargy, and being slow in their body movements (Edlin and Golanty, 2016). If the person is undergoing such changes, then they should be examined on whether they are depressed.

➢ **Inability to concentrate**—depression can make an individual experience a lack of concentration or become indecisive. This is another symptom a mental health practitioner should be observant about despite test results in the inflammatory markers in the blood that show no inflammation (Edlin and Golanty, 2016).

If some or all of these symptoms are in existence, a person could be having depression even though the patient's blood might not be showing any inflammatory markers and have no inflammation.

Inflammatory Medication as a Cure for Depression and Anxiety

Inflammation does not cause depression but can increase the risk an individual has in developing the disorder. The inflammation tends to bring changes in the functioning the brain or body, and it can lead to the development of various psychiatric disorders such as depression, but it is not the primary cause of depression (Dantzer and Capuron, 2017). Nevertheless, inflammation is one of the many factors that make an individual vulnerable to depression. When inflammation is the primary cause of depression, anti-inflammatory medications, non-steroidal inflammatory drugs can be used in the treatment of the disorder.

Depression is often connected to an increase in inflammatory cytokines in the brain and the peripheral blood in some of the people affected by the disorder. The pro-inflammatory cytokines may activate in the brain an inflammatory flow which incorporates the stimulation of cyclooxygenases, which are vital enzymes in prostaglandins production (Harden *et al.*, 2015). According to this observation, a treatment which targets the cyclooxygenases (COX-1) and (COX-2) can be useful for people affected by depression and have high levels of pro-inflammatory cytokines.

COX-1 tends to have a pro-inflammatory responsibility in the brain while COX-2 has both anti and pro-inflammatory reactions (Heinrich *et al.*, 2012). When COX-2 selective inhibitors are used in treating inflammation, the brain's inflammatory markers are reduced, which suggests that this may be applied to patients that are affected by depression.

There have been various studies that have investigated whether treating symptoms of depression with anti-inflammatory drugs such as TNF receptor antagonist, cyclooxygenase-2 inhibitors, and acetylsalicylic acid can reduce the symptoms of depression. Some of the non-steroidal anti-inflammatory drugs are more useful in the treatment of depression than placebo (Köhler *et al.*, 2014).

Non-steroidal anti-inflammatory drugs work by slowing down particular enzymes which are referred to as cyclooxygenase in the body which are released in the course of tissue damage (Bull and Creamer, 2006). The NSAIDS obstruct various kinds of cyclooxygenase such as COX- 1 and COX-2, which help in reducing inflammation. NSAIDS, when taken in the recommended dosage, are beneficial, but when a person exceeds the dosage, it can lead to various health complications such as high blood pressure and kidney problems.

Cytokine inhibitors and non-steroidal anti-inflammatory drugs, particularly cyclooxygenase 2 (COX-2) which hinders pro-inflammatory cytokines, tend to apply the anti-inflammatory effects. There are conflicting views regarding the impact of anti-inflammatory agents in the treatment of depression. Some studies have shown that the use of non-steroidal anti-inflammatory drugs tends to reduce some the symptoms of depression such as fatigue and anxiety while others show the opposite.

The benefits of using anti-inflammatory drugs should be weighed against the adverse effects that could arise. For instance, non-steroidal anti-inflammatory drugs can increase the risk of cardiovascular and gastrointestinal issues (de Abajo and Garcia-Rodriguez, 2008). The use of cytokine inhibitors in the treatment of anxiety and depression can raise the risk of various infections (Toussi *et al.*, 2013). Some of the selective cyclooxygenase 2 (COX-2) drugs have been removed from the market as they increase the risk of developing cardiovascular diseases.

Further studies have proposed that in comparison to other selective cyclooxygenase inhibitors, using celecoxib is safer in the early stage of antidepressant treatment (Müller *et al.*, 2006). However, the use of celecoxib should be approached carefully to avoid any adverse effect. Most of the non-steroidal anti-inflammatory drugs have been linked to a reduction in the symptoms of depression.

Non-steroidal anti-inflammatory drugs (NSAIDS) are believed to have a significant role in alleviating the anti-inflammatory effects of depression. For people who are eighteen years and above, NSAIDs tend to reduce the symptoms of bipolar disorder (Rosenblat *et al.*, 2016). A study was done in Australia for over five thousand men between the ages of 69–87 years examining the connection between aspirin which is an anti-inflammatory drug and depression showed that those who had used the drug previously but stopped were at a higher risk of developing symptoms linked to depression (Almeida *et al.*, 2010).

Non-steroid anti-inflammatory medications can reduce the risk of developing depression, especially during its early onset (Gibert Rahola, 2012).

Non-steroidal anti-inflammatory drugs are often used in the treatment of inflammation and pain. However, non-steroidal anti-inflammatory drugs tend to have several adverse effects, which include cardiovascular diseases and gastrointestinal bleeding. The side effects of COX-2 tend to increase with the age of the person (Bennett and Yuan, 2008).

Non-steroidal anti-inflammatory drugs can be used together with antidepressants as an additional treatment of depression because of anti-inflammatory mechanisms that are common (Kohler *et al.*, 2014). Anti-inflammatory drugs can help in the treatment of individuals affected by depression who have high levels of inflammatory biomarkers. The success of these treatments depends on measuring the peripheral inflammatory markers linked with a depressive score, and the information acquired should assist in establishing the period of the treatment.

Nevertheless, non-steroidal anti-inflammatory drugs are not the ultimate answer in the treatment of depression and can help only a small group of people affected by depression. Before prescribing any NSAID, various factors should be put into consideration. These factors include the cardiovascular and gastrointestinal risk factors involved.

Non-Steroidal Anti-Inflammatory Medications and How They Work

These are drugs that help in reducing inflammation but have no connection with steroids, which also alleviate inflammation. Non-steroidal anti-inflammatory medicines help in decreasing the production of the prostaglandins; these are chemicals which increase inflammation, fever, and pain (Golan, 2008). NSAIDs also safeguard the intestines and the stomach lining from the adverse acid effect, and by triggering blood, platelets enhance the clotting of blood. By doing this, the normal functioning of the kidneys is increased.

Prostaglandins are produced by cyclooxygenases (COX), which is an enzyme (Golan, 2008). COX enzymes are of two types, mainly COX-1 and COX-2, which both create prostaglandins which increase inflammation. Nonetheless, the prostaglandins that are produced by COX-1 stimulate platelets and shield the intestinal and stomach lining. By blocking COX enzymes, non-steroidal anti-inflammatory drugs lessen prostaglandins production, which helps in the reduction of fever, pain, and inflammation.

Non-steroidal anti-inflammatory drugs vary in the period of action and their effectiveness. Also, people tend to respond to NSAIDS differently (Walsh, 2009). They are used in the treatment of various conditions that cause inflammation, fever, and pain. Some of these conditions include headaches, rheumatoid arthritis, dental pain, backaches, and colds among others. Non-steroidal anti-inflammatory drugs work similarly to steroids but have fewer side effects than steroids. Some NSAIDs work faster in comparison to others, depending on the inflammation being treated.

There are various risks associated with taking NSAIDs, and they include among others:

> **Stomach problems**—the use of non-steroidal anti-inflammatory drugs can cause stomach problems, especially if a person has stomach ulcers. People that are sixty years and above or individuals who take alcohol and smoke often can also develop stomach problems when they take NSAIDs (Scully, 2010).

> **Heart problems**—researches have shown that all non-steroidal anti-inflammatory drugs except low doses of aspirin can raise the likelihood of getting a stroke or a heart attack.

> **Kidney problems**—NSAIDs impact the working of kidneys. People that are sixty years and above or are

dehydrated are at a higher of developing kidney problems when they use NSAIDs (Walsh, 2009).

➤ **Asthma**—non-steroidal anti-inflammatory drugs can make asthma symptoms such as shortness of breath, wheezing, or coughing to worsen.

➤ **Blood pressure**—the use of NSAIDs can increase blood pressure in some individuals.

➤ **Pregnancy**—during early pregnancy, NSAIDs can raise the possibility of miscarriage. It is recommended that a pregnant woman should avoid NSAIDs unless advised otherwise by their doctor.

Neurotoxins

This is a chemical that changes the function or structure of the nervous system. Neurotoxins can overstimulate nerve cells to death or interfere with their transmission process. Most neurotoxins come from environmental sources. On the other hand, other neurotoxins are internally produced and live in the body they include glutamate and neurotransmitters nitric oxide. The degree to which the neurotoxin affects the function of nerves is based on the person's health and age.

Furthermore, the frequency and level of contact one have with a particular chemical determines the extent to which the nerve function is affected. For example, vitamin B6 and A, are crucial; nevertheless, when consumed in large doses, they become neurotoxic. Also, treatments such as antipsychotic drugs and chemotherapy have a neurotoxic effect, but their benefits are more than their risks.

The absorption of neurotoxins can be through skin contact, inhalation, injection, or ingestion and might bring short or long-term effects by causing the malfunctioning of neurons or interrupting the communication of neurons (Dikshith, 2011).

Elderly and young people are most susceptible to neurotoxic

chemicals. Older adults, due to their age, often experience a decrease in the neural function, which hinders their capacity to manage with neurotoxins' effect. Exposure to chemicals in early childhood can lead to permanent brain damage (Roy, 2012). Some of the symptoms of neurotoxicity include a headache, paralysis in some limbs, the loss of memory, behavioural problems, compulsive behaviour, and depression among others.

Various researches have demonstrated that the lifespan of nerve cells can be shortened by neurotoxins, which can lead to mental disorders such as depression, insomnia, chronic fatigue, and anxiety (Berdanier, 2011).

CHAPTER 3

Correlation between Depression, Immune System, Inflammation, and Neurological Disorders

The previous chapter has explained the relationship between inflammation and depression and pointed out that inflammation does not cause depression even though most people affected by depression have inflammations. This chapter will be dedicated to looking at the impact which anxiety and depression have on the immune, neural, and endocrine systems.

What Is an Immune System?

The immune system can be described as the body's defence mechanism against germs and other intruders; it comprises of organs and cells (Sompayrac, 2011). The immune system fights germs and other infectious organisms attacking the body through what is referred to as the immune response. The immune system is further divided into two categories, namely the adaptive and innate immune systems.

The Innate Immune System

The innate immune system becomes effective from the start of a person's life; its operations are specified unto the genetic codes of a person (Sompayrac, 2011). The innate immune system acts in a non-specific or general manner, which means that whatever it recognises as an intruder becomes its target. This system comprises of barriers whose goal is to protect the body from parasites, viruses, bacteria, and other intruders. The physical barriers which are part of the innate system include the skin, the respiratory system, and body hairs such as eyelashes among others. Other defence mechanisms used by the innate system include the use of various bodily secretions like saliva, mucous, sweat, bile, and tears.

The skin protects the body in various ways such as blocking the entry of germs and other infectious organisms and also through the sweat glands which releases to the skin a substance that is slightly acidic and which inhibits bacterial growth (Sompayrac, 2011). Secretions such as tears act as a barrier against infection by washing away bacteria and keeping the eye from infection through lysozyme, which is an enzyme contained in tears. Saliva acts as a barrier against infection by washing away food particles, which are eaten by bacteria. Also, the saliva contains most of the body's protective antibodies.

In situations where the germs manage to get through the barriers and into the body, various immune responses occur. One of them is the defence mechanisms such as the white blood cells (leukocytes) which looks out for and ingests the germs or organisms that are attacking the body by causing diseases (Sompayrac, 2011). The white blood cells or leukocytes are formed and kept in various parts of the body, such as the bone marrow, spleen, and thymus. Owing to this, they are commonly referred to as the lymphoid organs.

In comparison to the adaptive immune system, the innate system retains no memory of earlier encounters with intruders (Sompayrac, 2011). Therefore, it does not guard the body against future infections like the adaptive immune system. The innate immune system comprises various kinds of white blood cells such as the monocytes, eosinophils, neutrophils, and basophils. The monocytes develop into macrophages whenever an infection takes place. After the monocytes move to the infected area, they enlarge and create granules that assist in destroying the foreign intruders or germs.

The neutrophils, on the other hand, consume intruders and bacteria and also strengthen the body's defence (Hartmann and Wagner, (2013). Eosinophils contain granules that release enzymes which target bacteria that cannot be ingested due to their large size. Eosinophils identify, stick to, and destroy the intruders. Basophils have granules that contain histamine, and when they come into contact with allergens, they discharge histamine to raise the flow of blood to the tissues that are damaged (Hartmann and Wagner, (2013). This process leads to swelling and inflammation as an allergic response.

The innate immune system is actively involved in the inflammation response by bringing in phagocytic cells to the infected area to prepare it for healing (Sompayrac, 2011). By bringing the cells of the innate immune system to the affected area, the pathogen is removed, and the affected area is isolated to restrict the pathogen from spreading. The innate immune responses are vital in managing infections early as a way of providing a physiological defence.

Innate responses happen fast but can be considered to be less efficient than adaptive immune responses. Various cells, antibacterial proteins, and mediators can cause innate immune responses (Hartmann and Wagner, 2013). After a few days of infection, other antibacterial proteins are stimulated which fight against the bacteria. The development of the adaptive immune response does not hinder the response of the innate immune system.

Adaptive/Acquired Immune System

The adaptive immune system comprises of lymphocytes and antibodies which are referred to as the cell-mediated response. The adaptive immune system modifies its response to the specific intruder

(Mak and Saunders, 2006). Unlike the innate immune system, the adaptive system retains memory regarding previous foreign intruders or infections. Therefore, the memory cells stay prepared to respond competently and promptly to an ensuing confrontation with a pathogen. Consequently, when a similar infection tries to re-occur, it is met by stiff resistance by the adaptive immune system (Mak and Saunders, 2006).

Immunological memory can be seen in vaccinations which copies the presence of a virus that is active to lead to an immune response although the vaccination poses no threat to the body. When a person receives a vaccination, they expose their immune system to an antigen that is needed to develop antibodies particular to that virus. Furthermore, the immune system obtains a remembrance of the virus devoid of experiencing the infection (Mak and Saunders, 2006).

The subsequent response tends to be stronger than the first reaction to an infection. As a result, the infections that occur in childhood tend to protect a person during their adulthood. In its response to infections and threats, the adaptive immune system tends to be slower than the innate immune system's response (Mak and Saunders, 2006). The response of the adaptive immune system is often perceived after several days of its encounter with the intruder or pathogen.

The T and B cells are the cellular components of the adaptive immune system. Memory and flexibility are the trademarks of the adaptive immune system (Kumar, 2013). The flexibility of the adaptive immune system is seen in the way through which the T and B lymphocytes identify antigens. T cells and B cells differ in various ways; the first is that T cells exist on the surface of cells and thus are not secreted. Another difference is that T cells identify peptides created by the antigens' proteolytic cleavage in contrast to the B cells, which tends to identify the native proteins (Kumar, 2013).

Another difference between the B and T cells includes T cells tend to identify the sequence of amino acids while B cells recognise a protein's tertiary structure. The other difference is that T cells can only identify antigenic peptides when they are on the cell surface, unlike the B cells (Kumar, 2013). The differentiation and proliferation of the naïve B cells in response to various antigens requires stimulation from helper T cells and CD4+, which is particular for the same antigen. When T cells encounter an antigen, their differentiation and proliferation necessitate the second signal.

The T cells that do not get this signal often have a higher likelihood of becoming unresponsive. Therefore, T cells govern the antigens, which B cells help to identify, which demonstrates that T and B cells engage together during immune responses (Kumar, 2013). It is possible for T cells to be divided into different subsets depending on their functional capacities and patterns of migration. Furthermore, memory T cells can be divided into effector and central memory cells (Sallusto, Geginat, and Lanzavecchia, 2004).

The central memory cells move between lymph nodes and the blood. When activated with antigen, memory cells rigger more effector, T, and memory cells. Effector memory T cells are aggressive, and their lifespan tends to be short (Sallusto, Geginat, and Lanzavecchia, 2004). Memory T cells could also be identified depending on the peripheral tissue they use for their entry. T cells that first come into contact with a particular antigen in the future recirculate through the tissue where the antigen was (Kupper and Fuhlbrigge, 2004).

Additionally, the adaptive immune system depends on a few cells, namely the T cells and the B cells, to carry out its duties. The B cells and T cells, which create antibodies, are obtained from the bone marrow (Kumar, 2013). The B cell mediates the humoral immunity while the T cells mediate the cell-mediated immunity. The humoral immunity is that part of the response of the adaptive immune system which the B cells cause (Mak and Saunders, 2006).

The humoral immunity can be active where an individual after being exposed to a foreign antigen makes an antibody (Mak and Saunders, 2006). This immunity can also be passive where a person receives an antigen produced by another person. For instance, antibodies passed to an unborn child from its mother through the placenta.

A person that has never been exposed to a particular disease can be administered with antibodies to get humoral immunity (Mak and Saunders, 2006). On the other hand, an individual can get cell-mediated immunity from a person that is immune to the particular infection or disease. The cell-mediated and humoral immune response depends on the host and the virus, and they are both vital in fighting viruses in the body. The adaptive immune system protects the body in circumstances that the innate immune system has failed. The adaptive immunity is activated once a pathogen escapes the innate immune system for long sufficient to create a threshold degree of an antigen.

Depression and anxiety tend to weaken the immune system and thus increases an individual's vulnerability to illnesses and diseases (Anisman, Hayley, and Kusnecov, 2018). Since anxiety or stress constantly activates the autonomic nervous system, the capacity of the immune system becomes diminished. One of the symptoms of depression is having a negative outlook on life (Anisman, Hayley, and Kusnecov, 2018). According to research, a negative outlook can weaken the immune's system capacity in fighting diseases. There is a correlation between the number of lymphocyte cells in an individual and their optimism's level.

Even in physical health conditions that are considered not dangerous such as common colds, a positive attitude is often linked with an enhanced capacity of fighting off the infection. Therefore, we can conclude that a person's immune system cannot be separated from their mental health (Anisman, Hayley, and Kusnecov, 2018).

T Cells

T cells are a type of white blood cells which are vital to the immune system. T cells act like soldiers that look for and eradicate the targeted intruders. These cells are produced in the bone marrow and develop in the thymus where the name T cell originates. Most of the T cells do not reach maturity since the body tends to be selective regarding the T cells that are formed to avoid damaging the cells in one's body (Eroschenko and Fiore, 2013). In the thymus, the T cells increase and separate into different kinds of mature T cells; they are also provided with various T-cell receptors.

After maturity, as a reaction to a hormone referred to as thymosin, among other factors, T cells tend to become actively involved in the immune system (Eroschenko and Fiore, 2013). When T cells become activated by the right antigen, they produce interleukins and cytokines, which are chemical messengers. T cells use cytokines to convey chemical commands to the immune system and increase its response.

T cells have various roles which include conveying information regarding the growth and stimulation of B cells. These cells also stimulate cells that ingest invaders. During an infection which is caused by a virus, T cells stimulate cytotoxic T cells. On their own, T cells cannot identify foreign intruders without receiving assistance from antigen-presenting cells which ingest the intruders (Hall and Guyton, 2011). These foreign substances are later introduced to the T cells by the antigen-presenting cells which initiate a response. After a response has been activated, numerous T cells of various kinds are released into the bloodstream (Hall and Guyton, 2011).

There are two kinds of T cells, the killer T cells and the helper T cells. The killer cells directly destroy cells which the intruders have infected. To function correctly, the T cells require distinguishing between cells that are infected and those that are healthy, and they do this with the assistance of antigens (Lotze and Thomson, 2010). Healthy cells have on their surface *self-antigens*, which allow the T cells to recognise that they are not invaders. On the contrary, cells that have a virus infection tend to have on their surface virus antigens; this acts as a signal to the killer T cells that these cells require destruction (Lotze and Thomson, 2010).

The helper T cells, on the other hand, influence the B cells into making antibodies and assist in the development of the killer cells (Boudewijn, 2018). The helper T cells do not fight intruders or produce toxins; instead, they act as coordinators in a team. These T cells provide instructions to other cells of the immune system through chemical messages. The instructions that are given assist the B cells and killer T cells in producing more cells to help fight infections efficiently. Helper T cells support other immune cells' activity through the release of cytokines (Boudewijn, 2018).

Additionally, the helper T cells aid in regulating or suppressing the immune responses. Whenever the helper T cells send a message, a killer T cell is made aware of the presence of a virus (Boudewijn, 2018). After the killer T cells have identified the infected cell, they destroy it (Boudewijn, 2018).

There are multiple kinds of T cells, each one produced to identify one specific antigen. T cells recognise the specific antigen by seeking two types of messages from the phagocyte which has destroyed the microbe. The first message is the part of antigen exhibited on the surface of the phagocyte (Boudewijn, 2018). The other signal is the red flag activated by the pattern-recognition receptors of the innate immune system's cells. This signal is vital since it communicates to the T cells the need to increase and ready itself to confront the foreign invaders.

When an antigen for the first time comes into contact with the T cells, these cells bind themselves on to an antigen receptor on the surface of the phagocyte (Rastogi, 2003). This action makes the T cells to begin producing copies that are similar to it and which can identify the particular antigen. After a few days, the number of T cells multiplies and categorises themselves to groups with allocated duties (Rastogi, 2003). Some of the T cells are designated with the task of destroying cells that are infected. Others are given the responsibility of remembering the antigen and waiting in case it comes back later (memory T cells).

There are also T cells which suppress or subdue the immune response to hinder the destruction of the normal cells after the immune response is completed. Suppressor cells have a significant role in guarding against autoimmune attacks (Jiang, 2008). There are also cytotoxic cells which guard against cells that have a viral infection. After the helper T cells have been activated, cytotoxic cells organise on how to destroy their target. The cytotoxic cells begin by latching on to the infected cell and then release an enzyme that destroys the structure of the cell (Acton, 2012). Nearby cells that are not infected are spared from the destruction.

The substances which the cytotoxic cell releases leads to the self-destruction of the infected cell and not an explosion (Acton, 2012). After the cell has been destroyed, the cytotoxic T cells disengage itself and go to eliminate other cells that are either damaged or infected. Depression and anxiety have been linked to a reduced number of cytotoxic T cell and less activity in the killer T cell.

Cytokines, which are produced when T cells become activated, tend to have a crucial role in the immune responses (Kim *et al.*, 2016). When the immune cytokines level is increased, this can lead to depression, and this may trigger the immune system, thereby releasing interleukins and cytokine (Eyre, Stuart, and Baune, 2014). High levels of cytokine and interleukins, which often are a result of trauma, and infections can lead to symptoms of depression (Dantzer *et al.*, 2008). According to research, low levels of regulatory T cells have been linked to depression among adolescents (Snijders *et al.*, 2016).

Cytokines and T Cells Helper

Cytokines are molecules that are involved in cell signalling and assist in sending information between cells in immune responses. Cytokines can be anti-inflammatory or pro-inflammatory. High levels of pro-inflammatory cytokines can lead to depression and its associated comorbid conditions (Dahl *et al.*, 2014).

Cytokines also activate cells movement towards areas where there is trauma, inflammation, or infection. Generally, cytokines tend to be anti or pro-inflammatory. The balance that occurs between the pro- and anti-inflammatory cytokines establishes the anti-inflammatory response outcome (Neurath, 2014).

Interferon and interleukin agents which regulate the response of the immune system to inflammation are examples of cytokines (Rubin and Tamaoki, 2005). Many cells in the body produce cytokines, but the principal producers are macrophages and the helper T cells. A cytokine is a common name as other names are described according to their presumed roles or objective of action. For instance, lymphokines refer to cytokines, which are made from lymphocytes.

A single cytokine can have multiple roles, and various cytokines can moderate similar roles (Rubin and Tamaoki, 2005). Cytokines can work against one another, work collectively, or act individually. Various aspects of immunity and inflammation involve cytokines. There are different kinds of cytokines whose functions are different. Chemokines are a kind of cytokine whose role is to call other cells to the area where there is an infection (Spellman, 2007). For instance, when an intruder is identified, chemical instructions are given out to the immune cells, which include white blood cells. Afterwards, the cells move to the area where there is an infection and get rid of the foreign substance (Spellman, 2007).

Interferons are another type of cytokines which hinder the duplication of viruses. Cells release interferons whenever they are attacked by a virus (Rubin and Tamaoki, 2005). This action informs other cells to guard against the spread of the virus; thus, interferons obstruct viruses from spreading. Additionally, interferons stimulate natural killer T cells which destroy the cells that are infected as a way of fighting the virus (Rubin and Tamaoki, 2005). Interleukins are another type of cytokines; they monitor the inflammatory and immune responses. Interleukins are primarily formed by white blood cells. Their central role is to assist in communication between white blood cells.

Cytokines are necessary for the development of the brain and can enhance the healthy functioning of the brain by reinforcing synaptic remodelling, neurogenesis, and neuronal integrity (Yirmiya and Goshen, 2011). Cytokines can also influence the neurotransmitter and neurocircuitry system to bring behavioural change (Harron *et al.*, 2012).

When cytokines are acutely administered a type of behaviour referred to as *sickness behaviour* is induced. This behaviour includes changes in sleep patterns, anhedonia, fever, reduction in social interactions, and anorexia (Dantzer and Kelly, 2007). The adaptive behavioural responses to cytokines can assist in improving the maintenance of energy and distribution of resources to fight infections or enhance recovery (Lotrich, 2012).

Nevertheless, when the body is exposed to high levels of inflammatory cytokines, the constant changes in the behaviour and function in the neurotransmitter can cause the development of mental disorders such as depression. For example, patients that have elevated inflammatory cytokines due to various health conditions tend to have higher depression rates in comparison to the general population. Additionally, when cytokines are administered to humans, it leads to neuropsychiatric symptoms and changes in behaviour, which can be linked to depression (Miller *et al.*, 2009). At this point, it is necessary to note that not all kinds of depressions are a result of cytokines.

Psychological and physical stressors can stimulate the immune cells in both the central nervous system and periphery to produce inflammatory cytokines that lead to neurotransmitters and behavioural alterations (Koo and Duman, 2008). Generally, cytokines are produced whenever a disease occurs as they trigger both physical and mental symptoms. When inflammation occurs, the immune cells as a response to cytokines enclose the infected area. This enclosure hinders the infection from spreading to other parts of the body, which confines the infection.

Cytokines can influence neurotransmitter and neurocircuitry systems to bring about behavioural change (Haroon *et al.*, 2012). Some of the behavioural changes include changes in sleep patterns, reduced social interactions, and fever among others (Dantzer and Kelley, 2007). Increased levels of inflammatory cytokines can lead to depression. For example, people that have elevated inflammatory cytokines owing to various medical conditions are at a higher risk of developing depression in comparison to the general public.

When cytokines are injected, they tend to bring alterations in the central nervous system. Also, when cytokines are internally produced in response to different issues such as stress they bring changes to the central nervous system. IL-1β, which is a pro-inflammatory cytokine, is elevated in elderly individuals that have depression (Thomas *et al.*, 2005). Other studies have also demonstrated that IL-1β levels are high in women who may be experiencing depressive symptoms (Corwin *et al.*, 2008).

Patients that are affected by depression tend to have increased inflammatory chemicals which are highly sensitive to stressful stimuli. People who have more marked inflammatory responses to illnesses that are chronic tend to be susceptible to depression and fatigue than other people (Khairova *et al.*, 2009). Therefore, people whose inflammatory cytokine levels are high are more prone to inflammatory illnesses.

During inflammation, cytokines can be used in the treatment of autoimmune disorders such as celiac disease, rheumatoid arthritis, and thyroid disease among others and also infections. The release of pro-inflammatory cytokines tends to affect an individual's mood (Khairova *et al.*, 2009). Cytokines trigger indoleamine, which reduces serotonin levels; this contributes to symptoms of depression. The release of cytokines into the blood can impact the function of all organs and tissues in the body, which includes the brain.

Cytokines can produce signs and symptoms of physical illness and can trigger the symptoms of various mental illnesses such as schizophrenia and depression (Melnyk and Beedy, 2012). Additionally, cytokines create physical symptoms often linked to depression, such as inflammation and abnormalities in hormones. Since cytokines are produced during illnesses, they tend to trigger many physical and mental symptoms (Melnyk and Beedy, 2012).

When inflammation occurs, immune cells as a response to cytokines encircle the area where the infection is and forms a surrounding wall which hinders the infection from spreading to other parts of the body. This action ensures that the infections remain in one place.

Cytokines can also lead to muscle wasting since when released into the blood, they move to every part of the body, including muscles (Melnyk and Beedy, 2012). Some cytokines activate enzymes which break down the muscles into an amino acid. The immune system engages in this kind of action when it requires more amino acids to fight against foreign substances.

Furthermore, antibodies which fight against intruders are created from amino acids. Muscles tend to act as storage of essential foods necessary for an immune system which is involved in fighting intruders. Cytokines can move to the brain and cause substantial changes in a person's mood, attitude, and behaviour (Melnyk and Beedy, 2012).

Cytokines are useful in treating medical illnesses such as leukaemia, hepatitis C, and multiple sclerosis. The cytokines which are commonly used are IL-2, IFNγ, IFNβ, and IFNα (Plotnikoff, 2007). These cytokines are reported to have different side effects like myalgia, confusion, and asthenia. The treatment that involves IL-2 and IFNα has been attributed to depression.

T-helper cell assists other cells by identifying foreign substances and producing cytokines, which stimulate band T cells. T-helper cells contain on their surface CD4 markers (Zhang, 2007). During an attack of the immune system, which might come from toxins, infections, or physical injuries, an inflammatory response is generated by the immune system. Inflammation leads to the production of cytokines.

T-helper cells are essential to human responses as they coordinate the immune system by managing other subsets of the T cells, innate human responses, and B cells. The T-helper cell responses are determined by two evident pathways comprising of two distinct subsets namely T-helper type 1 (Th1) and T-helper type 2 (Th2) cells (Sun, 2014). The Th1 target intravesicular pathogens like parasites and bacteria through macrophages that are infected. The Th2 cells, on the other hand, induce the production of antibodies in B cells, which deactivates extracellular toxins and pathogens.

The T-helper cells secrete cytokines, which are chemical messengers that activate the continuation of the non-specific immune response and enhance and strengthen the specific responses. In the immune system, the T-helper cells are referred to as *generals* since they gather cytotoxic T cells, B cells, and other T-helper cells to fight against foreign intruders (Renneberg and Demain, 2008). Macrophages warn T-helper cells regarding the presence of foreign agents. The macrophages envelop viruses and bacteria and may exhibit the foreign antigen on the exterior of their cell membrane.

The helper T cells attach to the intruder and the human leukocyte antigen (Renneberg and Demain, 2008). Only T-helper cells that have receptors that are identical with the foreign agents that are on the activated molecule can attach and respond. Some signals which the helper T cells send activate cytotoxic cells which are referred to as killer T cells. The cytotoxic T cells attach to cells that are already altered by various factors such as viral infection and avoid healthy cells (Renneberg and Demain, 2008). Surface antigens on the cell that is altered execute the binding. Furthermore, the cytotoxic cell concurrently binds the major histocompatibility complex molecule on the exterior of the infected cell. The cytotoxic cell then produces perforin a chemical that annihilates the offending cell.

Additionally, Helper T cells activate the manufacture of antibodies (Gandhi, 2004). Chemical signals originating from helper T cells activate the formation of B cells particular to pathogens that circulate in the lymph or blood. Antibodies act by hindering the receptors that permit pathogens to bind to target cells or by producing clusters of bacteria. Clumping or clustering simplifies the work of phagocytes since they readily swallow up bacteria in clusters (Gandhi, 2004).

Antibodies that have been bound at times act as labels referred to as opsonins, which increase phagocytosis. When antibodies are bound, biochemical reactions can be initiated, and this triggers chemicals which are referred to as complements. When complement components are activated, they may create holes in the bacterial membranes, and this may increase inflammation. Helper T cells are also vital on how the immune system operates; if destroyed, this cripples the immune system as a whole (Gandhi, 2004).

The immune system comprises of the cellular arm which relies on T cells to intervene attacks on cells that are cancerous or that have been infected by viruses. It also includes the humoral arm, which relies on antibodies to remove antigens that circulate in the lymph and blood (Gandhi, 2004).

Figure showing a cytotoxic cell fighting a host cell that is secreting foreign antigens

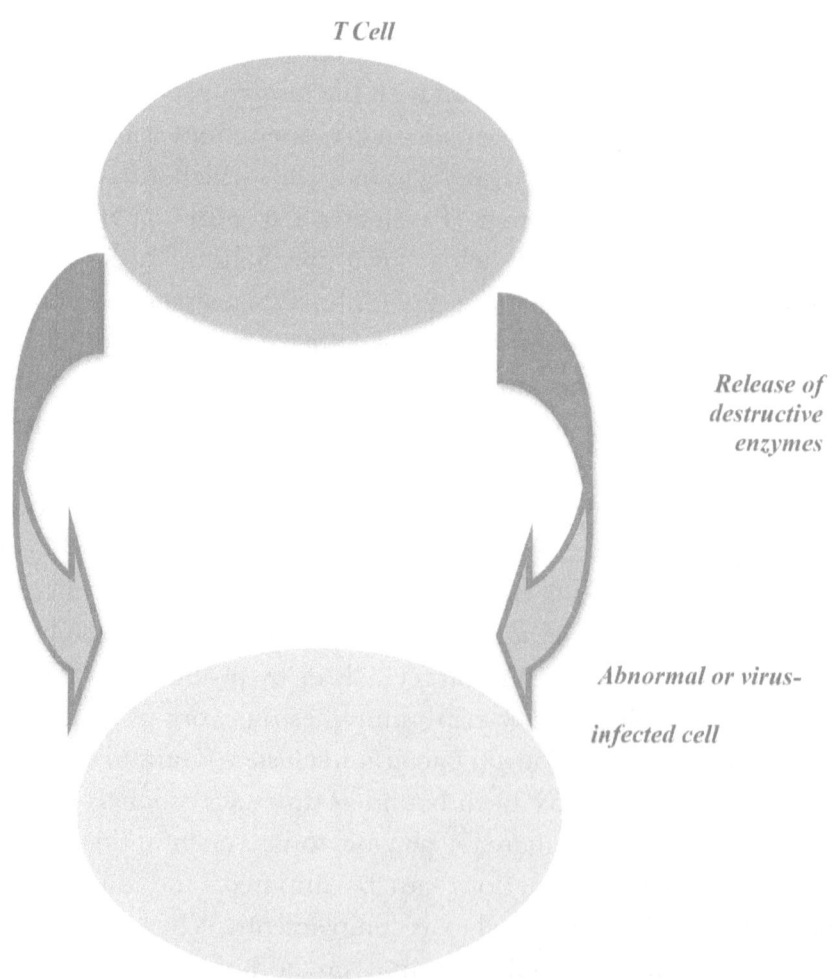

T Cell

Release of destructive enzymes

Abnormal or virus-infected cell

Interleukins

These are a group of cytokines which are involved in various functions such as the production, growth, relocation, and adhesion of cells. Interleukins are useful in moderating transmission between leukocytes and other cells which are involved in the immune response (Stewart, 2009). They are created by CD4 + helper T cells, endothelial cells, macrophages, and monocytes. Interleukins are vital in the functioning of both the adaptive and innate immune system (Young *et al.*, 2014). Interleukins begin their response by attaching themselves to receptors whose affinity is high and which are positioned on the cells' surface. Interleukins work in an autocrine or paracrine style, and not as an endocrine signal.

Unlike other cells, cytokines interleukins are stored away from cells and produced quickly when responding to a stimulus such as infectious substances. After the production of interleukin, it moves to its target cells and attaches to it through a receptor molecule, which is the cell's surface. Interleukins may have anti-inflammatory and inflammatory actions (Young *et al.*, 2014)

There are various types of interleukin, such as interleukin-1 which is produced by multiple by endothelial cells, macrophages, and fibroblasts among other cells (Abbas and Litchman, 2011). Since it is an agent that signals inflammation, endothelial cells tend to act in response to it by integrating unique receptors into the cell membrane. Afterwards, a leukocyte attaches to the receptor and moves into the injured tissue. The leukocyte then displaces and destroys cells; this is essential in fighting pathogens and cells that are defective.

Interleukin 1-α is formed by various types of cells but primarily produced by macrophages and monocytes (Abbas and Litchman, 2011). Interleukin 1-α plays a significant role in preserving the function of the skin as a barrier and assists other immune responses. The capacity of interleukin 1-α to enhance the manufacture of dermis elements to activate collagen has made it useful in the cosmetic industry.

In conditions that are not stressful IL-1 generates sickness behaviour while during stress, it generates hostile, anxious, and irritable behaviour (McMahon, 2013). This response is exceptionally critical since such behaviours are common among people that are affected by depression. Internal or external stressors can trigger behaviours that are depressive by increasing the release of pro-inflammatory cytokines interleukin-1 and interleukin-6.

There is also interleukin-2 which is primarily produced by T-lymphocytes. When the levels of IL-2 are low, often it leads to depressive symptoms such as irritability, becoming slow in responses, inability to concentrate, and the lack of interest in things around (Dowlati *et al.*, 2010). When IK-2 levels are high, it might trigger severe symptoms such as those linked to schizophrenia-like delusions, hallucinations, and disorientation. Interleukin-3 is useful in stimulating the formation of blood, particularly after chemotherapy or after a stem cell or bone marrow transplantation.

There is also the interleukin-12; a cytokine whose role is immunoregulatory and is critically involved in various infectious diseases. In various studies, IL-12 is needed in the early management of infections and at times for the maintenance of the adaptive protective immunity. When IL-12 is used as vaccine research has shown that diseases from similar infectious agents are prevented by activating innate resistance or enhancing particular reactivity.

IL-2 manages inflammation by hampering the differentiation of TH17; it does this by interrupting the signalling measures of IL-6 that are dependent. IL-2 by raising the volume of Treg cells and reducing the quantity of TFH and TH17 cells can put a stop to the unrestrained growth of immune responses thereby restricting general inflammation (Targan *et al.*, 2003). Even though the administration of IL-2 in high doses is an accepted therapy for metastatic cancer, its value clinically tends to be limited. On the contrary, when IL-2 is administered in low doses, it can reduce inflammation (Koreth *et al.*, 2011).

IL-6 reduces Treg cells and as a result, an individual's capacity to build tolerance for ingested proteins is inhibited, and this leads to allergies. IL-6 can also cause a person to have feelings of hopelessness, which may lead to changes in the brain (Mitchell *et al.*, 2013). Research has shown that IL-6 makes worse the impact of stress hormones in the gut mucosa and can also lead to a leaky gut (Al-Sadi *et al.*, 2014).

IL-6 is of two kinds namely the trans-signalling and class-signalling. Trans-signalling occurs when the IL-6 receptors which are in the blood attach to IL-6, and this leads to inflammatory issues (Rose-John, 2012). On the contrary, I-6 classic signalling is required for anti-inflammatory and regenerative functions.

There is also interleukin-6, which is a cytokine that has distinct anti- and pro-inflammatory agents (Wolf *et al.*, 2014). Interleukin-6 also controls the immune system and has a significant role in cognitive function. According to research, interleukin-6 has been associated with mental disorders such as anxiety and depression (Dowlati *et al.*, 2010). Studies have shown that patients with a major depressive disorder tend to have high levels of IL-6.

Furthermore, low levels of IL-6 can be lead to a negative mood. Individuals affected by a major depressive disorder tend to have high levels of IL-6 (Dowlati *et al.*, 2010). Whenever a person is sick or has engaged in exercise, their IL-6 levels tend to be high. Moreover, interleukin-6 subdues Th1 cells, stimulates Th2 cells, and raises B cells, which contributes to the production of antibodies and leads to various allergies and autoimmunity.

IL-6 is to blame for various autoimmune diseases as it reduces cells which prevent the immune system from attacking itself. Some of these autoimmune diseases that occur include rheumatoid arthritis, sclerosis, diabetes, pain, depression, and osteoporosis, among others. Post-menopausal women tend to have higher levels of IL-6 than men of their age (Endrighi, Hamer, and Steptoe, 2016).

The pro-inflammatory cytokines TNF, IL-6, and IL-1 are produced in response to a particular stressor; it triggers the HPA axis and stimulates the production of endogenous glucocorticoids which restrain the innate immune responses and HPA activity. When the production of immune intermediaries and pro-inflammatory cytokinesis increases, often it leads to glucocorticoid resistance, a condition often seen in patients that have depression (Pace and Miller, 2009).

During the first phase of inflammation, IL-6 is produced and through the bloodstream travels to the liver. What follows is the fast stimulation of a wide variety of acute proteins like the serum amyloid, haptoglobin, C-reactive protein, and fibrinogen. Additionally, IL-6 enhances the exact segregation of CD4+ cells, which helps in connecting the innate to the adaptive immune response.

Other benefits of IL-6 include enhancement of liver regeneration and assists a person in creating memories when they are sleeping. IL-6 also hinders tumour necrosis factor alpha, reduces resistance to insulin and breaking down of body fats, which is useful for people that want to reduce weight. IL-6 also assists in fighting infections from virus, bacteria, and fungi (Sompayrac, 2011). IL-6 can minimize fatigue by activating the HPA axis and repressing the tumour necrosis factor alpha, which leads to an increase in orexin. IL-6 activates the hypothalamus to release the corticotrophin-releasing hormone.

Various factors can be attributed to high IL-6 levels; they include among others a diet that has high levels of blood sugar and fat diet which often leads to inflammation (Kim, Kim, and Yun, 2012). There are some lifestyle issues such as insomnia, obesity, chronic stress, smoking, viruses, and infections that can increase il-6 levels (Rose-John, 2012). Low IL-6 levels can be achieved through positive emotions, eating healthy foods such as nuts, fish oil, vegetables, garlic, and oats among others (Salas-Salvadó et al., 2008).

In modern times there has been an increase in studying peripheral IL-6 as a system for treating depression among other mental disorders. Administering tricyclic antidepressants in high doses has been reported to enhance the stimulation of IL-6 in patients with depression.

IL-10 is produced by most kinds of cells of the immune system, which includes the innate immune system's cells and a large number of the lymphocyte cells. IL-10 restricts the response of the immune system when an infection occurs, thereby preventing the mediated injury to the host from the immune system (Li and Flavell, 2008).

IL-10 works in different phases of the immune response in a manner that efficiently controls the inflammatory process.

A wide range of illnesses are linked to the overproduction of IL-10; they include autoimmune diseases like melanoma cancers, systemic lupus, and other infectious illnesses like tuberculosis (O'garra *et al.*, 2008). There is a likelihood that administering I-10 correctly can aid in managing inflammatory diseases.

Tumour Necrosis Factor Alpha Protein

These are a group of cytokines which are produced primarily by macrophages and can lead to the death of particular tumour cell lines (Ritsner, 2009). Tumour necrosis factor was thus named for its capacity to eradicate tumours. These cytokines are useful in the body as they assist in regulating the immune response to an intruder or a foreign agent. Additionally, it enhances inflammation and helps in forming other cells that are beneficial in the inflammatory response and also assist in cell healing.

TNF-α protects the body against autoimmune diseases, parasitic, bacterial, and viral infections, autoimmune diseases. Macrophages and other white blood cells produce TNF-α. Tumour necrosis factor has a significant role in regulating the immune system; it can also cause fever. When the production of the tumour necrosis factor is dysregulated various diseases such as cancer, inflammatory bowel disease, Alzheimer's disease, and major depression can occur (Dowlati *et al.*, 2010).

Furthermore, changes in the tumour necrosis factor alpha (TNF-α) system have been attributed to various psychiatric disorders. Patients that have depression tend to have a dysfunction of the hypothalamic-pituitary-adrenocortical axis (Pratt and Stapelberg, 2018). Changes in the levels of the plasma cytokines are often observed in patients that have affective disorders which can be interpreted to mean that cytokines are responsible in the development of depression (Berthold-Losleben and Himmerich, 2008). Various studies have reported on the impact the cytokine system, which includes TNF-α has on the serotonin metabolism and the hypothalamic-pituitary-adrenocortical axis.

When the cytokine system is activated, it can lead to the stimulation of the hypothalamic-pituitary-adrenocortical system, which is considered to be one cause of depressive symptoms. This shows that there exists a direct link between the severity of depressive symptoms and TNF-α. Tumour necrosis factor can also stimulate neuronal serotonin transporters; when a patient is experiencing depressive symptoms, serotonin uptake tends to reduce. Therefore, drugs such as selective serotonin reuptake inhibitors tend to be useful when providing therapy in depression since it deactivates serotonin transporters (Berthold-Losleben and Himmerich, 2008).

Various kinds of tumour necrosis factor are linked to specific autoimmune diseases. High level of tumour necrosis factor (TNF) can lead to various adverse symptoms such as fever, loss of appetite, low blood pressure, and muscle aches. TNF has both useful and damaging functions in the body. For instance, TNF can lead to profound loss of weight in individuals that have parasitic and chronic bacterial infections and can also cause cancer (Miller et al., 2006).

Tumour necrosis factor can also cause shock in some individuals that have acute bacterial infections (Abbas, Litchman, and Pillai, 2012). On the positive side, TNF assists the body to guard itself against parasites that cause malaria. Also, research has demonstrated that TNF can destroy specific cancer cells. Tumour necrosis factor plays a significant role in the pathophysiology and neurodevelopment of different mental conditions.

Excess production of tumour necrosis factor has been linked to different inflammatory and autoimmune diseases like rheumatoid arthritis (Khardori and Khardori, 2012). When people are intravenously administered with TNF, they tend to develop various neuropsychiatric symptoms such as a headache, fatigue, muscle ache, and headaches. Tumour necrosis factor often makes an individual lousy as someone that is affected by depression. Patients with migraine tend to have a higher risk of depression and secrete more tumour necrosis factor.

Interferon Gamma Cells

Interferons can be described as proteins that create antiproliferative and antiviral responses in various cells (Ebadi, 2008). They are categorised into five groups namely α, α-ll, β, delta, and γ. Interferons have various roles, which include angiogenesis and reducing inflammation. Interferon-gamma is formed by natural killer cells and T cells (Boyer *et al.*, 2012). Interferon-gamma plays a significant role in allergic and cellular immunity. Interferon-gamma is useful in directly preventing viral reproduction as it stimulates the immune responses to assist in eliminating the viruses. This action helps in guarding the host from the viruses.

Interferon-gamma cells are also useful in inhibiting intracellular bacterial infection (Ebadi, 2008). This is a cytokine which is vital to both the adaptive and innate immunity. The primary role of the interferon-gamma includes stimulating and modulating various immune responses. Interferon-gamma can enhance macrophage stimulation, mediate antibacterial and antiviral immunity, organise stimulation of the innate immune system, and control the Th1 and Th2 balance. The primary producers of interferon-gamma are the activated T cells, CD8+ T cells, and natural killers.

Interferon-gamma has various effects on the immune system such as activating macrophages and monocytes to produce additional interleukin-1 and interleukin-2. Patients that have depression tend to produce more interferon-gamma than lymphocytes (Dowlati *et al.*, 2010). Interferon-gamma is a vital link of both the adaptive and immune responses and has a significant function in stressor-connected psychological pathology.

Various studies have demonstrated high levels of the interferon-gamma in patients that have depression (Schmidt, and Duman,

2010). Interferon-gamma is, in most circumstances, are antagonised by the frequent use of antidepressants.

Additionally, differences in the interferon-gamma gene in recent times have been reported to alter the risk of depression regarding IFN-treatment and the efficiency of antidepressants (Myint *et al.*, 2007). Interferon gamma has been linked to the treatment of multiple sclerosis, which is a condition that occurs when the body's immune system ambushes nerve fibres in the spinal cord and the brain.

Studies have reported that interferon gamma has a significant role in determining whether the immune cells fight and harm the central nervous system. Treating depression in such cases involves reducing the production of antigen-specific and non-specific interferon gamma (Myint *et al.*, 2007). Therefore, a reduction in the production of interferon gamma leads to a decrease in depressive symptoms.

The Anatomy of the Innate Immune Responses

The innate or natural immune system is one which a person is born with and which offers immediate defence against infections (Turner, 2012). Usually, it is recognised within a few hours but retains no memory and also it is not specific. Therefore, on its own, it cannot effectively manage infections (Turner, 2012). The innate immune response cells include phagocytes, which are a significant ingredient of the innate immune system as they help in new fighting infections.

Phagocytes include among others neutrophils, blood monocytes, tissue macrophages, and dendritic cells. Phagocytes are the initial line of immune protection against foreign substances that have broken the physical barriers and have penetrated the body tissues (Macintosh and Moore, 2011). After identifying the foreign agents, phagocytes engulf them, destroy them, and ingest them.

Afterwards, phagocytes take the protein antigens that have been digested to the adaptive immune system's cells through the histocompatibility complex, which works as a protective mechanism (Macintosh and Moore, 2011). This action hinders the over-activation of the immune system as it makes sure the T cells only respond to an antigen which has a histocompatibility complex.

Phagocytosis is a significant and efficient mechanism used during the responses of the innate system to destroy pathogens (Macintosh and Moore, 2011). Dendritic cells and neutrophils are the primary phagocytes of the immune system. Macrophages are the most flexible phagocyte which takes part in the innate immune responses and also collaborates with lymphocytes in their adaptive immune response. Macrophages are located in various body tissues where they are either fixed or are roaming freely; they are the ones first to offer protection to the body when the physical barriers are breached.

Neutrophils are phagocytic cells which move through chemotaxis to tissues that are infected (Macintosh and Moore, 2011). Neutrophils are always on the lookout against intruders and infections; they can be regarded as a military reinforcement which is always available to destroy the foreign substances. Monocytes, on the other hand, are circulating forerunner cells which divide into either a dendritic cell or a macrophage. Monocytes tend to speedily attracted to parts in the body that have inflammation or infection.

Natural killers, together with other phagocytes and neutrophils, tend to have a significant role during the early attack against an infection (Macintosh and Moore, 2011). Distinct from T cells, natural killers do not need stimulation by particular antigens; this enables them to have an instant response when they come into contact with a pathogen. According to research, a reduction in the function of the natural killer cells is often linked to depression. When the natural killer cell activity is decreased in conjunction with an elevated IL-6 level, this is an indication of the stimulation of the innate immune responses in depression (Blume, Douglas, and Evans, 2011).

Furthermore, when the activity of the natural killer is often reduced, it leads to symptoms closely linked to mood disorders like disturbances in a person's sleep. When changes in the sleep pattern occur, more pro-inflammatory cytokines are released (Clow and Hucklebridge, 2002). As a result, B and T cells might momentarily rise to get ready the body to battle against the foreign agent. In chronic depression, these processes might become harmful and maladaptive; this may inhibit the accessibility of messenger cells for the activation of T cells. This may lower the stimulation of leukocytes and reduce the body's immune system's regulation.

Cells that do not have a recognisable histocompatibility complex are probably *non-self* and are an easy target for destruction by the natural killers. Usually, natural killers cannot fight self (healthy) cells, but when cells have a viral infection or have cancer, the histocompatibility complex tends to be subdued. In such circumstances, natural killers can perform other crucial functions in viral immunity (Clow and Hucklebridge, 2002).

Innate immune response cells, natural killers, and cytotoxic cells identify the pattern of particular pathogen molecules using pattern-recognition receptors (Kimmel and Rosenberg, 2015). The receptors are usually on the surface of the cell always. However, their differences are restricted by two aspects namely since each receptor kind should be encoded by a particular gene this necessitates the cell to assign a large part of its DNA to ensure receptors can identify pathogens.

The second factor that determines the type of receptor is the surface area of the cell membrane (Kimmel and Rosenberg, 2015). Therefore, the innate immune system works using a limited amount of receptors which have to fight against a broad range of pathogens. This approach is different from the one the adaptive immune system employs, which uses various kinds of receptors, each targeting a specific pathogen, whenever the cells of the innate immune system come across a particular pathogen which they can identify, the cells attaches itself to it and begin phagocytosis to eliminate the foreign agent.

The innate chemical response involves pro-inflammatory cytokines, which are minute messenger proteins which the immune cells release in response to infection. There are diverse cytokine molecules which include tumour necrosis factors, interleukins, and chemokines. An inflammatory response is usually begun by the pro-inflammatory cytokines and the innate immune cells (Kimmel and Rosenberg, 2015).

Inflammation can be described as the primary role of the innate immune response. When the contents of damaged cellular are released into the injured area, it activates a response. The inflammatory response takes to the injured part, phagocytic cells to remove cellular remains and prepare the area for healing (Kimmel and Rosenberg, 2015). This response brings the innate immune system cells, permitting them to remove sources if a possible infection. The immune response brings cells and fluids to the injured area to eliminate the pathogen and take it away from the debris location. Additionally, the damaged area is isolated, which restricts the pathogens from spreading further.

The innate immune responses are vital to the early management of infections (Parrillo and Dellinger, 2013). Various cells, antibacterial proteins, and mediators can cause innate responses. A few days after an infection has occurred, other antibacterial proteins are stimulated which target specific bacteria (Parrillo and Dellinger, 2013). Furthermore, to guard cells against the surrounding viruses, interferons are activated. The response of the innate immune system does not end after the development of the adaptive system. Both the adaptive and immune response can work together in fighting pathogens.

B Cells

B cells are a type of white blood cells (lymphocytes); they form antibodies, which is one of the significant roles of the adaptive immune system (Cummings and Starr, 2003). B cells primary role is to protect the body from infections. The antibodies eliminate pathogens such as viruses and bacteria. The B cells have an outstanding function in the humoral immune response contrary to the T cells' response, which is cell-mediated (Cummings and Starr, 2003). The humoral response fights against viruses and bacteria in the body fluids through immunoglobulins, which the B cells produce. The body produces millions of different kinds of B cells daily, and each kind has a unique receptor (B-cell receptor). B cells are continually circulating in the lymph and blood but are not creating antibodies.

B cells are triggered when they encounter intruders or unknown antigens when an infection occurs (Cummings and Starr, 2003). As a response, the B cells divide into plasma cells, which are the primary producers of immunoglobulin which bind themselves on the exterior of the foreign agents. The antibodies or immunoglobulin enlist other molecules which are in the bloodstream to the area where there is an infection. The antibodies also incorporate other immune cells to help fight the intruders.

To provide immunity to the body, a B cell that is not mature moves in the bloodstream often winding up in the lymph nodes or the spleen. An antigen or any foreign substance then activates the B cell; during this process, T cells are also involved. The B cells then starts to change into a plasma B cell, whose primary role is to produce large amounts of antibodies which match the foreign substance (Cummings and Starr, 2003).

Every plasma B cell produces antibodies to a specific antigen only (Cummings and Starr, 2003). Some of the B cells that have been activated become memory cells which have a long lifespan. The memory B cells reside in the spleen, marrow, and lymph nodes. The memory B cells also retain the memory of an antigen they have encountered, and if they re-encounter it, their response tends to be swift. During the initial infection comprising of a specific antigen which has not previously been exposed to the antigen, cells reproduce to create a colony of cells.

B cells are the one that provides the body with long-lasting immunity. B cells are of various types, namely the plasma B cells, which are those that have antigen exposure and secrete large volumes of antibodies which help in microbes' destruction by attaching to them. This action makes the microbes an easy target for phagocytes. A high level of B cells is often witnessed among patients that have depression (Mikova *et al.*, 2001)

Tryptophan-Kynurenine Pathway and Inflammation of the Neurological System

A lot of attention has been given to the connection that exists between the kynurenine pathway, inflammation, neurological conditions, and the immune system. Tryptophan is an essential amino acid that is useful in developing proteins. It is well recognised as the first part for the biosynthesis of melatonin and serotonin. Kynurenine as a tryptophan pathway has been unknown in the past, but over time, it has gained attention. Kynurenine pathway came to the limelight in 1853 when it was detected in animal excretions. The serotonin hypothesis came to view as the connection between major depressive disorders, and kynurenine pathway became more evident.

This hypothesis states that when the kynurenine pathway is activated, it diverts the tryptophan that is available from the production of the serotonin. Various studies conducted recently have reported that the kynurenine pathway plays a significant role in depression (Myint, Schwarz, and Müller, 2012). Patients that have major depressive disorder tend to have elevated pro-inflammatory cytokines interleukins. Also, there exists a positive relationship between the kynurenine pathways with melancholia in adolescents that have a major depressive disorder (Gababy et al., 2010). Additionally, patients with a major depressive disorder who have a history of suicide tend to have a higher kynurenine pathway level than those who have no suicidal history (Sublette et al., 2011).

This demonstrates that in patients that have depression, the kynurenine pathway is imbalanced and this can lead to impairment of the glial-neuronal network which may increase the recurrence of major depressive disorder (Myint, Schwarz, and Müller, 2012). The tryptophan-kynurenine pathway connects the immune stimulation available in major depressive disorder and the cellular irregularity that has been credited to mood disorders.

The kynurenine pathway is also linked to other mental disorders such as bipolar disorder and schizophrenia. Patients with the two disorders tend to have elevated kynurenine acid in comparison to the general population (Kegel *et al.*, 2014). People affected by schizophrenia tend to have cognitive insufficiencies like impairment in learning and memory, the rate of information processing, and working memory. Studies have demonstrated that high kynurenine acid stimulates impairment in working memory and contextual processing (Alexander *et al.*, 2012). The results of these studies concur with the view that high kynurenine acid levels in patients that have bipolar disorder are linked with cognitive impairment (Sellgren *et al.*, 2015).

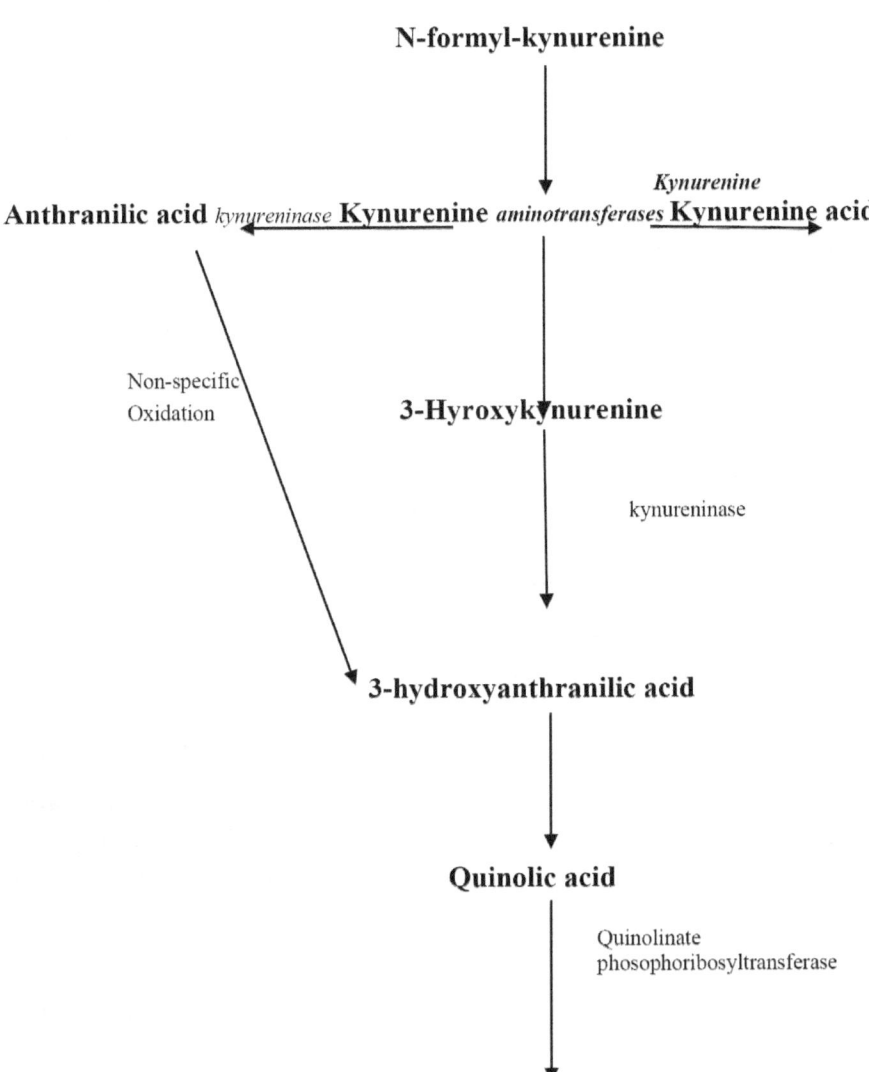

Tryptophan and Its Conversion to
Serotonin and Melatonin

Tryptophan is an essential amino acid in the body, which is often gotten from the diet a person, consumes (Richard *et al.*, 2007). Tryptophan is also directly used by the gut microbiota, which restricts its accessibility to the host (O'Mahony *et al.*, 2015). The human body is incapable of producing enough tryptophan on its own; therefore, the small intestine absorbs it from foods that are rich in protein (Friedman and Levin, 2012). After tryptophan is incorporated in the body, it is then converted to 5-hydroxytryptophan and later to into different essential amino acids such as melatonin and serotonin. Melatonin is necessary for sleep while serotonin assists in the transmission of information between nerve cells.

Though tryptophan converts to serotonin. Much of it tends to metabolise to various downstream metabolites, kynurenine, quinolinic acid, and kynurenic acid. The metabolism of tryptophan along the kynurenine pathway depends on the expression of indoleamine-2, 3-dioxygenase (Streilein, 2012). Furthermore, IL-4 and IL-10 tend to inhibit the metabolism of tryptophan in the kynurenine pathway.

The process of converting tryptophan into serotonin involves assistance from calcium, vitamin c, zinc, folate, iron, B6, and B3. Chronic stress can alter this process by triggering an immune response. At this point, an enzyme referred to as indoleamine, 3-dioxygenase (IDO) is stimulated (Streilein, 2012). This enzyme drives tryptophan along a path that might be unhealthy based on the level of antioxidant and anti-inflammatory reserves an individual possesses. Rather than tryptophan becoming converted to serotonin during this process, other compounds are produced. These compounds are the neurodegenerative quinolinic acid and the neuroprotective kynurenic acid. The quinolinic acid and N-methyl-D-aspartate increase inflammation, especially when kynurenic acid is absent.

Tryptophan has various functions wherein the brain its impact is notable. For instance, multiple studies have revealed that low levels of tryptophan can be linked to depression and anxiety (Schruers *et al.*, 2000). Tryptophan enhances sleep thereby improving an individual's general health. Lack of sleep can lead to health challenges such as depression, weight gain, reduced motor coordination, lack of concentration, and muscle aches, among others.

Furthermore, based on various studies, low tryptophan levels can also enhance aggressive and impulsive behaviour and mood disorders. When the tryptophan levels are below average, this can impair learning and memory. Studies have revealed that when the tryptophan levels are reduced, memory performance tends to be adversely affected. The memory associated with experiences and events might particularly be impaired. The reason for this is as the levels of tryptophan decrease, the production of serotonin also is reduced (Mendelsohn, Riedel, and Sambeth, 2009).

Tryptophan is necessary for cognitive processes due to its function in the production of serotonin. Therefore, low levels can impair an individual's cognition, including their memory of experiences and events. Five-hydroxytryptophan and serotonin impact many brain processes, and when their regular activity is interfered with, it may lead to anxiety and depression. Most drugs that are used in treating depression alter the serotonin's behaviour in the brain to enhance its activity treatment, which incorporates 5-hydroxytryptophan, elevates the serotonin level and improves panic and mood disorders.

Tryptophan supports the immune system as it heralds kynurenine, which helps in regulating inflammation and the immune system. Concerning depression, when tryptophan levels in the body are depleted, various studies have shown that this can lead to depressive symptoms. Additionally, during inflammation, extra tryptophan is converted into kynurenic, which reduces the amount of tryptophan and is converted into serotonin. Owing to the reduction in serotonin, a person tends to become unhappy.

Inflammatory cytokines can also interrupt the management of glutamate, which is a neurotransmitter that is related to excitement. When glutamate is not controlled, it can cause damage to the brain, which can lead to depression.

After tryptophan has produced serotonin, it is later converted to melatonin which is naturally found in the body. Melatonin can also be found in various types of food, such as grapes, strawberries, and tomatoes (Iriti, Varoni, and Vitalini, 2010). Melatonin influences the body's sleep-wake cycle, which affects various functions such as the immune system and nutrients' metabolism (Claustrat and Leston, 2015). Studies have revealed that when tryptophan is increased in an individual's diet, it can enhance sleep as melatonin is increased (Fukushige *et al.*, 2014).

The production of melatonin in the brain requires moving tryptophan via the blood-brain barrier into the brain. After tryptophan has passed the blood-brain barrier, it fights against large neural amino acids. Thus, the more the plasma level, the better it is for the transportation of tryptophan through the blood-brain barrier (Markus *et al.*, 2010).

Studies have also revealed that eating at breakfast, and dinner cereal that is rich in tryptophan has assisted adults in sleeping quickly and for a long time in comparison to when only standard cereals are consumed (Bravo *et al.*, 2013). Melatonin has also been shown to be useful in reducing the symptoms of anxiety and depression. Tryptophan can be got from various foods that contain protein such as egg shrimp, white, spirulina, fish, crab, poultry, and sesame flour among others. A person can also decide to take supplement molecules which are obtained from tryptophan.

Tryptophan does not only lead to mood disorders and depression but has been found to have the same benefits in the treatment of depression as antidepressants (Richard *et al.*, 2009). Studies have also revealed that tryptophan can decrease symptoms of social and general anxiety disorders as well as panic attack disorders. Supplements that contain tryptophan have according to different research been found useful in treating the depression that comes due to bipolar disorder.

Tryptophan can also lessen the adverse side effects of antipsychotic drugs (Leavitt, 2003). Furthermore, tryptophan boosts the impact of selective serotonin reuptake inhibitors. Tryptophan is most effective when taken together with vitamin B6 and niacin. Symptoms of the seasonal affective disorder are also reduced when tryptophan is combined with light therapy. Tryptophan supplements should be taken with caution due to the various side effects that can occur. Some of the side effects include drowsiness, digestion problems, headache, and loss of appetite.

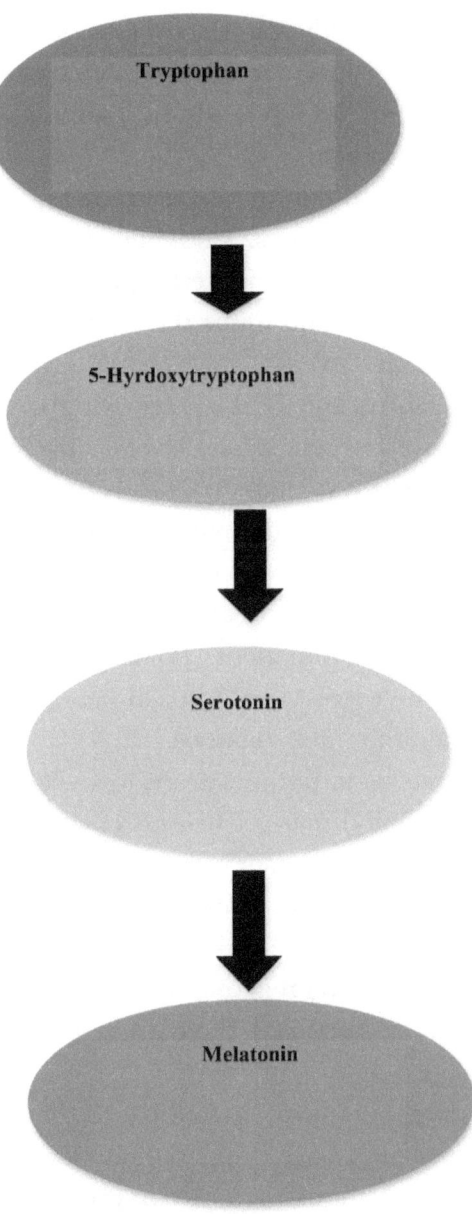

Oxidative Stress Response

Oxidative stress is the imbalance that occurs in the body between free radicals and antioxidants (Kohlstadt, 2006). Free radicals can be defined as molecules that contain oxygen that have an imbalanced amount of electrons. This imbalance often causes free radicals to react with other molecules readily. On the other hand, antioxidants refer to molecules which can provide a free radical an electron without causing any instability, which leads to stabilisation and reduced reactivity to the free radicals.

Some environmental causes of free radicals include pollution, some chemicals and pesticides, smoking of cigarette, and ozone (Ming *et al.*, 2011). Smoking of cigarettes produces in the body large quantities of free radicals and limits the circulation of antioxidants, which leads to oxidative stress.

In normal circumstances, the anti-oxidative defence system balances the reactive oxygen species levels. This interferes with the ability of the biological system to effortlessly repair the damage that may have resulted and also detoxify the reactive intermediaries. When the tissues' normal redox position is interrupted, it can bring toxic impact since free radicals and peroxides are produced and which tend to harm cell components, lipids, DNA, and proteins. The occurrence of oxidative stress begins to counter the resultant oxidant effects and reinstate the redox balance.

The oxidative stress in humans leads to various diseases such as heart failure, sickle cell disease, schizophrenia, Parkinson's disease, bipolar disorder, and Alzheimer's disease among others (Alcaraz *et al.*, 2013). On the contrary, temporary oxidative stress can assist in arresting the ageing process through a process referred to as mitohormesis. Additionally, reactive oxygen species may be useful since the immune system uses them in fighting and destroying pathogens.

Brain cells are particularly susceptible to the damaging impact of oxidative stress, which occurs due to their elevated metabolic rate (Gadoth and Göbel). Although reactive oxygen species are regarded as toxic products which result from cellular metabolism, they are also vital components of various neurobiological processes. Some of these processes include cell growth, production, differentiation, and immune responses

The brain, due to its large capacity of consuming large quantities of oxygen and the creation of free radicals, is regarded particularly susceptible to oxidative damage (Halliwell, 2006). Consequently, oxidative stress is associated with various mental and neurodegenerative disorders (Reynolds *et al.*, 2007). This link is often due to the brain's vulnerability to oxidative load (Ng *et al.*, 2008).

Studies have also linked various anxiety disorders such as panic and obsessive compulsive disorders to oxidative stress. Some of these studies have reported that oxidative metabolism can impact the management of anxiety. Oxidative stress has also been linked to depression (Ng *et al.*, 2008). Elevated levels of reactive oxygen species and reactive nitrogen species have been associated with a major depressive disorder (Ray, Huang, and Tsuji, 2012). The body has an inbuilt mechanism which fights unwarranted production of reactive oxygen species and reactive nitrogen species.

The mechanism that is used to fight this includes putting a stop to the formation of free radicals such as an enzyme that inhibits the catalysing of free radicals formation. If these defence mechanisms are inadequate and the reactive oxygen species and free radicals have already formed, the free radicals become trapped and reactive oxygen species are eliminated by changing them into non-toxic and non-radical metabolites. If at this point, the organism protection fails, systems of repair identify molecules that have been impaired and cause their decomposition. Inflammation and depression can lead to an alteration of the oxidative stress enzymes.

It is difficult to control oxidative stress; nevertheless, there are some things which an individual can do to minimise the effect of this process. Some of these things include enhancing the antioxidant levels, which will reduce the production of free radicals (Levin *et al.*, 2008). A healthy diet can also minimise the oxidative stress; some of the foods which can help in this include consumption of vegetables and fruits. Some of the vegetables and fruits include cherries, prunes, carrots, prunes, olives, citrus, and tomatoes. Other antioxidant foods are onions, nuts, fish, turmeric, onion, and green tea (Levin *et al.*, 2008).

Besides diet, maintaining a healthy lifestyle can also hinder or minimise oxidative stress. Some of the healthy lifestyles which can assist this include engaging in regular exercise which has been linked to higher levels of the natural antioxidant and a reduction of the harm which oxidative stress causes (Gogus, 2011). Smoking can also lead to oxidative stress; therefore, avoiding this habit can prove beneficial to an individual. Some chemicals such as those used in cleaning should be avoided as they might contain harmful chemicals (Gogus, 2011). When in contact with the direct sun, it is advisable to wear sunscreen to protect oneself from the skin damage which may be caused through exposure to ultraviolet light.

Getting adequate sleep is also necessary for enhancing a balance between the various systems of the body (Gogus, 2011). During sleep, various functions such as those related to the brain, the production of hormones, and the stabilisation of free radicals and antioxidants are affected. Various studies have reported that overeating may cause the body to stay in a position of oxidative stress. Therefore, a person should eat moderate or small portions at intervals.

Additionally, stress reduction techniques such as meditation can reduce chronic stress, which often is responsible for oxidative stress. Also, infections should be treated promptly since they have a strong link to oxidative stress and should be dealt with to hinder the progression of free radicals (Gogus, 2011).

Quinolinic Acid

This refers to a product that comes from the kynurenine pathway and which metabolises the tryptophan amino acid. Alone, quinolinic acid cannot go through the blood-brain barrier. It therefore has to be formed within the macrophages or microglial cells that have gone through the blood-brain barrier (Guillemin, 2012). After its production, the quinolinic acid is released and activates the N-methyl-D-aspartate receptors, and this causes excitatory neurotoxicity (Schwarcz *et al.*, 2012). During an immune response, the production of quinolinic acid by macrophages and microglia is increased. The production of quinolinic acid levels also tends to become elevated when inflammation occurs.

Studies have shown that patients with depression tend to have high quinolinic acid levels, which build up in some parts of the brain and could lead to neuronal damage (Steiner *et al.*, 2012). One symptom of depression includes suicidal thoughts or attempts; research has demonstrated that people with depression tend to have high quinolinic levels enclosing their central nervous system. This discovery may clarify the connection between mental disorders and inflammation. When quinolinic acid levels are elevated, this might also lead to forgetfulness and the feeling of having a foggy head.

Quinolinic acid can also lead to inflammation since microglia helps in the formation of quinolinic acid and generally leads to inflammatory responses in the central nervous system and also has a significant role in changed quinolinic acid levels. Kynurenic acid often hampers the quinolinic acid neuronal excitotoxic action (Myint *et al.*, 2007). Therefore, kynurenine downstream metabolites do not directly link to depression; nevertheless, they impact the body in both harmful and beneficial ways.

Oxidative stress and the generation of free radical are often involved in quinolinic induced toxicity. Nevertheless, these mechanisms can act independently of the quinolinic. In line with this, research has demonstrated that quinolinic acid can lead to oxidative damage away from its activity in the N-methyl-D-aspartate receptor. Microglial which takes care of the inflammatory responses in the central nervous system plays a significant role in modified levels of quinolinic acid. The reason behind this is that quinolinic acid is increased when indolamine 2, 3- dioxygenase is induced by lipopolysaccharide (Guillemin *et al.*, 2005).

Quinolinic Acid Concentration in Cerebrospinal Fluid and Neurological Diseases

The kynurenine pathway is located in the circulatory inflammatory cells and the glial cells of the central nervous system. The regulation of the kynurenine pathway often is usually done by redox and inflammatory components. When the kynurenine pathway is inappropriately stimulated, it can lead to high quinolinic acid levels. The change in the levels of quinolinic acid has been attributed to various neurological diseases such as Huntington's, Parkinson's, and Alzheimer's diseases (Maiese, 2008). The high levels of quinolinic acid in the central nervous system are fundamental to the development of these disorders through its action mode at the N-methyl-D-aspartate receptor.

In both neurological and inflammatory diseases kynurenic, L-kynurenine, and quinolinic acid tend to be the neuroactive kynurenine pathway metabolites, which accumulate in these disorders. The indoleamine -2, dioxygenase induction is linked to the elevated levels of these acids. When there is inflammation in the central nervous system, the brain tissue directly converts L-tryptophan into quinolinic acid (Patarca-Montero, 2004).

Quinolinic acid can also stimulate toxicity in the brain cells through the production of exogenous free radicals (Gendelman *et al.*, 2006). On the other hand, when the levels of kynurenine acid are low, neurological diseases like Alzheimer's and Huntington's diseases tend to develop. There has been the view that neuropathology that is inflammatory mediated is connected to alterations in the quinolinic and kynurenine acid and not just the quinolinic acid only.

People with neurological diseases tend to have elevated levels of cerebrospinal fluid (Wood, 2013). Thus, this can be used as an inflammation marker and can help in determining prognosis. One of the neurological diseases where the patient has high levels of quinolinic acid is Huntington's disease. When the quinolinic acid levels are high, this may lead to excitotoxic neuronal damage (Schwarcz *et al.*, 2012). Additionally, children that are infected by various bacterial infections of the central nervous system also tend to have elevated quinolinic acid levels. High quinolinic levels are also found in patients that have experienced trauma in their central nervous system.

How Kynurenine Pathways and the Production of Quinolinic Acid Contributes to Inflammations and Neurological Diseases

In recent times, the relationship between neurological diseases and inflammation and the production of quinolinic acid and kynurenine pathways has been critically reviewed (Schwartz *et al.*, 2012). Various kynurenine derived metabolites tend to cross the blood-brain barrier poorly; this implies that the kynurenine metabolites of the central nervous system tend to be controlled by the activity of the local enzyme. Nevertheless, kynurenine is transported by the large neutral amino acid transporter into the brain. During conditions that are regarded as being physiologically normal, the brain is brained from surrounding sources.

During inflammation, when the expression of indole-2, 3-dioxygenase tends to be high, most kynurenine in the central nervous system tends to come from the surrounding areas (Macchiarulo *et al.*, 2009). The dysregulation of kynurenine metabolism has often been linked to various central nervous system disorders. An example of a neurological disorder is Alzheimer's disease, which is characterised by low tryptophan levels and elevated kynurenine levels. Furthermore, quinolinic and N-methyl-D-aspartate tend to be high in the hippocampus of patients with Alzheimer's disease.

Quinolinic and Kynurenic Acids and Suicidality

Suicide has become a major global crisis, which claims over eight hundred thousand lives every year. Suicidal patients are often reported to have high inflammation levels in the peripheral blood and the central nervous system. Various studies have indicated that in suicidal patients, inflammation is linked to the dysregulation of the kynurenine pathway, particularly enhanced quinolinic acid level, which is an N-methyl-D-aspartic acid receptor agonist.

Suicide is regarded as the fourteenth cause of lives that are lost according to the World Health Organization statistics (World Health Organization, 2014). Most of the suicide cases remain unreported due to the stigma and illegality that is attached to it in various countries (Varnik, 2012). Suicide and attempts bring significant economic and psychological burdens for families, individuals, and countries. In the United States alone, the financial cost of death through suicide is estimated to be around forty-four billion per year (Centers for Disease Control and Prevention, 2010).

Although there has been an increase in treatment alternatives for suicidality, which includes electroconvulsive and pharmacological treatment, the rate of suicide in many countries is increasing (World Health Organization, 2014). Even though most suicidal patients tend to have contact with their primary and mental health care providers a short time before the act, the healthcare system has not been able to correctly identify and stop suicide (Da Cruz et al., 2011). Proper identification of patients that have suicidal intentions is often a challenge, since most of them may hide their plan from both their family and health care providers.

Most patients that commit suicide tend to have various psychiatric disorders such as depression, schizophrenia, bipolar, and mood disorders. The suicidality treatment options offered are dependent on psychiatric diagnosis and comprises of anxiolytics and antidepressants (Wasserman et al., 2012). The most used antidepressants include SNRIs and SSRIs which take a while before a patient develops beneficial mood-enhancing impact; this increases the suicidal risk in the first few weeks during treatment (Wasserman et al., 2012). Pharmacological treatment using clozapine in schizophrenia and lithium in mood disorders has proven beneficial in reducing suicidal behaviour (Guzzetta et al., 2007).

Various risk factors are linked to suicidal behaviour, and they can either be environmental or genetic (Roy *et al.*, 2009). Research has demonstrated that genetic factors contribute to around 40% of suicide attempt and completion (McGuffin *et al.*, 2010). The most significant factor that can be used to predict death by suicide is where an individual may have previously attempted self-harm (Hawton and van Heeringen, 2009). Various studies have also reported that around ninety per cent (90%) of people that complete suicides have bipolar disorder and major depressive disorder.

There are individual traits that have been viewed as further risk factors in persons who have or do not have psychiatric disorders. These traits include, among others, aggression, hopelessness, and elevated impulsivity levels, particularly in young suicide victims (Perroud *et al.*, 2011). The neurobiological variance witnessed in suicidal behaviour remains mostly unknown. Serotonergic neurotransmission and dysregulation of the hypothalamic-pituitary-adrenal (HPA) axis are often identified in persons that display suicidal behaviour (Dwivedi, 2012).

Inflammation is also regarded as a factor in suicidal behaviour since inflammatory markers like cytokines directly interact with the serotonin system and HPA axis. Furthermore, inflammation causes the degradation of the kynurenine pathway of tryptophan, which can lead to neurobiological modification often witnessed in suicidal patients.

When tryptophan is converted to N-formylkynurenine by various enzymes such as tryptophan 2, 3-dioxygenase or indoleamine 2, 3-dioxygenase it initiates kynurenine pathway. The N-formylkynurenine that results from this process further degenerates to kynurenine, which precedes bioactive compounds that include kynurenic, quinolinic, and picolinic acids (Schwartz *et al.*, 2012).

Given the fact that tryptophan is a precursor for serotonin, it is believed that the stimulation of kynurenine pathway through inflammation can decrease the accessibility of tryptophan which can limit the serotonin production (Maes *et al.*, 2011). Theoretically, this can lead to low levels of 5-hydroyxyindoleacetic acid, which is serotonin's central metabolite that has been noticed in the cerebrospinal fluid of people that had attempted suicide.

A study conducted in the year 2011, reported that patients with depression who had attempted suicide had high kynurenine levels in comparison to those with depression but who had no history of suicide (Sublette *et al.*, 2011). More current studies have reported reduced tryptophan plasma levels and a forty per cent (40%) increase in the tryptophan/kynurenine ratio in adolescents with a major depressive disorder that had suicide ideation (Bradley *et al.*, 2015). Both tryptophan and kynurenine enter the brain through the blood-brain barrier (Schwartz *et al.*, 2012). After the kynurenine is in the brain, it may be processed differently by either the microglia or astrocytes to form evident neuroactive compounds.

Quinolinic acid is regarded as a significant kynurenine pathway metabolite in connection to its biological activity. Quinolinic acid is created by unplanned conversion form the 2-amino-3-carboxymuconic-6-semialdehyde (ACMSD). Pyrazinamide, which is an anti-tuberculosis drug and contamination in the environment, can hamper the ACMSD activity and as the quinolinic acid level is increased (Fukuwatari *et al.*, 2004). Diseases such as renal failure and diabetes and dietary changes can also change the activity and expression of ACMSD (Egashira *et al.*, 2007). ACMSD saturation takes place when there are high levels of the upstream ACMS precursor, which occurs in various circumstances like when the inflammation level is high, and this causes more quinolinic acid to be produced.

Quinolinic acid can only last for around twenty minutes only as the quinolinate phosphoribosyl transferase (QPRT) which is a subsequent enzyme in the kynurenine pathway breaks it down rapidly (Schwartz *et al.*, 2012). Consequently, the QPRT activity and levels control the quinolinic acid concentration. The brain through macrophages and microglial cells produce quinolinic acid. The cerebrospinal fluids of patients that have attempted suicide tend to contain over 300% of quinolinic acid levels in comparison to individuals that have not (Erhardt *et al.*, 2013).

A positive correlation is found to exist between quinolinic acid, cerebrospinal fluids, and suicidal intentions. Even if the levels of quinolinic acid are highest during a suicide attempt, they tend to remain high for two years before the attempt (Bay-Richter *et al.*, 2015). Theoretically, the high quinolinic acid and the resulting neurotoxic impact can cause functional alterations in patients with psychiatric conditions who have suicidal behaviours (van Heeringen *et al.*, 2014).

Other studies have also reported that the quinolinic acid-reactive microglia cells' density in some parts of the anterior cingulate cortex is observed in patients that are depressed and whose death was a result of suicide (Steiner *et al.*, 2011). The kynurenic acid is formed in the central nervous system by kynurenine aminotransferase, and it is synthesised in neurons and astrocytes (Wejksza *et al.*, 2005). The psychological role of kynurenic acid is both anticonvulsive and neuroprotective. Nevertheless, high kynurenic acid levels correlate with psychosis and cognitive deficits (Erhardt, Olsson, and Engberg, 2009).

A study conducted on patients that had schizophrenia and were suicidal showed that they had reduced kynurenic acid levels in comparison to patients that were not suicidal (Carlborg *et al.*, 2013). During this study, it was observed that cerebrospinal fluids kynurenic acid levels reduced by around thirty-five per cent (35%) two years after a suicide attempt. The decreased levels corresponded with suicidal behaviour and severe depression (Bay-Richter *et al.*, 2015).

There is growing evidence which shows that inflammation exists in patients with suicidal ideation and behaviour. The kynurenine pathway tends to be activated by inflammation by producing metabolites that affect the glutamate neurotransmission. To establish the right treatment for suicidal symptoms would require first identifying the upstream causes of inflammation, the downstream neurobiological effectors and the moderators that communicate resilience or susceptibility. Additionally, there are various anti-inflammatory treatments which are clinically accepted that can be used.

CHAPTER 4

Kappa-Opioid Receptors—
Cure for Depression

Opioids refer to chemicals which create in the body effects that are morphine-like that often are barred by morphine antagonists like naloxone. Opioids tend to have a significant role in the immune functions, respiration, stress reactions, processing of pain, and the endocrine system (Bodnar, 2011). The dysregulation of opioids has a significant role in anhedonia, loss, attachment, and major depressive disorder (Scherrer *et al.*, 2014).

Opioid receptors antagonists comprise of several neuropeptides such as endomorphin, beta-endorphin, enkephalins, and dynorphins. Opioid receptors belong to the family of G-protein coupled receptors which tend to impede adenylate cyclase, thus decreasing the intracellular volume of cyclic adenosine monophosphate. Other direct roles of opioids can also include passages.

Opioid receptors are mostly located in the spinal cord, gut, brain, cardiac, some immune system cells, and the lung airway. The opioid system comprises of three G-protein receptors, namely the mu-, delta-, and kappa-opioid receptors. The mu receptors are believed to provide much of their analgesic impact in the central nervous system. The delta-opioid receptor, on the other hand, tends to be more dominant regarding analgesia in the peripheral nervous system.

The three receptors tend to act similarly at the cellular level although how they are distributed in the body and their reaction to different opioid medication impacts various tissues at differing levels. Opioid receptors tend to control motivational procedures and often play a significant role in mental disorders caused by incentive dysfunction like depression and addiction (Le Merrer *et al.*, 2009). Opioids are categorised as being either antagonists or agonists on their target receptors. Most opioids are agonists and produce their impact by activating the opioid receptors.

Full agonists refer to drugs that stimulate the brain; they tend to attach to receptors and activate them (Lessa and Scanlon, 2006). Antagonists too attach to opioid receptors; however, rather than stimulating receptors, they tend to obstruct them. Additionally, antagonists tend to hinder receptors from being stimulated by agonist compounds (McEvoy, Rabrich and Murphy, 2018). Antagonists can be likened to a key which fits into a particular lock, except it does not unlock it and stops other keys from being inserted. Naloxone and naltrexone are some opioid antagonists' examples.

In some circumstances, an opioid may act fully as an agonist on a particular receptor and as a partial agonist or an antagonist on another receptor. These opioids are categorised as agonists-antagonists due to their unsatisfactory mu-opioid receptor usefulness (McEvoy, Rabrich and Murphy, 2018). This may cause these opioids to functionally act as mu-opioid receptors while possessing kappa agonistic properties. The opioid agonists-antagonists can be used as analgesics though they tend to have a ceiling effect regarding their analgesic impact. This means that increasing the dosage past a particular level can only produce more opioid side effect, thereby reducing the opioids' potential to be abused.

Research conducted in mice showed that kappa-, mu-, and delta-opioid receptors have a well-defined role in processes that are mood-related (Lutz and Kieffer, 2013). For instance, mu-opioid receptors through which buprenorphine acts as partial agonist is a primary molecular player in the circuit that processes reward and often leads to addictive behaviours. The delta-opioid receptor, which is often antagonised by buprenorphine, tends to enhance a person's mood. Kappa-opioid receptor, which is buprenorphine antagonised in contrast to the mu-opioid receptor, portrays a significant anti-reward role in contrast to Mu opioid receptor (Wee and Koob, 2010).

The kappa-opioid receptor, which is our primary interest in this chapter, leads to analgesia in the spine and can portray sedation and dysphoria (Dean, Bilsky, and Negus, 2009). Kappa-opioid receptors refer to brain proteins which hinder the neurotransmitter glutamate release in a region of the brain which controls emotions. Kappa-opioid receptors can be found in the brain, peripheral tissues, and the spinal cord. These are the areas that are frequently linked to emotional responses and motivation. Kappa-opioid receptors are situated in both ends of the mesolimbic DA system (Dean, Bilsky, and Negus, 2009).

The kappa-opioid receptors are part of the opioid system and are commonly found in the peripheral and central nervous systems. High concentrations of the kappa-opioid receptor have been found in the ventral tegmental area, prefrontal cortex, amygdala, hippocampus, and the hypothalamus (Wang et al., 2010). The inactivation of the kappa-opioid receptors often activate the release of glutamate, and this reduces anxiety, which is one of the symptoms of depression. On the contrary, the activation of kappa-opioid receptors leads to less release of glutamate, thereby increasing the symptoms associated with depression.

Studies have revealed that kappa-opioid receptors tend to regulate emotional reactions, especially when an individual is experiencing stress. Stress is one of the risk factors which can lead to the development of various mental disorders among them being depression (Charney and Manji, 2004). When the brain is exposed to stress, it releases a hormone that directly works together with the kappa-opioid receptors. As a result, the kappa-opioid receptors activate p38α MAPK protein, which then communicates with the serotonin carrier in the cells to decrease the quantity of available serotonin.

In situations where an opioid attaches to kappa-opioid receptor as an antagonist, it tends to have an analgesic impact, which includes respiratory depression, constipation, and nausea. On the contrary, when antagonists attach to receptors, they do not produce any analgesic effect. The presence of an antagonist leads to competition with opioid molecules for connecting position on the receptors (Marie, 2010). During that time, analgesia, among other effects, is hindered. For instance, naloxone, which is an opioid antagonist, may attach to mu site and alter analgesia among other opioid-negative effects like sedation and respiratory depression.

Opioid medications that create analgesia tend to have an agonist impact in either one or more opioid receptor location; they are categorised according to the receptor they attach and act on (Marie, 2010). A majority of the opioid analgesics that are clinically helpful attach first and foremost to mu-opioid receptor location (Gutskein and Akil, 2006). The administration of the Mu receptor can be through various paths, and the analgesia onset could occur within a short period.

A study done on mice that were exposed to stress showed that their brain activates the p38α MAPK protein, which reduced the serotonin levels and triggered behaviours that were related to depression. The mice became withdrawn and did not want interactions with other mice (Bruchas et al., 2011). When the p38α MAPK protein was disabled in the brain's serotonin system, the mice that had been exposed to stress no longer withdrew from other mice.

According to research, the brain's flow of events that lead to a reduction in serotonin seems to be the same in both humans and mice (Bruchas et al., 2011). Based on the study on mice, the involvement of kappa-opioid receptors and p38α MAPK protein demonstrates a significant finding in establishing how cells control addictive and depressive behaviours.

Various mediators tend to be linked in the way the body reacts to stress, including vasopressin, corticotrophin-releasing factor, glucocorticoids and adrenocorticotrophic, which moderate the hypothalamic-pituitary-adrenal axis' actions. Various recommendations have been made regarding the counter-regulatory role of opioids in regulating the stress response of HPA during stressful conditions (Zhou *et al.*, 2013).

Dynorphin and β-endorphin stimulate the activity of HPA and apply tonic hindrance by acting on kappa and mu-opioid receptors, respectively. Kappa-opioid receptors (KOP) and dynorphin tend to be produced in limbic brain parts that are linked with mood regulation. Symptoms of depression are often enhanced by dynorphin, which is a kappa-opioid receptor agonist in the brain.

Stress can be considered as one of the significant risk factors which could lead to psychiatric disorders that are stress-induced such as depression. When kappa-opioid receptors are activated, behavioural reactions to stress are facilitated (Land *et al.*, 2008). During stressful events, the corticotropin-releasing factor is released, which can increase the release of dynorphin and ensuing activation of kappa-opioid receptors in particular circuits of the brain (Land *et al.*, 2008).

Stress tends to affect the brain's ventral tegmental area; this is an area of the brain that is involved in the reward process. Stress, in a way, increases the ventral tegmental area activity by activating the kappa-opioid receptors. Unpleasant or stressful experiences make the brain to release dynorphin, which activates and attaches itself to kappa-opioid receptors. Stressful experiences often make receptors to become active; when this activity is blocked, it hinders stress. Kappa-opioid receptors are developed on the presynaptic terminals of the ventral tegmental area and the ventral tegmental area cell bodies.

Studies have shown that when kappa-opioid receptor antagonists are administered before a stressful experience, it tends to block the impact of stress on an individual's behaviour (Chartoff *et al.*, 2012). Short-acting kappa-opioid receptor antagonists tend to have a more significant potential when used in an approach that is prophylactic before stressful events and not afterwards (Van't Veer and Carlexon, 2013). Therefore, activating kappa-opioid receptor during stressful events can lead to behavioural changes that are long-term in both females and males (Donahue *et al.*, 2015).

When kappa-opioid receptors are inhibited, symptoms of

depression, such as becoming socially withdrawn and portraying stress-seeking behaviours, can be reduced (Bruchas *et al.*, 2011). When the kappa-opioid receptors are activated, the release of dopamine is decreased, which leads to a dysphoric impact. Therefore, these receptors could represent a likely molecular target in treating mood disorders in people, especially for episodes that are a result of life stresses.

By reducing the transmission of dopamine, most kappa-opioid receptors agonists act as sedatives and reduce locomotion. Studies have further demonstrated that the kappa-opioid receptor agonists create psychotomimetic and dysphoric reactions in humans (Taylor and Manzella, 2016). Such findings demonstrate that kappa-opioid receptors antagonists could be used as antidepressant medication. Furthermore, research has shown that kappa-opioid agonists may be used to treat manic depression (Dean, Bilsky, and Negus, 2009).

Kappa-opioid receptor antagonists have proved useful in the treatment of the post-traumatic disorder, a bipolar disorder, which is also referred to as manic depression, dysthymia, and major depression. Recent studies have concentrated on the usefulness of kappa-opioid receptor antagonists in the treatment of depression. The administration of kappa receptor antagonists can be done systemically, for instance by subcutaneous, intramuscular, or intravenous injections. The receptor can also be administered through transdermal or topical application or orally as long as the receptor can penetrate the blood-brain barrier successfully.

Kappa receptor antagonists can either competitively or non-competitively inhibit the binding of dynorphin, which tends to selectively attach to the kappa-opioid receptor, causing a downstream impact on neurochemical systems linked to major depressive disorder. Additionally, inverse agonists, which might have a reverse impact of the agonist, could be applied instead of the kappa antagonists. Kappa-opioid antagonists tend to be more useful when administered before experiences, which can trigger stress (Land *et al.*, 2008). Studies have demonstrated that when kappa-opioid receptors are activated during times of stress, it could lead to behavioural change that is long-term in both females and males (Laman-Maharg *et al.*, 2017).

Kappa-opioid receptor antagonists, just like other antidepressants, tend to bring actions that are similar to those of acute anxiolytic. However, unlike other antidepressants, kappa-opioid antidepressants do not require a period of constant treatment for these impacts to be realised. Studies have even demonstrated that people who use antidepressants such as selective serotonin reuptake inhibitors (SSRI) at first have anxiogenic impacts, which may affect their adherence adversely (Drapier *et al.*, 2007). Therefore, the existence of an acute anxiolytic-like impact differentiates kappa-opioid receptor antagonists from other antidepressants.

Currently, kappa-opioid receptor antagonists are the single group of agents where critical treatment creates both anxiolytic and antidepressant-like effects simultaneously. Consequently, it can be considered that kappa-opioid receptor antagonists may epitomise an upgrading over the current treatment as can show that that they do not have anxiogenesis (side effect) which makes patients not to adhere to their medication routine. Preclinical studies have demonstrated that kappa-opioid receptor antagonists tend to be predominantly useful in alleviating the impact of stress (Carlezon and George, 2015). This is useful in the long-term as a preventive measure against the adverse effects of stress, which include depression.

The view that kappa antagonists may prove helpful in treating depression has come from studies which have demonstrated that constant exposure to abuse of drugs and stress can trigger depressive symptoms in humans. In rodents, kappa antagonists tend to obstruct signs of despair, anhedonia, and dysphoria (Dean, Bilsky, and Negus, 2009). Pharmacological research on rodents showed that the kappa-opioid receptor/dynorphin system controls behaviours that are mood-related (López *et al.*, 2016). Additionally, in rats administering kappa-opioid receptor agonists and antagonists systemically led to antidepressant-like impact. Fascinatingly, the kappa-opioid receptor-dependent pro-depressant-like impact can be influenced by an individual's gender (López *et al.*, 2016).

Buprenorphine and How It Works

Buprenorphine is a synthetic, analgesic drug that is often used in the treatment of opioid dependence. In the United States, this drug was approved by the Food and Drug Administration in October 2002 as a treatment for opioid addiction in men and also women who are not pregnant. The pharmacological attributes of buprenorphine lead to a lower risk of euphoria and dependence in comparison to other opioids like heroin, methadone, or morphine. Nevertheless, similar to other opioids, buprenorphine causes significant impact by interrelating with the mu-opioid receptor, which is a structure found on the nerve cells (McCann, 2008).

Buprenorphine also refers to a limited agonist, which means that similar to other opioids, the drug tends to stimulate receptors in the brain. However, its maximal impact tends to be less in comparison to that of a full agonist. Buprenorphine is a part of a family of drugs referred to as diverse opioid agonist-antagonists and is usually sold under the brand name Subutex or Suboxone (Obemebe, 2012). The drug is approved for detoxification in individuals who have an opioid dependence and also for analgesia (Howland, 2010).

The drug is primarily used in the treatment of opioid dependence; such opioids comprise, among others, heroin or prescription pain relievers like fentanyl, morphine, and oxycodone (Fisher and Roget, 2009). Moreover, the drug is utilised in medication-assisted treatment in assisting individuals in abandoning or lessening their use of opiates like morphine and also heroin.

When an individual uses opioid-like prescription painkillers or heroin, when ingested by the body, the opioids' molecular element binds itself to the brain's opioid receptors. The opioid receptors in the brain are primarily for controlling pain among other pathophysiological activities, which makes it an endogenous portion of the brain. After an opioid has attached itself to a receptor, it over-activates it and starts saturating the brain with false signs which produce the effects commonly referred to as *high*.

Buprenorphine is a kappa-opioid receptor antagonist and also a partial mu-opioid receptor. The drug tends to have an elevated affinity and little inherent activity towards the mu receptor. This means that buprenorphine attaches firmly to the mu receptor more than other opioids. Therefore, when a patient abuses a particular opioid in addition to buprenorphine, the drug tends to block the opioid from reaching the receptors, thereby hindering the expected outcome (Jones, 2004).

Additionally, if buprenorphine is administered to a person who already has taken another opioid, it replaces the opioid from the receptors. Owing to this, a clinician should be careful when beginning the buprenorphine treatment depending on the patient's degree of physical dependence and buprenorphine dosage. Other factors which the clinician should consider before beginning the buprenorphine therapy include, the last time the patient had abused the opioid. It is important also to realise that buprenorphine disengages slowly from the mu-opioid receptor. This trait can be linked to buprenorphine's extended period of activity during the treatment of patients who have an opioid dependence (Jones, 2004).

Dopamine is primarily the chemical which is saturated in the brain receptors that are overstimulated (Fink, 2010). Dopamine is a neurotransmitter that is accountable for pleasurable feelings, motivation, and emotions. The persistent stimulation of the brain's opioid receptors regularly conditions the person towards behaviour that is repetitive, which usually causes addiction. When buprenorphine us taken, it imitates the molecular configuration of opioids that bind to the opioid receptor. Through this action, buprenorphine can activate attachment to the brain's opioid receptors.

Buprenorphine is recognised as a partial opioid agonist, and in comparison to drugs such as methadone and heroin, its side effects tend to be weaker (Rapeli et al., 2007). The drug is referred to as a partial agonist since it attaches to the mu-opioid receptors as an agonist though it has restricted inherent efficacy. Furthermore, buprenorphine has a strong bond with the mu receptor, and it is not easily altered by opioid antagonists like naloxone which means that the drug delinks at a slow pace from the mu receptor locations (Gutsken and Akil, 2006).

Image showing the impact of buprenorphine
introduction on other opioids

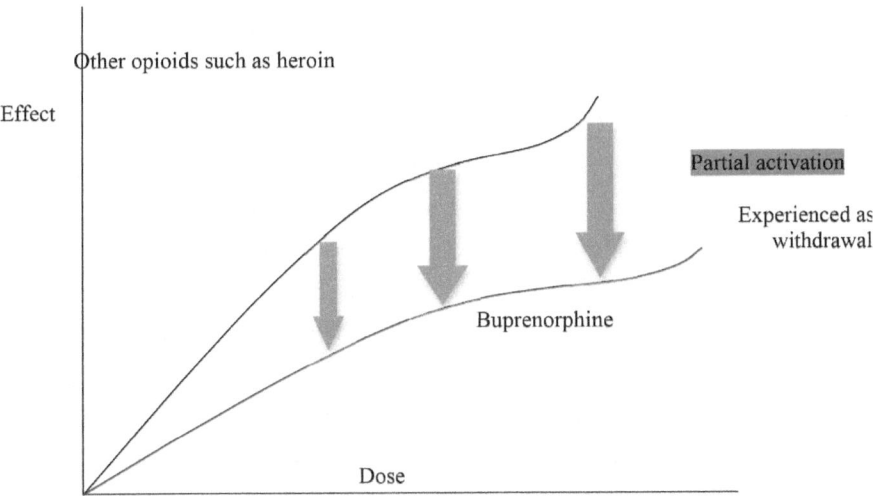

Before a physician prescribes buprenorphine, the patient should be exhibiting signs of opioid dependence. These symptoms include, among others, the incapacity to stop using opioids regardless of relationships and health challenges. Other symptoms include the desire for more opioids to sustain the same impact. Additionally, when an individual gives up activities they previously enjoyed to have more time to use opioids, this could be a sign of opioid dependence (Fisher, and Roget, 2009). People that have an opioid dependence may at times portray the desire to reduce the quantity of opioids used but cannot. After a physician finds that the patient has an opioid dependence, they then establish when the treatment should ensue.

Contrary to the treatment with methadone, which is administered in clinics that are vastly structured, buprenorphine is used to treat opioid dependency, and physicians can prescribe and dispense it (Rapeli *et al.*, 2007). Nevertheless, before the physicians prescribe buprenorphine, they ought to get acquainted with the State's and federal regulations, treatment guidelines, information on how to prescribe the drug, and requirements regarding their training (Cruciani and Knotkova, 2013). These physicians are required first to attend a special training where they receive a certificate which permits them to prescribe opioids for the treatment of addictions.

Moreover, the physicians, together with their staff, ought to create a working procedure that is standardised in caring for their buprenorphine patients (Cruciani and Knotkova, 2013). This care can comprise assembling a record of accessible psychosocial and community services such as group and individual counselling, homeless shelters, and case management among others. It is necessary when buprenorphine is prescribed that the patient should not mix it with alcohol to avoid adverse effects. The reason being that slowed breathing and also death can occur when buprenorphine is combined with other alcohol or antidepressants.

Previously, methadone was the only drug that was being used in the treatment of opioid dependence. Methadone's availability was limited since it could be dispensed only in clinics which were specialized in the treatment of addictions (Rapeli *et al.*, 2007). It is necessary to note that methadone is a full agonist. Also, since it is a full mu-opioid agonist and it tends to affect receptors up to a point there is a complete activation of all the effects, or the ceiling impact is attained. On the contrary, buprenorphine, which is a partial agonist, does not stimulate mu receptors to a similar degree as methadone.

The impact of buprenorphine tends to increase up to the ceiling level. In this level, patients who have an opioid dependence can stop the use of buprenorphine without any withdrawal symptoms. Other differences between buprenorphine and methadone include the duration of their half-life; methadone lasts for a period of eight to fifty-nine hours while buprenorphine half-life lasts between twenty-four to sixty hours (Rapeli *et al.*, 2007). The other difference between the two is that buprenorphine has a ceiling effect while methadone does not have the same effect.

The introduction of buprenorphine changed this since any licensed physician can dispense the drug. This means that buprenorphine can be used to treat opiate addiction by physicians who are qualified in their offices, unlike methadone which requires the patient to be enrolled in a treatment program (Nathan and Gorman, 2007). Buprenorphine also does not necessitate in-clinic administration. The fact that the drug is a combination of both an agonist and antagonist tends to lower its risk of overdose and abuse.

The pharmacological content in buprenorphine assists in circumstances when there is a likelihood of the drug's misuse. Additionally, the drug reduces the impact of opioid's physical dependency like cravings and withdrawal symptoms. Buprenorphine enhances safety in circumstances when there is an overdose. The effects of buprenorphine tend to intensify with each dosage up until at moderate doses where a ceiling effect is reached (Dahan, Aarts, and Smith, 2010). At this stage, a patient may cease the usage of opioids without undergoing any withdrawal.

With constant use, buprenorphine can lead to physical dependence, but since it is a partial agonist, the level of physical dependence tends to be lower in comparison to that produced by a full agonist (Cruciani and Knotkova, 2013). The use of buprenorphine by people who are physically reliant on full opioids such as methadone, morphine, and heroin can lead to withdrawal tends to be less severe in comparison to full mu-opioid agonists (Cruciani and Knotkova, 2013).

Buprenorphine, as an opioid, binds to opioid receptors, thereby substituting and hindering other opioids whereby they are rendered ineffective (Fisher, and Roget, 2009). By attaching to receptors, buprenorphine tricks the receptor to believing that its need for opioids has been met without creating euphoric feelings or leading to respiratory depression. By doing this, the receptor is hindered from connecting with full opioids; hence if a person uses painkillers or heroin, it would not be possible to experience other effects.

Buprenorphine by attaching to receptors tends to block them for a longer period than other opioids. As a partial agonist, buprenorphine tends to have restricted pleasurable impacts which assist in preventing the withdrawal symptoms (Boone et al., 2004). Moreover, buprenorphine does not stimulate mu receptors to the same degree as methadone since buprenorphine is a partial opioid agonist which means that it works on some opioid receptors that are in the brain, thereby giving a reprieve from opioid withdrawal symptoms and pain.

Buprenorphine tends to attach with a high affinity to kappa and mu-opioid receptors but attaches to delta-opioid receptor with a lower affinity (McCann, 2008). As a result, if an individual consumes an abused opioid in addition to buprenorphine, the opioid tends to be blocked before getting to the receptors and creating the desired strong effects. Furthermore, if a person takes an opioid and later takes buprenorphine, the latter replaces from the receptors the other opioids.

Buprenorphine tends to detach slowly from the mu-opioid receptor. This feature can be linked to buprenorphine's extended period of action when a patient is receiving treatment for opioid dependence. It is necessary to note that buprenorphine is an antagonist of the kappa-opioid receptor, which means that it hinders stimulation. Activation of the kappa-opioid receptors plays a significant role in causing some of the key symptoms linked to opioid withdrawal-like chronic depression. The attachment of buprenorphine to the kappa-opioid receptor, which slows its activity can create feelings of wellness and enhance positive mood (Kaye and Shah, 2015).

Additionally, since buprenorphine is a partial agonist, it stimulates the mu receptor which tends to activate various activities of the nerve cells that underlie a majority of the well-known opioid effects such as respiratory suppression, reducing pain, or feelings of pleasure. When the mu receptor becomes partially activated, buprenorphine produces similar effects though with less intensity in comparison to other opioids. Drugs such as methadone, heroin, or morphine can lead to euphoria, leading to continuous abuse of the drug. On the contrary, buprenorphine gives a moderate and positive psychosocial effect. This effect lessens cravings and assists patients to adhere to their medication schedule.

A study was conducted among incarcerated men that were addicted to heroin. These men were divided into two groups; one group was assigned buprenorphine and the other methadone. The patients that were assigned buprenorphine reported that they would willingly propose the treatment to others and ninety-three per cent (93%) of these men intended to continue with the treatment after their release. Furthermore, a quarter of the patients that were assigned methadone for their treatment opted to change to buprenorphine treatment. Research has also shown that buprenorphine can improve the quality of life that is health-related.

Moreover, as buprenorphine is slow in dissolving, it produces a firmer impact on the receptors. Fundamentally, by taking buprenorphine, the need for other unsafe opioids is reduced. Therefore, a person can participate in their daily activities without experiencing any highs or withdrawals. Also, there is a likelihood of reducing the dosage with time to take back the brain to its normal state.

Buprenorphine, when administered at low dosage, has a better medicinal value, which assists individuals who are addicted to opioids to stop abusing opioids and the accompanying withdrawal symptoms (Fisher, and Roget, 2009). Buprenorphine is often administered through intravenous transfusion, sublingual tablets, and ethanolic liquid oral solution. When an individual takes buprenorphine as prescribed, it tends to have a balancing effect on their brain and often works in the first few days after the initial dose.

After a patient has been examined and found fitting to begin buprenorphine treatment, there is need to advise the patient that at the initial stages of the treatment that he or she may be required to be at the clinic for monitoring. Before beginning the treatment, the physician and the patient should agree with the treatment plans, goals, and termination.

Before the first buprenorphine dose, the patient should abstain from the usage of other opioids such as heroin for a period of twelve to twenty-four hours (Cruciani and Knotkova, 2013). This means that treatment with buprenorphine should be initiated during withdrawal. In situations where people that are addicted to various opioids start the treatment when they are not experiencing withdrawal symptoms, then buprenorphine tends to activate withdrawal symptoms.

The treatment with buprenorphine commonly occurs in three stages. The first is the induction stage, which is medically observed start-up treatment with the drug, which is conducted in the office of a qualified physician (Cruciani and Knotkova, 2013). During this phase, the person should be in the initial stages of opioid withdrawal for buprenorphine treatment to be administered (Cruciani and Knotkova, 2013). It is necessary to realise that buprenorphine can cause severe withdrawal for individuals that are not in initial phases of withdrawal and who could be having in their bloodstream other opioids.

Image demonstrating the process undertaken
during the induction phase

- The phase lasts between two to ten days
- Before the first dose, the physician should ensure that the patient last dose of illicit opioid was between twelve to twenty-four hours

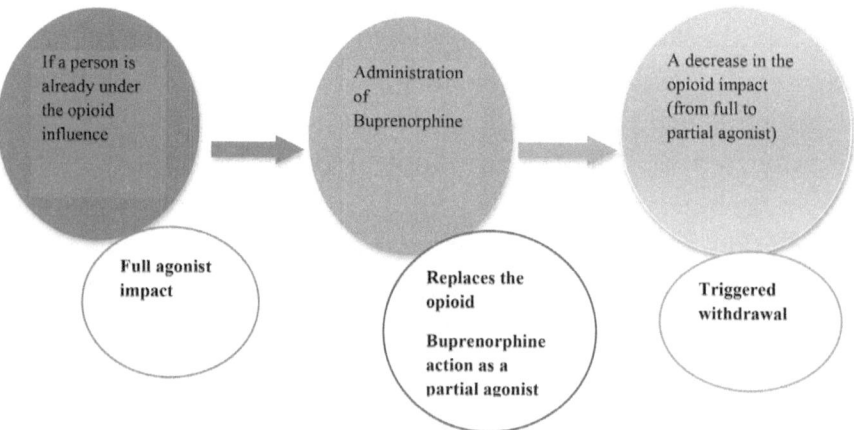

The second phase is the stabilisation stage, which starts after an individual has suspended or decreased their abuse of the opioid, and their craving is no longer in existence. In this stage, the dosage of buprenorphine requires adjustment. In some circumstances, after the patient has stabilised, the daily dosage can be adjusted to alternate daily dosage.

The third phase is the maintenance stage and ensues when an individual is recovering and is on a steady buprenorphine dose. After the person is steadied, a different strategy can involve going into a withdrawal that is medically supervised, which would make the switch from physical dependence on the opioids smoother.

Treating opioid dependence with buprenorphine is effective, reducing death by around 50%. Individuals who are treated with buprenorphine tend to demonstrate enhanced social functioning, decreased criminal behaviour, and reduced substance abuse disorder. Buprenorphine is an effective pain reliever, especially for people that have chronic pain or pain caused by an opioid dependence (Berland et al., 2013).

A patient should not cease taking buprenorphine when they feel better but should wait for the healthcare provider to determine the extent of the treatment that is appropriate. In situations when a patient stops taking buprenorphine suddenly, the person may experience withdrawal symptoms. Additionally, the person should take buprenorphine as prescribed and avoid missing doses to prevent the risk of a relapse.

Buprenorphine should not be injected to avoid withdrawal symptom, slowed breathing, or even death caused by overdose in an individual that has an opioid dependence. Furthermore, buprenorphine is not to be used in relieving pain or by individuals that have acute liver disease. In most circumstances, buprenorphine is available in the form of a film or tablet that melts in the mouth. A person should avoid swallowing buprenorphine, but instead, they ought to dissolve it under their tongue.

The drug should not be chewed, crushed, broken, or cut. Additionally, if the patient requires more than one tablet at a time, both should be placed under the tongue simultaneously. On the other hand, the patient can put one tablet first under the language, and after it has dissolved immediately, place the other tablet. The patient should also avoid drinking or eating until the buprenorphine tablet has completely dissolved.

The adult liver effectively metabolises buprenorphine, which explains why it is more effective when it dissolves in the mouth rather than it being swallowed. The person should not drink or eat anything until buprenorphine is dissolved. Often buprenorphine effects tend to occur around one and a half hours after its administration. Usually, buprenorphine is taken once per day since the effects typically last for twenty-four hours. Physicians often advise the patient to stick to a daily routine when taking buprenorphine to enhance maximum benefits of the drug (Cruciani and Knotkova, 2013).

Buprenorphine effects tend to be on the brain's opioid receptors and the spinal cord. The drug tends to have a depressing effect on the brain's respiratory centres. Buprenorphine also decreases gut motility, which may lead to constipation. Since buprenorphine is a vasodilator, it may cause the feeling of fainting, sweating, and having a flushed skin when the patient either sits or lies down.

In circumstances where the physician administers an incorrect dose, the patient should be notified immediately. The pharmacist should also warn the patient of possible consequences of the drug such as drowsiness.

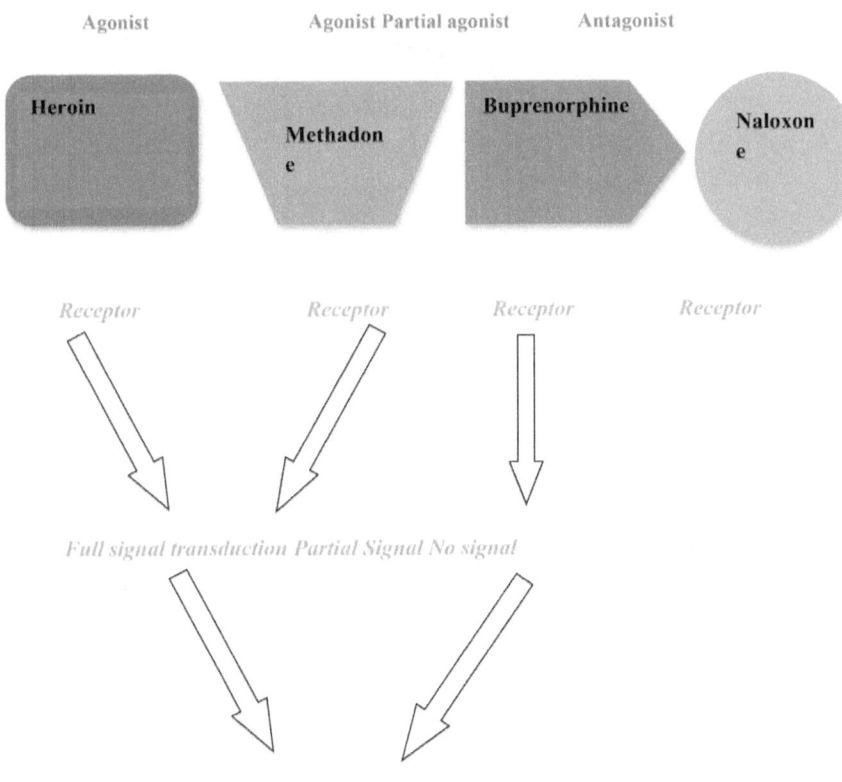

Image 2

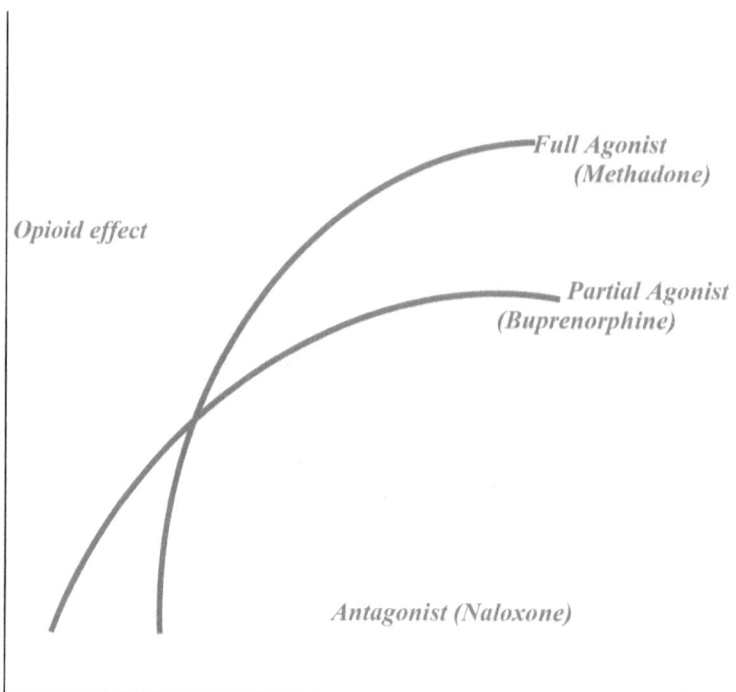

Buprenorphine as a Cure for Depression

In 2015, in the United States alone, an estimated 6.7% of adults were diagnosed with a major depressive disorder. A significant percentage of these individuals do not respond to various antidepressant treatment, which leads to the treatment of resistant depression; this shows the need for a different kind of treatment. Most antidepressants tend to regulate monoamines neuronal transmission by increasing the serotonin, dopamine, and norepinephrine synaptic levels. The currently used antidepressants like serotonin-norepinephrine reuptake inhibitors and selective serotonin reuptake inhibitors tend to have a high degree of mechanistic overlap that targets monoamine (Deardorff and Grossberg, 2014).

Additionally, based on the World Health Organization (WHO) statistics, over three hundred and twenty million individuals are affected by depression globally. The WHO statistics further state that depression has increased between the years 2005–2015 by 18.4% (Vos et al., 2016). The study also demonstrated that around 50% of individuals affected by major depressive disorder often respond to the initial treatment. On the other hand, only thirty per cent of individuals affected by the disorder attain total remission while the remaining individuals have to get additional treatment to enhance response (Valenstein, 2006).

The degree of remission tends to be low in depression that is resistant to treatment; this is often linked to a high rate of recurrence, suicidal behaviour, and substance abuse (Serafini et al., 2018). The major depressive disorder usually tends to cause frequent episodes with a growing severity and a decreased response to therapy (Sibille and French, 2013). In such circumstances, it is necessary to attain total remission or learn to treat and adequately manage the remaining symptoms of the disorder to avoid relapse (Serafine et al., 2018).

There are several risk factors which may trigger depression that is resistant to treatment. One of the factors includes the length of the depression episode if it is longer the more the degeneration in some parts of the brain such as the hippocampus. The behavioural and cognitive changes which occur during the extended episode can hinder these regions of the brain from returning to their previous form. Another risk factor which can predispose a person to this kind of depression includes the severity of the episode. Severe episodes can be linked to biological imbalances and mild depression.

Melancholic traits can also trigger the treatment of resistant depression. Anxiety and personality disorders can also trigger the development of this depression. Additionally, old age can increase the risk of developing a depression that is resistant to treatment. Some symptoms of the treatment-resistant depression include, among others, suicidal thoughts, feelings of hopelessness, and isolation. Other symptoms include inadequate response to various treatment trials or those prescribed. Another symptom of the treatment of resistant depression consists of the worsening of symptoms after failed treatment. The incapacity to put up with antidepressants treatment doses owing to severe side effects can also indicate the existence of this kind of depression.

The fact that depression that is resistant to treatment rarely responds to conventional antidepressants led to studies with the sole purpose of seeking alternative medicine. During the 1950s, opioids were frequently used in the treatment of various forms of depression (Tenore, 2008). Presently, selective serotonin reuptake inhibitors (SSRIs) are often regarded as the first line of treatment for depression (Cleare *et al.*, 2015). Regrettably, selective serotonin reuptake inhibitors tend to be successful in only forty to fifty per cent of individuals affected by depression.

SSRIs among other antidepressants are founded on the monoamine hypothesis and tend to modulate dopamine, norepinephrine, and serotonin. These traits are not useful in the treatment of depression that is resistant to treatment or major depression since the mechanism of the disorder tends to be complex. Therefore, presently, opioids are being explored as an option in treating major depression. The opioids that are being considered include samidorphan and naloxone, which tends to have a low chance of being abused (Jordan and Morrisonponce, 2018).

Naloxone is often added to buprenorphine to avert the misuse of buprenorphine, which means preventing the patient from injecting it into their vein. Naloxone tends to have no side effects when the patient does not inject it but rather allows the drug to dissolve under the tongue. In circumstances where naloxone is injected, it blocks the buprenorphine effect, thereby causing withdrawal symptoms.

Treating major depressive disorder with conventional methods frequently requires a long period and can be linked to constant depressive symptoms and a higher risk of suicide. More than fifty per cent of older adults and those in midlife are not responsive to conventional antidepressants (Dew *et al.*, 2007).

Depression that is resistant to treatment and which is often unresponsive to conventional antidepressants such as SNRIs and SSRIs regularly pose a therapeutic predicament due to the insufficient evidence-based substitute treatment. At times, aggressive treatments such as magnetic seizure, deep brain stimulation, and ketamine infusion have been used in treating depression that is resistant to treatment.

In such cases, buprenorphine which is both a kappa-opioid receptor antagonist and a partial mu-opioid receptor agonist can be useful as a cure to depression that is resistant to treatment (Richards and Hara, 2014). This kind of depression is diagnosed when the depressive symptoms in patient do not lessen following two antidepressant trials (Knoth *et al.*, 2010). Studies on both humans and animals have shown that buprenorphine is a synthetic opiate which has an effect that is similar to the one triggered by antidepressants and leads to a decrease in suicidal behaviours (Sher, 2016).

Furthermore, since buprenorphine is a partial mu-opioid agonist, it is considered as a preferable approach to suicidal behaviour in patients who have both mood and opioid use disorder. The pharmacological grounds for the anti-depressive and anti-suicidal impact of buprenorphine are often since the drug is a potent kappa-opioid antagonist and a μ opioid agonist. Kappa antagonists contain anti-anxiety, anti-suicidal, anti-depressive properties.

Furthermore, a study that was conducted among forty individuals that were addicted to opioids and were treated with buprenorphine had their depressive symptoms considerably reduce in the nineteen patients that were initially depressed.

Moreover, fast mood improvement was observed among the seven to ten individuals who did not have opioid dependence but was depressed after the buprenorphine treatment. There was also a considerable improvement in four of the patients who had depressive symptoms (Richards and Hara, 2014).

Other studies conducted have demonstrated that between sixty to seventy per cent (60%–70%) of individuals with depression especially major depressive disorders tend to have an unsatisfactory reaction to the treatment they are initially given (Trivedi, 2007). Based on various researches that have been conducted, buprenorphine can be useful in patients that have depression that is resistant to treatment and who may not be responding to other forms of medications.

A study conducted on the impact of buprenorphine on emotion processing among healthy volunteers showed that the drug enhanced memory (Syal *et al.*, 2015). Buprenorphine, as a medication that is used in treating opioid addiction, is also useful in treating depression that is resistant to treatment. This drug is a mu-opioid receptor partial antagonist and also a kappa-opioid antagonist.

Various studies have been conducted concerning the usefulness of buprenorphine in treating mental health conditions. The results have shown that symptoms of depression tend to improve with the use of buprenorphine, particularly for patients that have opioid dependence. Patients that were resistant to either electroconvulsive therapy or antidepressant medications seemed to respond positively to buprenorphine treatment (Karp *et al.*, 2014). It is also necessary to note that buprenorphine reduces the response of an individual to stress, which, as discussed above, often leads to depression (Bershad *et al.*, 2015).

Buprenorphine can also mitigate the impact of stress and may have a therapeutic impact on individuals that have mood disorders (Kaye and Shah, 2015). However, buprenorphine should not be confused with selective kappa-opioid receptor antagonist as the two are different. At times, to achieve more pharmacological selectivity, buprenorphine is combined with other agents such as naltrexone (Almatroudi *et al.*, 2015).

Another useful antidepressant therapy includes combining buprenorphine and samidorphan. In this combination, buprenorphine brings an antidepressant relief, whereas samidorphan cancels any extreme pleasure reaction as it causes discriminatory antagonism of the mu receptor. This leads to insignificant pleasurable impact from buprenorphine. This treatment is currently being developed as an additional treatment for individuals who have been affected by depression that is resistant to treatment. The combination of buprenorphine and samidorphan is presently being promoted as a supplementary treatment for individuals who have a treatment-resistant kind of depression (Fava *et al.*, 2016).

Due to the increased mortality risk connected with the treatment of resistant depression, there is a need to explore other medications that target new treatment pathways in conjunction with norepinephrine and serotonin. The buprenorphine/samidorphan combination is a new antidepressant which works through the opioid receptor pathway to enhance dopaminergic channelling in the mesolimbic pathway.

Buprenorphine can also be combined with tramadol in treating patients who have neurodegenerative diseases, which include chronic pain and depression. Studies have shown that treatment with buprenorphine often leads to an enhancement of the regional cerebral perfusion abnormalities. On the other hand, tramadol remarkably reduces histological, biochemical, and behavioural alterations (Murray *et al.* 2018). Care is required when administering tramadol since its chronic use can be linked to the neuronal deterioration of the brain and eventually, cerebral palsy (Faria *et al.*, 2017).

Studies have also shown that suicide ideations, which are one of the symptoms of depression, tend to be reduced in adults that are suicidal (Karp *et al.*, 2014). Additionally, buprenorphine decreases the capacity to identify fearful faces and improves memory for valenced emotional stimuli that are positive (Syal *et al.*, 2015). Buprenorphine can also reduce responses to various negative stimuli and other psychosocial stress (Bershad *et al.*, 2014).

Buprenorphine alone has shown clinical usefulness in treating depression that is resistant to treatment and in a study conducted on rats and mice it showed decreased anxiety and depressive behaviours in them (Browne, van Nest, and Lucki, 2015). Initially, there was the belief that the efficacy of buprenorphine in treating patients that were depressed was as a result of its partial mu-opioid receptor agonist activity. Over the years, this view has been challenged, and evidence has shown that buprenorphine's behavioural effect can be credited to its kappa-opioid receptor antagonism (Falcon *et al.*, 2015).

Interestingly, current studies have shown that in situations where the motivational component is present, mu-opioid receptor antagonists tend to impact the behavioural reaction of buprenorphine (Browne at al., 2017). Consequently, it seems that both mu and kappa-opioid antagonisms could be significant for buprenorphine capacity to regulate the emotional state of an individual.

Buprenorphine seems to be useful in individuals who do not have opioid dependence. In treating the symptoms of depression, the initial administration of buprenorphine can be at 0.1–0.2 mg per day. Where necessary, the physician can advise the patient to gradually titrate the drug, to keep away from its adverse side effects; this will assist in giving time for an adequate clinical reaction.

Older adults and those in midlife who are affected by treatment-resistant depression have been found to tolerate low doses of buprenorphine. Studies have demonstrated that more than fifty per cent of older adults or those in midlife affected by depression rarely respond to conventional antidepressants (Dew *et al.*, 2007).

Exposing the older adults and those in midlife who are affected by depression to buprenorphine often shows a remarkable improvement in a short period. When buprenorphine is provided to these adults in low doses, its antidepressant usefulness can only be achieved when the drug is taken for long-term. Opioid dependence in older adults and those in midlife can cause degeneration to their cognitive function.

On the contrary, adults who do not have an opioid dependence may benefit more from the administration of buprenorphine (Dagtekin *et al.*, 2007). Buprenorphine, when administered in high doses, can help in the treatment of suicide and refractory depression. Buprenorphine can reduce suicidal tendencies and the degree of depression fast (Osório *et al.*, 2016).

Studies have shown that the administration buprenorphine in low doses tends to reduce the severity of the symptoms linked to major depression within the initial three weeks of treatment. Additionally, the research demonstrated that patients' learning and executive functioning were enhanced (Fava *et al.*, 2016).

Despite the usefulness of buprenorphine in treating opioid dependence, there are some likely side effects (Ducharme, Fraser, and Gill, 2012). Some of them include vomiting, insomnia, nausea, swelling of the legs and arms, constipation, drowsiness after taking the drug, and headache. Other common side effects that might occur while using buprenorphine include redness and numbness of the user's mouth or having one's tongue burning or paining.

Buprenorphine's adverse side effects tend to be mild and usually happen at the time of the initial treatment where the symptoms may subside with time. Managing the side effects of the drug often depend on their severity. Side effects such as nausea can be controlled by avoiding fast increases of the dose given, also reducing the dosage can help in managing nausea. Constipation, which is common in all opioids, can be controlled by a regular intake of fibre and fluids. Insomnia, which is another side effect of buprenorphine, can be managed by avoiding stimulants such as amphetamines, nicotine, and coffee and having a regular sleep schedule.

If a patient is experiencing drowsiness after taking buprenorphine, the clinician can reduce the maintenance dose and also evaluate other medications being taken by the patient. The patient should also not participate in activities which may require them to be active such as driving. Headache, which tends to be common in the initial stages of buprenorphine treatment, can be managed by taking paracetamol. Additionally, the physician may check if there are other issues which could be causing the headache.

A combination of buprenorphine and naloxone may increase pressure in the head. Severe injuries in the head and other conditions that can increase pressure in the head should first be discussed with the doctor before the administration of buprenorphine. By doing this, the physician can administer the right dose, which will be useful to the patient. Issues which may affect the kidney or liver functioning should also be notified to the physician before the administration of buprenorphine. In situations where a patient has breathing problems such as those caused by respiratory depression or asthma, he or she ought to inform the doctor since such conditions can affect the success of buprenorphine.

Whenever a patient visits the pharmacy to get more of the drug, they should be evaluated for buprenorphine toxicity. The clinician should obtain the patient's vital signs, mental and physical health condition. If the patient is intoxicated or lethargic, buprenorphine ought not to be dispensed to them. Buprenorphine can be withdrawn for a few days with no side effects since its half-life is long. In circumstances where the patient could be demonstrating symptoms of respiratory depression, he ought to be examined in the emergency room where they receive treatment for opioid overdose.

Before a patient takes medication of any kind including buprenorphine, he or she should inform the physician regarding any allergies or medical condition they could be having, for instance, if a woman is pregnant or breastfeeding. Also, if a woman becomes pregnant while taking buprenorphine, they should immediately contact their doctor to avoid harming the unborn baby. Buprenorphine can easily pass into the breast milk; therefore, breastfeeding mother should avoid the drug.

Moreover, buprenorphine should also not be combined with medications such as serotonin reuptake inhibitors and tricyclic antidepressants, which are often used in the treatment of depression (Jones, 2004). Some reactions which can result from such a combination can include experiencing difficulties in moving, muscle spasms and rigidity, and changes in mental condition including agitation and delirium. Furthermore, coma or death can come as a result of combining buprenorphine with other medications that are used in treating depression. Therefore, though buprenorphine can be used in managing the symptoms of the treatment-resistant depression, it should be administered by a physician who has adequate training regarding the administration of buprenorphine.

Developing a new drug close enough to buprenorphine to manage the symptoms of depression should be made of the benzene ring, carbon connector and a tertiary amine.

Benzene ring   Carbon bridges   Tertiary amine buprenorphine

In general, developing a new drug can be costly and usually takes some times before the perfectly metabolised molecule is found (lead) and ready to trails. Considering the pain and suffering caused by untreated depression to our communities, development of an improved and strongest kappa-opioid and mu-receptor antagonist with antidepressant effects should be seriously considered regardless of the costs.

I am currently working on a new chemical structure that will potentially be used to develop a new medication based on a very similar chemical structure of buprenorphine. I will talk more about it in one of my next books. It is worth to mention that an amino acid called taurine has significantly improved symptoms of depression during the 6 months trial I have conducted with my clients (1g of taurine per 20kg of body weight has shown the best results). However, I have strong beliefs that kappa-opioid receptors antagonists combined together with transcranial magnetic stimulation therapy is the key to control depression and many other mental episodic illnesses such as borderline personality and bipolar disorders.

CHAPTER 5

Lifestyle and Depression

Individuals who are not healthy physically tend to be at a higher risk of developing depression and other mental illnesses. Individuals are involved in lifestyle habits which are considered unhealthy tend to experience challenges when trying to overcome symptoms of depression. Some of the adverse lifestyle factors which may lead to depression include physical inactivity, lack of sleep (insomnia), poor diet, overwork, substance and alcohol abuse, environmental factors, and lack of recreational activities and leisure time among others. In this chapter each one of these factors and their association with depression will be discussed.

Physical Activity and Depression

Physical inactivity has been linked to the increase which has been witnesses of most physical and mental health conditions. According to the World Health Organization, physical inactivity is one of the leading causes of death globally (Alwan, 2010). Physical exercise can be classified as either aerobic or anaerobic. Lack of physical activity has been often linked to disability and depressive symptoms. Physical activity includes lifestyle activities which are either modest or intense and also physical exercises.

Evidence has shown that constant physical exercises or activity is useful in the prevention and management of depression and other illnesses. Engaging constantly in physical activity can enhance the quality of life and health among individuals of all ages despite the existence of a disability or a chronic disease. Research has demonstrated that in adults, physical activity may reduce the likelihood of developing depression (Mafra and Fouque, 2014). Nevertheless, most people are not physically active which can be linked to the increased rate of mental and other physical illnesses.

Participating regularly in physical activities enhances long- and short-term psychosocial health thereby decreasing feelings of depression, anxiety, and stress. Studies have shown that physical activity can reduce mild or moderate unipolar depression (Mafra and Fouque, 2014). Exercises such as walking, cycling, running, and jogging can also act as therapy for individuals who have been diagnosed with depression.

The benefits of exercise and physical activity on general mood and depression have been established in all age groups. Studies have demonstrated that when an individual exercises, his or her state is enhanced. Several clinical trials have shown that interventions which involve physical activity can considerably lessen depressive symptoms in comparison to conventional treatment. The impact of physical activity on people affected by depression has been compared to that of cognitive therapy and antidepressants (Beaulac *et al.*, 2011). Based on some studies, engaging in constant exercises can reduce the symptoms of depression, and the impact may be long lasting.

When an individual is affected by depression, the last thing in their mind is to engage in any physical exercise or activity. However, physical activity can help in enhancing an individual's mood and reducing anxiety. Exercise assists in producing endorphins which enhance a sense of well-being, thereby reducing stress. Additionally, physical activity assists in taking off a person's mind away from negative thoughts which feed anxiety and depression (Beaulac *et al.*, 2011).

Some symptoms of depression include social isolation; physical activity or exercise can provide the affected person with an opportunity to socialise with other people. Additionally, exercise may become among people affected by depression a healthy coping mechanism. Exercise such as aerobics tends to reduce general stress levels. Physical activity provides individuals opportunities to interact socially with others and this can enhance moods for those affected by depression. The completion of a particular physical activity produces a sense of achievement and this enhances self-efficacy which can cause the individual who is affected by depression to start believing in their abilities.

Low-intensity exercise or physical activities tend to release neurotrophic factors which lead to the growth of nerve cells in the hippocampus region. This helps in relieving the symptoms of depression. It is believed that stress can inhibit the development of neurons which are new nerve cells, a process referred to as neurogenesis. Exercise releases not just endorphins but other neurotransmitters such as serotonin, a chemical which helps in enhancing a person's mood, sleep, and appetite. Serotonin, which is a neurotransmitter located in the gut and the brain, has an impact on a person's mood.

Serotonin is directly linked to the level of happiness and sadness an individual experiences. Studies have shown that people who are affected by depression tend to have low serotonin levels. Additionally, dopamine, which plays a critical role in how an individual views reality and stays motivated, is also released through exercise or physical activity (Burchard, 2017). Norepinephrine which helps in raising the blood pressure and constricting blood vessels is also produced during physical exercises (Wolfe, 2010). Furthermore, physical activities decrease chemicals in the immune system which could be aggravating the depressive symptoms.

Various physical and mental health issues which include depression, eating disorders, and hypertension among others can be caused by low levels of serotonin (Pytliak *et al.*, 2011). When serotonin levels are low, individuals may encounter challenges controlling their impulses, become annoyed easily, or be sluggish which are some of the symptoms of depression. Exercises such as swimming, biking, running, and walking often are useful in enhancing the serotonin levels in the brain.

Insomnia and depression tend to be closely related to each other. A constant lack of sleep can make the affected individual to lack pleasure in life's activities which is another symptom of depression. Studies have demonstrated that treating insomnia may lessen the symptoms of depression. Low melatonin levels have frequently been linked to the loss of sleep. Low melatonin levels are also associated with constant fatigue and absent-mindedness which are other symptoms of depression (D S M V, 2013). Exercises especially when done in morning hours are one way through which melatonin levels can be increased. Melatonin does not only regulate an individual's sleep pattern but also positively impacts on the person's mood and immune system.

Physical inactivity can also lead to obesity and depression, and these two have become serious health issues in modern times (Ng et al., 2014). Based on the World Health Organization statistics, approximately three hundred and fifty million individuals are affected by depression and six hundred million are obese (WHO, 2016). Studies have shown that globally 20% of adults tend to be physically inactive which increases the risk of obesity and other physical and mental health conditions (Herring et al., 2012). According to research, obesity can increase the risk of developing depression (Rhew et al., 2008).

Loss of energy and fatigue are some the symptoms of depressions; people with this kind of symptoms rarely engage in physical activity, and this increases the risk of obesity (D S M V, 2013). Undeniably, symptoms of depression are often linked to very little or no physical exercises. Studies have demonstrated that physical activity or exercises can prevent the development of symptoms of depression in individuals with obesity (Dankel et al., 2016) Individuals who have obesity tend to be diagnosed more with major depression in comparison to those whose weight is normal (Ma and Xiao, 2010).

Studies have also shown that obesity among adolescence is often related to symptoms of depression later in adulthood (Jerstad *et al.*, 2010). This can be linked to the stigma which a child with obesity experiences, and this includes social isolation by peers and ridicule. Additionally, men who are obese were found to have a higher risk of developing depression. People with obesity tend to suffer discrimination in society, and this can lead to depressive symptoms. Depression and obesity can increase the risk of an individual developing other chronic diseases (Ma and Xiao, 2010).

Both obesity and depression can be treated through physical activity or exercise. Various studies have compared physical activity to psychotherapy and pharmacological treatment for depression (Blumenthal *et al.*, 2007). The side effects of pharmacological treatment which include diarrhoea can be avoided when exercise is used as therapy in the treatment of both obesity and depression. Furthermore, physical activity or exercise does not attract social stigmas as compared to psychotherapy or pharmacological treatment. Therefore, it may be more affordable, readily accessible, and an acceptable treatment choice for those affected by depression (Dinas *et al.*, 2011).

Studies have shown that patients affected by major depression who participated in aerobic exercises had their depressive symptoms reduce in comparison to those who took conventional medications only (Blumenthal *et al.*, 2007). Thus, exercises can be used as a form of therapy in treating patients affected by chronic depression. Starting and maintaining a consistent physical activity routine can be difficult especially for people affected by depression. As a result, it is necessary to follow a few steps such as determining what one enjoys doing first. An individual should assess the kind of physical activities they like. An example is if a person enjoys evening walks, going for bike rides, swimming, or gardening.

After establishing what one enjoys the person should then engage and continue with the preferred physical activities. For individuals who have already been diagnosed with depression, it is important to consult first with their mental health provider. The person should discuss the physical activity which he or she desires to engage in and ways in which it can fit in their general treatment regimen. It is necessary to put in place goals that are both realistic and attainable.

The exercise program should be tailored to meet an individual's abilities and needs. A person should avoid viewing physical activity or exercise as a duty. Instead, he or she should view the physical activity program just the same as therapy sessions or medications. Before beginning the physical activity, it is essential to consider the hindrances. For instance, a person who is self-conscious and plans to walk as a part of his or her exercise may need to consider engaging in this physical activity at home.

A person should also applaud their achievements however small; engaging in any physical activity is considered better than living a sedentary lifestyle. For instance, substituting sleeping all day due to depression with walking for twenty minutes can reduce depressive symptoms. Such physical activities despite their low intensity can enhance the individual's mood which may assist him or her to sleep better.

Additionally, if an individual does not have sufficient money to use on exercise gear, he or she may consider engaging in something which is cost-free. By looking at the hindrances to exercising or physical activity, it is possible to get a different solution. Obstacles are bound to occur in any new venture in life and that includes exercising; therefore, a person should be ready for any setback. It is important to maintain a positive attitude and recognise every step one makes, no matter its magnitude. Outdoor exercises have an additional benefit since the person is exposed to sunlight which impacts the pineal glands thereby enhancing one's moods.

Sleep and Depression

There exists a strong connection between mental health and sleep. Deprivation of sleep can lead to depression and the reverse is true. Lack of sleep can affect an individual's mental health and psychological condition (Taylor *et al.*, 2008). People who have already been diagnosed with a mental health condition are more susceptible to sleep disorders or insomnia. Traditionally, health professionals treating people affected by various mental health disorders have regarded insomnia as only a symptom of the disorder. Sleep deprivation or insomnia tends to come first before depression in some individuals. At times it becomes difficult to determine which comes first, whether it is insomnia or depression.

Nevertheless, studies have revealed that sleep issues can increase the risk of developing psychiatric disorders such as depression. Neurochemistry and neuroimaging studies have shown that when a person has adequate sleep, it can enhance emotional and mental resilience. On the contrary, insomnia can lead to emotional vulnerability and negative thoughts.

Mental illnesses such as depression can lead to a lack of sleep (insomnia) and vice versa. It is necessary to note that whether depression is leading to insomnia or the reverse is happening both can worsen the situation. During sleep, a person's mind and body are repaired and made ready for the following day. Insomnia or lack of sleep can lead to irritability and fatigue, and this may worsen the quality of an individual's life. People, who have been diagnosed with depression and have insomnia, rarely respond positively to treatment and are at a higher risk of a relapse (Carney *et al.*, 2007).

The lack of sleep is known to cause harm to various functions such as neurocognitive processes which include memory and learning, metabolic control, and immune regulation. Studies have shown that emotions and sleep are related; almost all psychiatric disorders which include a lack of sleep demonstrate related signs of affective imbalance. Insomnia or sleep problems can impact the outcome of individuals who have been diagnosed with depression (Taylor *et al.*, 2008).

Studies have reported that patients affected by depression who constantly experience sleep issues often remain unresponsive to treatment in comparison to those who do not have insomnia (Taylor *et al.*, 2008). These patients have a higher probability of having suicidal thoughts than individuals affected by depression who have adequate sleep (McCall *et al.*, 2010).

Depression and insomnia often have symptoms that are similar such as lack of concentration, inability to make decisions, suicidal thoughts, restlessness, lack of concentration, and forgetting details. Healthcare providers who are involved in the treatment of depression and insomnia should be aware of the likely association between the two. This will assist them in providing comprehensive health care to those affected (Taylor *et al.*, 2007). Moreover, due to the relationship which exists between depression and insomnia, individuals with depression should be screened first for insomnia and vice versa.

Having established that insomnia can cause depression and vice versa, both conditions should be treated concurrently. Some interventions which can be used in treating these conditions include cognitive behavioural therapy (Taylor *et al.*, 2007). This therapy assists individuals affected by these two conditions to acquire healthier behaviours which can assist them in developing realistic positive thought patterns regarding sleep. Moreover, treating insomnia before depression tends to be less stigmatising; therefore, those affected may be encouraged to seek additional help. For instance, individuals affected by depression are unlikely to respond to therapy if they are experiencing insomnia (Taylor *et al.*, 2008).

Techniques used to reduce worry and enhance relaxation may be applied to deal with the symptoms of depression. Individuals who are experiencing insomnia due to depression can benefit from regulating their sleep pattern. One way the person may enhance his or her sleep is by ensuring that the bedroom or the sleeping area is free from distractions. Light, extreme heat or cold, or noise can interrupt sleep. The person may use earplugs to mask noise or a fan to maintain coolness in the room.

Maintaining a regular time for sleeping can be another way of enhancing sleep. For instance, the person may establish a routine where he wakes up at a particular time since this can assist in getting back to a regular pattern of sleep. At times it is difficult for individuals affected by depression to maintain a regular sleep routine.

Nevertheless, the benefits of such a routine are enormous; they include among others waking up in the morning feeling refreshed, being focused and energised during the day.

Studies have shown that maintaining a regular sleeping time is as essential as the duration an individual sleeps. The human brain has a better response to routines; therefore, maintaining the same practice can assist in fighting lethargic feelings which are often linked to depression. Exercise is another way which can assist the person that is affected by depression to establish a regular bedtime routine. Meditation may also assist in enhancing sleep for those affected by depression and insomnia. Constant naps can interfere with sleep pattern; therefore, a person that is struggling with insomnia due to depression should limit their napping time.

Additionally, it is necessary to avoid engaging in stressful or difficult tasks when it is almost bedtime. A person should at least slow down an hour or so before going to sleep. The stressful activities can include watching television before bedtime since the blue light emitted by the screen tends to overstimulate the brain, thereby suppressing the melatonin production which is a hormone that enhances sleep.

Meditation in Treating Depression

Depression often tends to lead to a recurring and relapsing trend (Richards, Derek, 2011). Lack of constant treatment can lead those affected by depression to have an elevated risk of recurring episodes of depression. Interventions which may prevent recurrence and relapse in individuals who are at high risk are therefore required. At present, depression is treated through antidepressants in preventing recurrence or relapse. Nevertheless, the rate of adherence tends to be low; antidepressants are helpful only when taken regularly (National Institute for Clinical Excellence, 2009).

Anxiety and stress can trigger depression; meditation may change the response an individual has regarding such feelings. Meditation helps the brain to attain continuous focus, especially when the individual experiences negative emotions and thoughts which often occur due to depression. Studies have shown that meditation may alter some parts of the brain which are related to depression. An example is the medial prefrontal cortex which tends to become hyperactive for those diagnosed with depression.

The medial prefrontal cortex part is where information processing takes place; consequently, when an individual has life stresses, the medial prefrontal cortex is over-activated. Meditation helps in the development of the prefrontal cortex. Studies have shown that the grey matter in the prefrontal cortex of people who engage in meditation tends to be thick (Fraser, 2013). This means that the constant engagement in the practice of meditation leads to a stronger prefrontal cortex and as a result better emotional well-being.

The amygdala is another region of the brain which is linked to depression. This region of the brain is associated with the fight-or-flight response which stimulates the adrenal gland to produce cortisol which is a stress hormone. Both the medial prefrontal cortex and amygdala can trigger the symptoms associated with depression. The medial prefrontal cortex gets over-activated in response to anxiety and stress and the response of the fear centre increases the levels of cortisol to fight imagined danger. Mediation helps in ignoring the adverse emotions of anxiety and stress; this may explain why the levels of stress go down after meditation (Fraser, 2013).

Meditation protects the hippocampus, a region of the brain that regulates emotions and memory. Studies have shown that meditating for only half an hour a day for a period of eight weeks increases the amount of grey matter in the hippocampus. Other studies have shown that people affected by persistent depression have a hippocampus that is small; therefore, they can benefit from meditation (Arden, 2015). Studies have demonstrated that people who practise meditation tend to have stronger and bigger hippocampus. This can mean that the more meditation an individual engages in, the stronger the hippocampus becomes and this helps the brain to overcome depression

The purpose of meditation is to help a person identify their negative feelings and thoughts and avoid acting on them (Goyal *et al.*, 2010). Meditation may also assist in preparing the brain to handle situations that are stressful. Depression is often based on fears concerning the future and disappointments regarding the past; meditation helps an individual to focus more on the present. Meditation reinstates the focus of the mind to the present, allowing an individual to recognise the good moments in their life.

Meditation opens the mind to new stimuli where even things that are routine feel alive and fresh; this can help in eliminating the symptoms of depression. Meditation assists in identifying negative thoughts, thereby reducing their effect. By watching what a one is thinking, it may aid in recognising that thoughts and reality are different (Goyal *et al.*, 2010). Therefore, thoughts should not influence an individual's emotional state or mood.

Studies have shown that meditation can utilise the power of neurogenesis in developing a happier and healthier brain. Antidepressants such as the selective serotonin reuptake inhibitors tend to fight the death of brain cells which eventually causes depression. On the contrary, meditation is a superior alternative which has no side effects. Thoughts are temporary. Hence, it is not necessary to become fixated on them (Goyal *et al.*, 2010).

Rather than negative thoughts escalating beyond one's control, meditation hinders these thoughts triggering depression (Goyal *et al.*, 2010). Meditation helps in understanding how emotions and thoughts are related to each other and the control an individual has over his or her thought pattern. Meditation can assist a person to maintain a focused, calm, and well-balanced state of mind.

Meditation can also help an individual who is affected by depression to re-channel his or her focus to issues that matter, thereby restoring his or her life back to balance and allowing the person to feel whole. When this practice is done on a regular basis, the individual tends to experience a sense of calmness. The person's mood becomes enhanced which leads to relaxation and focus. Research has demonstrated that mindfulness meditation is as helpful as drugs in treating depression (Rapgay and Bystrisky, 2009). One symptom of depression is the practice of negative thinking; mindfulness mediation trains individuals to easily identify such thoughts and avoid them (McManus *et al.*, 2012).

Mindfulness which is one technique of meditation entails identifying feelings and thoughts and not getting caught in them (Brewer *et al.*, 2010). During this kind of meditation, the person identifies his or her thoughts and the direction they are taking. After this, the person calmly retreats back to the present moment through techniques such as yoga and deep breathing. Mindfulness tends to activate senses which are dull due to depression. When an individual changes his or her negative thoughts with positive ones, the brain becomes transformed.

Another form of meditation which can be used as a cure for depression is the mindfulness-based cognitive therapy (MBCT). This treatment is a combination of cognitive behavioural therapy and mindfulness. Through mindfulness, a person can identify his or her feelings with the use the cognitive behavioural therapy which will assist the individual to learn how they can manage feelings. MBCT integrates mindfulness practices like breathing exercises and meditation. Through the mindfulness-based cognitive therapy, a person who is struggling with negative thoughts due to depression learns how to stop the thought pattern which is negative (Brewer *et al.*, 2010).

MBCT is mostly used for individuals who have recurring symptoms of depression to avoid relapse (Piet and Hougaard, 2011). The goal of MBCT is to enhance the mindfulness skills in people by assisting them to view thoughts not as commands which require their response but only as thoughts. These skills assist individuals to identify the tendency they have to fall into a negative thought pattern. Identifying such thoughts is crucial in being able to draw back instead of having an emotional response towards such thoughts.

Studies have shown that MBCT tends to reduce some symptoms of depression in individuals who have physical health conditions like traumatic brain injury and vascular diseases (Abbott *et al.*, 2014). Through MBCT, the patient learns meditation practices and fundamental cognition principles which include the link between feelings and thoughts.

MBCT helps people affected by depression not to do away with negative feelings but instead change the association they have with them through the practice of mindfulness exercises. For instance, the person may develop a practice of not allowing negative thoughts from taking over by counteracting them with facts which states that these thoughts are not true (Michalak *et al.*, 2008). Such actions bring a balance to the neural networks which help the individual to depart from involuntary negative reactions and realise that there are better ways to act in response to circumstances.

MBCT tends to be successful when practised with a spirit of compassion towards oneself. With depression comes the tendency to become harsh on oneself, develop self-judgement and self-criticism. The practice of compassion makes it easier to integrate compassion even as the depressive symptoms worsen. By maintaining a regular meditation routine, the person can apply the techniques learned when negative emotions recur (Michalak *et al.*, 2008).

The mindfulness-based cognitive therapy came into being as a psychosocial intervention to educate individuals affected by recurrent depression (Williams and Kuyken, 2012). Mindfulness may assist with depression since the person learns how to redirect his attention from negative thoughts by starving them. Becoming mindful of what one is doing is one technique of weakening the hold of the negative thought pattern thereby enhancing one's mood. When this habit is engaged in constantly the person tends to live more in the reality of the current moment and less in the past or being anxious about the future.

When an individual becomes deliberately mindful of what he or she is doing, it helps in shifting of mental gears. It is possible for the brain to fall unconsciously into a negative thought pattern which may increase the symptoms of depression. Becoming intentionally mindful of what one is doing can lead to a different way of thinking. When this happens, the individual is unlikely to get trapped in negative or destructive thoughts. Mindfulness assists a person to pay more attention to their experiences instead of becoming lost in them (Michalak *et al.*, 2008). By doing this, the individual is able to relate to challenging experiences differently.

Mindfulness can also assist the person that is struggling with depression to view negative thoughts as patterns in their mind which come and go and not as *the truth* of the kind of individual they are or will be in the future (Brewer *et al.*, 2010). Therefore, practising mindfulness can assist in weakening the power of the negative thoughts; this helps to manage the symptoms linked to depression. Additionally, engaging in the practice of identifying what one is doing when doing it helps a person to recognise what he or she is feeling and thinking at every moment.

Understanding the feelings and thoughts one has is necessary for dealing swiftly and successfully with depressive symptoms which may arise (Brewer *et al.*, 2010). A person who has previously been depressed at times may be unwilling to admit the symptoms of another depressive episode. The person may wait until the symptoms have worsened before dealing with their condition. On the contrary, when an individual is more in tune with their experience every moment, they are in a better position to recognise when the depressive symptoms begin. The person will therefore take the necessary actions to deal with the depressive symptoms before the situation worsens (Piet and Hougaard, 2011).

Mindfulness can assist in managing the symptoms linked with depression, but it is often faced with some challenges. One of the obstacles include forgetting to be mindful; the mind can become used to a particular way of thinking, that it becomes hard to remember to be mindful. Also, the mode the mind operates in may oppose the change to a mode that is different, emphasising its precedence over that of the mindfulness approach.

When one is depressed, the feelings and thoughts one has keep him or her stuck in a negative thought pattern which makes it hard to recall being mindful (Brewer *et al.*, 2010). Therefore, allocating time to become mindful is necessary since this will aid in developing a mental pattern which is positive. MBCT alters the way an individual thinks which may decrease his or her risk of having a relapse. This therapy achieves this through indirect mechanisms which entail decreasing a person's emotional response towards negative feelings and thoughts which may be triggered by the environment.

Social Interaction and Depression

Depressive disorders have been linked to social deficits. Lack of social interaction among people affected by depression can account for the worsening of the disorder and brings other physical health conditions. Currently, studies are showing that social interactions can reduce the symptoms of depression and can avert a relapse (Holt-Lunstad, 2018). People who have been diagnosed with depression are less likely to socially interact with other people. These individuals have few if any intimate relationships since they tend to expect rejection from others.

Depression makes who have been diagnosed with the condition experience challenges in managing social interactions (Gopinath *et al.*, 2012). Individuals affected by depression tend to benefit less from positive social interactions. These people are often socially withdrawn; they also fear becoming socially rejected by others and rarely expect others to be kind to them (Overall and Hammond, 2013).

Depression makes those affected to have a distorted view of themselves and others, which often leads them to have a wrong interpretation of social interactions (Gopinath *et al.*, 2012). For instance, an individual due to depression may interpret short conversations from friends as evidence that they are disliked. It is necessary that the individual understand that not everyone is out to harm him or her since they too have personal issues. Although there are awful people in society, they are the minority; therefore, the person who is affected by depression should not be afraid to interact socially with others.

Furthermore, the inability for those diagnosed with depression to disengage from their feelings and thoughts can make them be viewed by others as being rude and annoying, further worsening their interpersonal relationships (Schwartz-Mette and Rose, 2015). These people may also be unresponsive to social interactions to avoid scorn, rejection, or anticipated disappointment (Girard *et al.*, 2013)

At times, the person may be experiencing low self-esteem due to depression, and he or she may have the belief that other people are having a similar view. For instance, the individual may believe that when they enter a room, they are being judged by everyone (Overall and Hammond, 2013). It is vital that such an individual develops a way of managing the fears he or she could be having regarding social interactions. Additionally, it is important that the person avoids assuming what other people are thinking about him or her during social interactions. It would be useful that the person take what others say at face value, and if need be, seek for clarification.

Mind reading which can refer to an involuntary negative thought may lead to social anxiety; therefore, the individual who is affected by depression and is afraid of social interaction should avoid this habit (Overall and Hammond, 2013). When a person is afraid of social interaction, he or she may believe that other people are judging him or her negatively. Social isolation or the lack of social interaction may worsen the symptoms of depression.

A lack of social interaction can be caused by negative thoughts such as the belief that one does not deserve to be happy. Other negative thoughts which can cause an individual affected by depression to become socially withdrawn include viewing other people as being better in comparison to the person (Overall and Hammond, 2013). To some degree considering others as better is good but when this leads to low self-esteem then this should be addressed.

Having looked at how depression impacts adversely on social interaction, it is necessary for the affected to develop ways of becoming socially active. Some of the ways include

> ➤ ***getting out of the house***—when people are depressed, the last thing they want to do is to get out of the house. Most

of these individuals prefer to stay in bed throughout. The reason being, it is more comfortable to stay at home since one can easily control their environment. It is necessary for the individual to get out of the house and engage in exercises like walking which have both psychological and physical benefits (Burchard, 2017).

➤ *regularly connecting with family and friends*—family and friends are critical in enhancing social interaction. If the person who has been diagnosed with depression finds it difficult to get out of the house, he/she can invite a family member or friend to their place. This may help in overcoming the habit of becoming socially withdrawn or isolated.

➤ *joining a social support group*—meeting people who have similar issues can assist in overcoming social isolation. Support groups bring together people who have experienced or are experiencing similar issues. A support group gives chance for individuals to share their feelings, experiences, and coping strategies they have used and succeeded.

Participating in a support group gives a person the chance to be with individuals who understand each other. By participating in a group, a person may feel less judged, isolated, or lonely. Furthermore, a support group can assist in reducing anxiety, depression, or distress.

In a support group, an individual can honestly talk about his or her feelings and can also enhance their skills on how to manage challenges. A support group also offers a sense of hope, empowerment, or control to the members.

➤ *taking the focus from yourself to others*—social intercalation requires that a person shows interest to other people. Depression can make a person be self-focused where everything revolves around the person. Overcoming the fear of social interaction would require the person to deliberately show interest to other people (Overall and Hammond, 2013). It is easy to make friends by demonstrating interest in others rather than waiting for people to show interest in you. One can make friends by volunteering, joining a club, taking walks, or attending various social events.

➤ *having social skills training*—this is a kind of psychotherapy which helps in enhancing social skills. Social skills training is a cognitive therapy which can be done in a group or a one-on-one situation. People who have been diagnosed with depression and have problems in socially interacting with others can benefit from this therapy. SST may be efficient in assisting such individuals to learn the crucial skills required in social interactions.

SST tends to be combined with other kinds of psychotherapies which include cognitive behavioural therapy. The time required to complete the social skills training programs differs depending on how the individual is learning the techniques being taught and the confidence he has in applying the skills.

There are several steps which are involved in the social skills training program. The first step is identifying the social problem. For instance, does the person fear socialising with large groups of people? To identify the problem, the psychologist and patient need to work together. The underlying problem which in this case is depression needs to be determined. The psychologist then can establish what skills the person requires most, and what other therapies are needful.

After identifying the problem, specific goals for the therapy should be set. The goals may either be broad or focused, and they may also change from one session to another. For social skills training, broad overall goals can include the capacity to comfortably socialise. On the other hand, individual goals are skill-specific such as learning ways of greeting a person and also how to respond properly (Overall and Hammond, 2013).

After the goals have been set, the psychologist will model the skills so that the person can understand what they are expected to do. After the psychologist has modelled the skill, the person will be requested to role play. This is a crucial feature of social skills training. It can feel awkward to role play, but the skills need to be practised to enable one to use it outside the confinement of the therapy sessions.

At the end of each session, the psychologist gives feedback to assist in identifying the person's strengths and weaknesses and what he/she needs to practice. The psychologist also in between sessions assigns challenges in form of *homework* to the person. The homework can be carried out immediately after the session to help the individual to practice the learnt skills. The success the person has in meeting the challenge determines the skill he/she will learn in the next session.

➢ *having cognitive behavioural therapy*—this psychotherapy is useful in understanding how people's thoughts impact on their behaviour and feelings (Johnco, Wuthrich, and Rapee, 2014). Since the fear of social interaction is founded on fears which are irrational, cognitive behavioural therapies can assist in developing a rational thought pattern. Therefore, rather than picturing negative scenarios regarding social settings, the person through CBT learns how to focus on outcomes which are realistic.

An unfounded fear can include thoughts such as 'No one wants to interact with me,' or 'People hate me.' A rational thought pattern may include thoughts such as 'Everyone in the room is nervous and preoccupied with their looks, thus are not too concerned about me.'

➤ **taking medication**—depression which is accompanied by social anxiety can be treated using antidepressants such as selective serotonin reuptake inhibitors or benzodiazepines (Acton, 2012).

Diet and Depression

What we eat affects not only our physical health but also mental health but a few people seem to be aware of this (Rao *et al.*, 2008). Although depression has been viewed as being emotionally or biochemically based, nutrition plays a significant role in its development. Nutritional neuroscience is a new field which is demonstrating that nutrition is linked to human emotions, behaviour, and cognition (Rao *et al.*, 2008). Most of the diet which people takes especially in the developed world lacks vital nutrients such as minerals and essential vitamins (American Psychiatric Association, 2013).

Studies conducted on people who have been diagnosed with depression report that most of their diet lack nutritional value. These people were found to have a poor choice of the food they take which has been linked to depression. The foods a person eats have a significant impact on their emotional state and mind. Studies have demonstrated that there is a relationship between what a person eats and their risk of developing depression (Li *et al.*, 2017).

Food can be described as the best medicine. The tissues, bones, and cells in the body are built from what a person eats. For instance, dietary fats help in developing the brain tissue and balancing hormones; muscles, on the other hand, are built from proteins. Various minerals and vitamins produce energy and transmit electrical impulses along the neurons to assist in movement, thoughts, and feelings (Rao *et al.*, 2008).

The food which a person eats influences the feelings one has since serotonin which regulates moods, appetite, and sleep is produced in the gastrointestinal tract. The interior workings of the digestive system not only help in digesting food but also guiding one's emotions. Furthermore, neurons and the creation of neurotransmitters such as serotonin tend to be influenced by the *good bacteria* which comprise the intestinal microbiome. These bacteria guard the intestines' lining and protect against *bad* bacteria and toxins. The bacteria also enhance how well nutrients from food are absorbed and limit inflammation.

The bacteria also stimulate the neural pathways which move between the gut and the brain. Studies have shown that when probiotics which are supplements that contain good bacteria are taken, an individual's mental outlook is enhanced, and the anxiety stress levels are reduced. Studies have shown that people who take traditional diets in comparison to Western diets have a lower risk of developing depression (Hechtman, 2018). The reason being traditional diets have more fruits, seafood, vegetables, fish, and unprocessed grains. Moreover, most of these foods tend to be fermented and unprocessed; hence, they act as natural probiotics (Hechtman, 2018).

Fermentation utilises yeast and bacteria to change the sugar in various foods to lactic acid, alcohol, and carbon dioxide. Fermentation ensures that food does not spoil, and it can also add a pleasant texture and taste to the food (Hechtman, 2018). Food can be regarded as medicine since tissues, signalling molecules, and cell bones are developed from what a person eats. For instance, dietary fats are involved in building the brain tissue and assist in balancing hormones; proteins, on the other hand, build muscles.

Different minerals and vitamins help in creating energy and transmitting along the neurons electrical impulses. These impulses help in movement, feelings, and thought. Therefore, a balanced diet can be used to prevent or cure depression. Food which a person eats has an impact on the microbial and human cells. Studies show that food alters the useful bacteria in the gut which is referred to as the microbiome. Out of habit, most people daily consume inflammatory foods which lead to a leaky gut, thereby harming the microbiome

(Hechtman, 2018). This leads to chronic inflammation which can eventually cause depression.

Studies have demonstrated that individuals who consume an anti-inflammatory diet tend to have a significantly reduced risk of developing depression (Hechtman, 2018). An anti-inflammatory diet comprises of antioxidants, vitamins, healthy fats, and high-quality proteins. Studies have also shown that a diet consisting of vegetables, fish, fruits, and low-fat dairy can enhance the risk of developing depression. The risk of developing depression according to the study can be increased by a high intake of red meat either processed or unprocessed.

Other unhealthy diets such as sweets, butter, refined grains, and dairy products with high-fat content can also increase the risk of developing depression (Hechtman, 2018). Inflammatory foods such as those containing gluten can lead to inflammation through inflaming the gut, microbes, and intestinal tissues. Gluten can adversely affect an individual leading to depression.

Carbohydrates and Depression

Carbohydrates play a significant role in the function and structure of an organism. In humans, carbohydrates have been found to have an impact on behaviour and mood. Diets with a high level of carbohydrate activate the production of insulin in the human body. Insulin assists cells to get the blood sugar which is required for energy. Insulin also activates the transmission of tryptophan to the brain, and this affects the level of neurotransmitters in the brain. On the contrary, consuming a diet with a low level of carbohydrates can trigger depression because brain chemicals such as tryptophan and serotonin which enhance the feeling of wellness are lacking.

Proteins and Depression

Proteins are composed of amino acids which are essential building blocks in the body. Most amino acids are produced by the body while others have to be provided through diet. People who have been diagnosed with depression often have insufficient amino acids. Most neurotransmitters in the brain such as dopamine and tryptophan comprise of amino acids. The lack of these neurotransmitters can be linked to aggression and low moods. On the contrary, excess amino acids can damage the brain leading to mental retardation (Rao *et al.*, 2008).

Foods which are considered to be rich in protein and which can enhance the level of amino acids in the body include eggs, milk, fish, and meat. The intake of proteins can impact the functioning of the brain and also the mental health condition of an individual. The lack of sufficient proteins in the body can lead to depression.

Iron and Depression

Oxygenation and the production of energy in the cerebral parenchyma are dependent on iron. Studies have reported that women are more vulnerable to depression than men; this difference often begins in adolescence and becomes noticeable when the woman begins to bear children (Tait *et al.*, 2012). Insufficient iron in the body is often linked to depression, fatigue, and apathy (Bourre, 2006). Research has demonstrated that supplementing iron has considerably improved postpartum depression among new mothers (Sheikh *et al.*, 2017).

Iodine and Depression

Iodine plays a significant role in mental health; too much or too little iodine can adversely impact the functioning of the thyroid gland and eventually the manufacture of the thyroid hormone (Katagiri *et al.*, 2017). Studies show that when the thyroid is impaired, it increases the risk of developing depression (Hage and Azar, 2012). To ensure the level of iodine in the body is regulated, a person can include in their diet iodised salt, seaweed, and sea vegetables.

Sugar and Depression

The intake of sugar is also harmful to a person's health as it quickly increases the blood sugar. The rapid increase spikes up insulin which can lead to a blood sugar crash. Cortisol then compensates by trying to remove the sugar from the storage and into the bloodstream, a process, referred to as hypoglycaemia. This process leads to a craving for sugar and carbohydrates since the brain requires constant sugar for it to function properly. This often leads to irritability, headaches, anxiety, and eventually depression. High levels of blood sugar lead to inflammation, one of the key risk factors linked to depression. Balancing of blood sugar is one way of treating anxiety and depression.

Sugar adversely impact the brain. For instance, it causes inflammation by damaging the gut microbiome and by increasing insulin. Furthermore, sugars distract various hormones and eventually raise the levels of cortisol which is a stress hormone. Sugar also starves the brain and harms significant structures in the body such as blood vessels and the cell membrane which can cause depression. Excess sugar in the brain according to research reduces (BDNF) brain-derived neurotrophic factor which leads to anxiety and depression.

Fighting Depression through Nutrition

It is necessary to note that the food a person eats influences the structure of the gut microbiota. The microorganisms in the gut can communicate with the systems in the body including the brain which can lead to anxiety and depression. The microorganisms which reside in the gut can interact with the brain among other systems in the body which plays a significant role in anxiety and depression.

Studies of animals have reported that foods that are plant-based can enhance the microbial structure in the gut (Hechtman, 2018). On the other hand, a diet with high levels of fats destabilises the microbial balance. Such an imbalance can lead to the permeability of the intestines thereby letting large molecules which interfere with the functioning of the brain into the bloodstream. A person can benefit more from the diet as a therapy for depression rather than medication.

Nevertheless, it is necessary to note that there is no diet which can substitute conventional treatment for depression. However, a nutritional diet can assist in preventing and fighting depression. A diet which can help in fighting depression consists of vegetables, fish, and meat which help in ensuring adequate intake of vital nutrients such as amino acids, vitamins, and Omega-3. Moreover, one should avoid diets which can raise their risk of developing depression. For example, a high intake of refined carbohydrates and sugars according to studies can increase the risk of depression (Gangwisch *et al.*, 2015).

Omega 3 which is found in fish has also been found to enhance mood. Therefore, consuming fish can improve the mental health of an individual including alleviating the symptoms linked to depression. Omega 3 can be found in oily fish, for example, salmon, mackerel, and tuna. Vitamin B which is found in greens is believed to be critical in preventing depression (Hechtman, 2018). Studies show that this vitamin has the potential to decrease the level of homocysteine which is an amino acid that is linked to depression. Foods that contain folic acid include pulses, beans, and green vegetables which are slightly cooked.

A person can develop depression due to low levels of tryptophan which is a vital amino acid in the body that is converted to serotonin a neurotransmitter in the brain. When the level of serotonin is low, a person is at a higher risk of developing depression. The body cannot manufacture tryptophan; therefore, one can only get it through foods such as beans, tuna, turkey, and salmon.

Research has associated depression with low levels of selenium. This mineral according to studies enhances a person's mood and reduces depressive symptoms among the elderly (Gao *et al.*, 2012). Foods that contain selenium include meat, fish, and Brazil nuts (Sánchez *et al.*, 2009). Drinking water is another essential factor for every person especially those diagnosed with depression. Lack of enough water in the body can lead to a chemical imbalance. Dehydration can affect an individual's mood making him or her irritable and eventually depressed. Although no single treatment or intervention works for every person, combining nutrition and conventional medicine can boost improvement.

The Impact of Alcohol, Cigarettes, Illegal Drugs, and Coffee on Depression

Alcohol, caffeine, and nicotine are basically consumed by different people but more so by psychiatric patients. These substances are regarded as a significant part of today's culture and viewed as tools for social interaction.

Alcohol and Depression

The relationship between alcohol and depression is complex; the question which frequently arises is whether alcohol causes depression or vice versa. Alcohol abuse and depression are both psychiatric conditions. The two conditions are linked and it is difficult to determine which comes first. Studies have reported that the consumption of alcohol increases the risk of developing depression and vice versa (Boden and Fergusson, 2011). Additionally, studies have demonstrated that higher rates of depression are common in people who abuse or are dependent on alcohol (Boden and Fergusson, 2011).

When an individual is depressed, often they become desperate, and they can do anything to take away the depressive symptoms. It is at this point that the person may resort to alcohol. Drinking alcohol leads to a feeling of relaxation, but for most people, it helps them to temporarily forget their sadness and problems. For people diagnosed with depression, this oblivion can serve as an escape route for the issues they are facing. This can lead to more drinking to escape from the symptoms associated with depression. This leads to a cycle of depression and alcoholism which is hard to break.

Although the consumption of alcohol does not directly cause depression, it significantly influences the development of depression among other mental health conditions. A person with an alcohol disorder can develop depression, and one who has already been diagnosed with depression can have their symptoms become worse (Boden and Fergusson, 2011). People who are considered heavy drinkers tend to experience mood disturbances, especially during withdrawal.

Individuals who consume alcohol are at a higher risk of developing depression than those who do not since alcohol impacts adversely on the neurotransmitters in the brain (Boden and Fergusson, 2011). Alcoholics when not drunk often report anxiety, depression, poor concentration, and irritability. Just like any other substance, alcohol affects brain chemicals such as dopamine and serotonin. When drinking, a person may experience an initial boost of excitement, but the next day become depressed or anxious.

Alcohol intake can also impede the development of healthy coping techniques. When a person who has been diagnosed with depression does not have healthy coping techniques, he or she cannot adequately manage the disorder. The psychosocial issues linked to alcohol such as deterioration of the relationship, loss of a job, and problems with the law can lead to depression (Rognmo et al., 2013). Alcohol abuse can lead to poor economic, social and health issues which may trigger depressive symptoms.

When alcohol is consumed and it enters into the bloodstream, feelings of pleasure are increased. In the initial stages, as the alcohol level in the blood increases, the person may feel excited. This occurs due to an increase in neurotransmitters like dopamine which are linked to good feelings. Nevertheless, as the alcohol level in the blood reduces, more of its suppressive traits take hold off the person. Alcohol suppresses excitatory neurotransmitters such as glutamate (Patten, 2009).

A person may drink to ease his mind from despondency, fear, sorrow, or to fight loneliness. The absorption of alcohol can enhance a person's mood although the benefits are short-term. The long-term use of alcohol can lead to more withdrawal, anxiety, and depression. Regular intake of alcohol can reduce the serotonin levels in the brain; this chemical helps in regulating moods. Some individuals drink to manage depressive symptoms. Whereas alcohol can temporarily alleviate some of the depressive symptoms, eventually it worsens the depression (Patten, 2009).

Researchers have tried to enlighten the link between depressive symptoms and alcohol use. One of the explanations given by the researchers is that the pharmacological impact of alcohol can lead to depressive symptoms, intoxication, or withdrawal. People who have been diagnosed with depression can resort to drinking to cope with the symptoms of the disorder.

The abuse of alcohol has many adverse effects such as financial distress and relationship problems. This frequently leads to a destructive cycle of alcohol abuse as a way of dealing with depressive symptoms which further worsen depression. There is a higher likelihood of divorce among couples whose consumption of alcohol is high. Studies have shown that high levels of alcohol consumption increase the probability of divorce which aggravates the symptoms of depression (Rognmo et al., 2013).

Some individuals are genetically predisposed to both depression and alcohol. People who, due to depression, are taking alcohol can lessen the effectiveness of the antidepressants through the intake of alcohol. If an individual develops depression due to alcohol abuse, there is a likelihood that these symptoms will fade away after one ceases to consume alcohol (Patten, 2009).

Alcohol can reduce the norepinephrine and serotonin levels, chemicals that are involved in regulating a person's mood. When the levels of these chemicals in the brain are reduced, a person who has been diagnosed with depression becomes even more depressed. Furthermore, alcohol momentarily discontinues the impact of the stress hormone; this can amplify the symptoms of depression. Alcohol use can also reduce folic acid levels; this deficiency often triggers depressive symptoms. Additionally, alcohol alters the sleep pattern of an individual and this can increase the depressive symptoms.

People diagnosed with major depression when they use alcohol can develop symptoms such as intensified hopelessness, increased risk of suicide, poor adherence to treatment, high risk of relapse, and limited options of treatment (Suter *et al.*, 2011). The intake of alcohol increases the risk of suicide since it can lead to impaired judgement, lowered inhibitions, and increased impulsivity.

Combining alcohol with antidepressants for people diagnosed with depression is dangerous for several reasons. The first is depression becomes difficult to treat when there is alcohol intake. Additionally, some antidepressants such as monoamine oxidase inhibitors when combined with alcohol can lead to a drastic rise in the blood pressure. When antidepressants are accompanied by alcohol intake, physical coordination and judgement may be impaired which can be dangerous when working or driving. Some patients might also opt to stop taking antidepressants to drink.

Alcoholism and depression can occur together, and this is referred to as dual diagnosis (DeVido and Weiss, 2012). The treatment of dual diagnosis can be difficult since it is a challenge to determine which came first, alcohol or depression. If a person has both depression and alcoholism, the two conditions should be treated concurrently. If alcoholism is treated and depression ignored, then the likelihood of self-medication will be increased. On the contrary, if depression is treated without addressing alcoholism, then the impact of the treatment is likely to be negated.

A person who wants to recover from both alcoholism and depression should seek treatment from a facility which treats both conditions. Treatment programs dealing with dual diagnosis have now become more available and common since there is an increased awareness of collaboration between mental health care providers and programs dealing with addictions. At times it is challenging to treat depression co-occurring with alcoholism (DeVido and Weiss, 2012).

Various approaches have been used to address this co-occurring disorder; they include parallel, sequential, and integrated. The sequential approach is where the symptoms of depression are not addressed until the person has had a period of abstinence from alcohol. Consequently, in this approach, treatment is provided for one disorder at a time and begins by addressing the more acute disorder. The parallel approach addresses the two disorders concurrently although different clinicians are used to treat both disorders. In the integrated approach, one treatment team or clinician manages the two disorders concurrently (DeVido and Weiss, 2012).

The integrated approach is considered to be the best in treating both disorders since having one treatment team working simultaneously with the patient can enhance communication leading to a better diagnosis and treatments. Furthermore, this model can provide better treatment flexibility to the patient. Components of the integrated approach for patients that have been diagnosed with both depression and alcohol use disorder include pharmacotherapy and psychosocial therapies (Popova *et al.*, 2011).

Pharmacotherapy

Studies have been conducted trying to examine the efficiency of co-administering antidepressant medicines and pharmacological alcohol use disorder treatment. For instance, a number of studies have evaluated the effect of SSRI drugs and opioid antagonist medications in treating the two disorders (Balaratnasingam and Janca, 2011). These studies hold the view that combining both treatments may lead to more alcohol abstinence, experiencing a longer period before relapse and enhancing the mood of the affected individual.

Adequate measures should be taken when prescribing medication to people who are affected by the two disorders. Alcoholic patients require close attention regarding their interactions with drugs (Balaratnasingam and Janca, 2011). For instance, to attain therapeutic levels, these people might need higher doses of tricyclic antidepressants. Suicide ideations, side effects, and medication history should be factored when selecting the medication.

Additionally, for diagnostic clarification, it is necessary to monitor the patient for a minimum period of abstinence from alcohol of two weeks. After this, a comprehensive assessment of depression can be more precise (DeVido and Weiss, 2012).

Psychosocial Therapy

The association between substance use and mood disorders such as depression is dynamic and complex. There are different stages involved in the treatment of each patient. Effective management of the two disorders requires collaboration between the patient and clinician (DeVido and Weiss, 2012). Recovery from alcohol use disorder and depression is an active process whose goal is to educate the patient regarding his or her illness and the impact it has on those around them (DeVido and Weiss, 2012).

Psychotherapy stabilises the patient from the severe impacts of either of the disorder. Additionally, through psychotherapy, the patient learns strategies and skills to help him or her in managing the symptoms of both disorders. Some of the psychosocial therapies that have been used in treating alcohol use disorder include motivational enhancement therapy, cognitive behavioural therapy, contingency management, and relapse prevention therapy among others.

> ➤ *Motivational enhancement therapy*—this is an evidence-based approach used to engage patients to assist them in self-motivation as this would help them in changing their negative behaviour. This therapy is based on the idea that an individual's motivation level for change is flexible (Broody, 2009). Studies show that motivational enhancement therapy has led to a decline in substance use, number of

hospitalisations, and enhances the possibility of making the change to outpatient treatment for patients with the two disorders (Baker *et al.*, 2012).

➢ ***Cognitive behavioural therapy***—after the patient has begun his or her treatment through the motivational enhancement therapy, investigating the dysfunctional beliefs and thoughts which patients have regarding themselves and the world around them should be done. Cognitive behavioural therapy can be used for this purpose. CBT can enhance the period the person abstains from alcohol and also reduce the severity of the depressive symptoms (Brown *et al.*, 2011).

➢ ***Contingency management***—this therapy is founded on the view that substance use is linked to particular rewards. Therefore, alternative rewards should be provided to replace the rewards obtained from the use of these substances. For instance, voucher-reinforcement therapy is given to people who abstain from alcohol use or giving services and goods for a negative alcohol screen.

➢ ***Relapse prevention***—the goal of this therapy is to recognise the nature of the relapse and develop strategies to manage situations of potential relapse. Relapse prevention therapy investigates and classifies people who are at a high risk of relapse. Cognitive behavioural therapy is then applied to assist these people to keep away from triggers and effectively manage them by enhancing self-efficacy.

➢ ***Twelve-step facilitation***—this is a professionally led therapy intended to promote engagement in alcoholic anonymous and other twelve-step groups. In the twelve-step facilitation, the physician works together with the patient to evaluate the alcohol disorder and educate patients regarding the need for abstinence and encourage them to actively participate in self-group activities (Lydecker *et al.*, 2010).

Cigarette and Depression

Smoking is common among people who have been diagnosed with various mental disorders such as depression. In developed countries, smoking of cigarettes has been classified as a primary preventable cause of morbidity and mortality. Smoking is associated with various physical and mental health problems. For instance, adults who smoke cigarettes have been reported to have a higher probability of developing psychiatric disorders such as depression (Smith *et al.*, 2014). Studies in the United States have shown that people with mental disorders are more likely to smoke than those who do not have a history of mental disorders (Smith eta l., 2014). The co-occurrence of mental illnesses such as depression and smoking has become a significant issue in public health.

Studies show that a positive relationship exists between mental illness and smoking. People with mental illness including depression often begin to smoke at a young age, smoke more intensely, and are more addicted to smoking than the general public (Smith *et al.*, 2014). For instance, a recent study has reported that 42% of the cigarettes consumed in England are by people diagnosed with various mental illnesses (McManus *et al.*, 2010). Furthermore, whereas the rate of smoking cigarettes in the general public has declined over the last 20 years, smoking among people with various mental illnesses has remained unchanged (Fluharty *et al.*, 2016).

Another study has reported that 44% of cigarettes that are consumed annually in the United States are by people who have been diagnosed with psychiatric disorders such as depression. Adults who have been diagnosed with depression and also smoke tend to respond highly to smoking prompts. Studies show that this group of people report receiving more benefits from smoking.

There are several theories which have been used to explain

the relationship between smoking and depression. The first is the self-medication theory which suggests that those diagnosed with depression smoke to lessen the symptoms associated with the disorder (Chaiton *et al.*, 2009). For instance, nicotine produces dopamine which elevates the mood and well-being of the affected individual. Additionally, nicotine enhances serotonin's supply similar to that which is provided by antidepressant medications. Another theory holds the view that smoking can cause depression through its effect on a person's neurocircuitry; this increases vulnerability to environmental stressors. Most people diagnosed with depression use smoking as a dysfunctional self-care technique based on the emotional rewards they get.

Smoking stimulates the brain's pleasure centre and temporarily enhances an indivdiual's mood. Nicotine triggers a dopamine release which enhances positive emotions; people diagnosed with depression may resort to smoking to enhance their dopamine level. Nevertheless, smoking can make the brain to stop its own dopamine production and begin to rely on cigarettes for the supply. Nicotine smoking changes the brain after some time, and this leads to withdrawal symptoms when nicotine supply reduces, trying to stop smoking leads to various emotional issues (Weinberger *et al.*, 2012).

Additionally, adults who have depression and smoke according to studies experience more withdrawal symptoms when trying to quit the habit. These people are also reported to have little confidence in their ability to stop smoking (Siru *et al.*, 2009). There are several mechanisms which people who have been diagnosed with depression and are involved in smoking can use to quit the habit; they include among others:

> **Looking for ways to manage stress**—people diagnosed with mental illnesses such as depression use smoking as a way of dealing with the symptoms of the disorder or stress. Therefore, there is a need for such people to look for other mechanisms to deal with stress which may include exercise, meditation, and counselling among others. Talking with

friends and family can also help in stopping the habit of smoking. It is necessary to note that making any changes takes effort and time; hence, the person should be patient with their progress however slow it may appear. One might not fully identify the factors which lead to stress and thereby depression, but recognising the source of the problem can help.

➢ **Receiving support from friends and family**—a person can quit the habit of smoking by involving friends, family, or support groups. Interacting with people who have been smokers and have conquered the habit or are in the process of doing so can assist the person who is trying to quit smoking.

➢ **Keep away from things that trigger smoking**—taking away tobacco products from one's environment can assist in reducing some of the nicotine cravings. People who smoke often do so after meals or in pubs; therefore, avoiding such situations could reduce the chance of a relapse. For instance, the person can arrange to meet with friends in smoke-free locations such as restaurants or movies.

➢ **Prepare for withdrawal symptoms**—quitting smoking is usually accompanied by withdrawal symptoms such as anxiety, headaches, feeling miserable, drowsiness, and poor concentration among others. The person can drink more water, consume foods with high-fibre content, and reduce sugar and caffeine in the diet as a way of managing the withdrawal symptoms.

➢ **Therapy**—group or individual therapy can assist in stopping the habit of smoking. One type of therapy which has been found to be helpful is where the person talks with a trained therapist (referred to as talking therapy). Cognitive behavioural therapy is also useful since it helps in changing the thought pattern of the affected person and helps in adopting positive thoughts which can help in overcoming the habit of smoking.

> **Nicotine replacement therapy**—this therapy is used for people who have been unable to quit. Nicotine patches, mouth sprays, lozenges, or gums are often used in this therapy. The nicotine replacement products used do not contain dangerous chemicals; therefore, they are much safer to use.

Caffeine, Coffee, and Depression

Coffee is one of the drinks that is widely consumed globally. Studies have demonstrated that too much coffee can adversely impact a person's health. Caffeine can disrupt a person's sleep pattern thereby affecting his or her moods (Chokroverty, 2010). Caffeine can make it difficult for a person to sleep or stay awake. Inadequate sleep can aggravate the symptoms of depression. Additionally, depression and anxiety may occur concurrently; in such circumstances, caffeine may exacerbate the anxiety.

When caffeine is consumed together with antidepressants, it can amplify their negative effects. Antidepressants such as selective serotonin reuptake inhibitors can minimise the breakdown of caffeine thereby enhancing the half-life of caffeine; this can lead to anxiety and restlessness. Since caffeine is an addictive substance, it impacts on a person's mood when using it and also after quitting (Miller, 2013). When a person who is addicted to caffeine quits taking it, his or her serotonin level drops, and this has an instant effect on their mood eventually leading to depression.

Caffeine reduces vitamin B which is essential for the serotonin synthesis. The constant consumption of coffee can be addictive, and this overworks and exhausts the adrenal glands (Miller, 2013). The person will then experience constant fatigue and this becomes a vicious cycle. Although drinking coffee can provide energy, it only lasts for a short period only. A person's natural response would be to look for something sweet to maintain the same energy; this may cause depression and high blood sugar. Addiction to coffee can lead to excessive production of adrenaline which reduces serotonin or *the happy hormone*, and this leads to depression.

Although caffeine has been linked to an increase of the depressive symptoms, studies show that when taken moderately it can relieve some of these symptoms (Miller, 2013). After the consumption of coffee, caffeine is absorbed into the person's bloodstream and later into the brain. Due to this, the quantity of other neurotransmitters such as dopamine and norepinephrine increases. Coffee enhances various features of the brain function such as vigilance, mood, memory, and the general functioning of the mind.

Substance Use and Depression

The link between substance abuse and depression is bidirectional. People who have been diagnosed with depression are at a higher likelihood of using illegal drugs. Studies estimate that 90% of people who abuse drugs are also affected by various mood disorders such as depression, stress, and anxiety (Hunter *et al.*, 2012). Additionally, individuals with addictions have a greater risk of developing depression. Addiction to illegal drugs can negatively affect a person's behaviour, thereby disrupting his or her intellectual and social life. Addiction may also reduce the economic efficiency of a person and this can lead to crime and at times death (Volkow, 2014).

Most people who are living with depression often use various substances to enhance their mood (Swendsen *et al.*, 2010). Nevertheless, most illegal drugs contain depressant properties which can enhance the feelings of sadness and other symptoms associated with depression. Therefore, using illegal drugs to manage the negative emotions can become a cycle, hampering the person's capacity to be successfully treated.

People who abuse various substances and illegal drugs are frequently reported to develop depression. The two disorders often lead to increased mortality and morbidity and also poorer treatment results (Clar, Samnaliev, and McGovern, 2009). In most situations, depression precedes substance abuse, and this is an indication that the two are co-occurring disorders. This shows that individuals affected by the two disorders might require treatment which handles both issues concurrently.

The use of illicit drugs can make a person believe that their depressive symptoms are improving, which is not true (Swendsen *et al.*, 2010). Depression increases a person's risk of self-harm, accidental injuries, and other physical health conditions. When a person begins to use illegal drugs, his or her emotional and physical health may become worse. For instance, marijuana also referred to as cannabis generates chemical properties which affect the behaviour, emotions, and cognition of a person. This drug might provisionally alleviate the depressive symptoms but might lead to negative feelings such as sadness after the high has subsided.

The constant use of marijuana has been linked to depression and anxiety. People who have been diagnosed with depression and also use marijuana, studies show that they are often ineffective when handling life stressors. Stimulants such as cocaine also are known to increase the symptoms of depression. Given that most people who have been diagnosed with depression have traumatic histories, stimulants may trigger complex reactions. The trauma can enhance the desire for the stimulant which can be particularly difficult for individuals with depression.

Stimulants rarely relax a person but can lead to short-lived energy and happiness. Once the high is over, the person may experience depression and might use extra stimulants to achieve the same high. This cycle can lead to drug addiction which may interrupt the person's life and might hinder him or her from getting the right treatment required for complete recovery.

Research has shown that depression is the most common mental health condition among people with substance use (Chan *et al.*, 2008).

Individuals who have co-occurring disorders like depression and substance use experience adverse outcomes compared to those who have only one of the two disorders (Kofler *et al.*, 2011). Females, according to studies, are at greater risk of co-occurring disorders involving substance use and depression than males (Sihvola *et al.*, 2008). For instance, one study reported that depression among female adolescents often led to substance use, smoking, and alcohol which was not the case among males (Sihvola *et al.*, 2008). Most people who use illegal drugs may continue with the habit as a way of managing the depressive symptoms (Clark *et al.*, 2011).

Owing to similar or overlapping symptoms between depression and those illegal substances, it can be difficult to diagnose the co-occurring disorder. As a result, people who have been diagnosed with depression might fail to receive treatment for substance abuse. Additionally, those diagnosed with depression and engage in substance abuse are at a higher risk of developing an addiction which may expose them to the criminal justice system (Volkow, 2014). In jail at times it might be difficult for the person to be diagnosed and treated for both conditions.

Furthermore, patients who have been diagnosed with depression and are using illegal drugs often have a greater risk of a delayed diagnosis, are less compliant with treatment, have suicidal ideations, and their social functioning is more impaired. Such individuals are also often unemployed, homeless, and frequently become involved in violent and criminal activities (Goldstein and Levitt, 2008).

Studies show that the use of illegal drugs tends to be more among adolescents who are also reported to have high rates of depression (Townsend *et al.*, 2006). Regrettably, adolescents with depression tend in comparison to adults to be less responsive to antidepressant medications which worsen their depressive symptoms (Andersen and Teicher, 2008). Studies show that the rate of substance use among depressed adolescents is twice as high in comparison to their non-depressed counterparts (Goldsten *et al.*, 2009).

Most people turn to drugs as a way of managing stress (Andreou *et al.*, 2011). Studies report that there exists a relationship between external and internal stress and addiction (Wand, 2008). A person might want to avoid an unpleasant situation by turning to drugs. It is crucial for people who have been diagnosed with depression to develop healthy coping mechanisms of dealing with stress to avoid turning to illegal drugs. The person should first identify the cause of the stress although it might be easy.

Managing stress may entail taking control of one's environment, for instance, turning off the TV if what is being aired is bringing stress. It is also necessary to avoid bottling emotions up; a person should learn how to openly communicate the concerns he or she has to others. Sharing one's feelings can be cathartic despite the fact that the stressful situation might remain unchanged (Verderber *et al.*, 2013). Viewing stressful situations positively can help in avoiding substance abuse. The individual can also view the bigger picture regarding the stressful issue. If a situation cannot be controlled, a person should avoid controlling it since this can lead to stress and eventually substance abuse. One should focus on situations which he or she can control or manage.

Studies show that co-occurring disorders such as depression and substance abuse require to be treated by a mental health professional at the same time. Mental health practitioners should provide integrated treatment to those affected (Lydecker *et al.*, 2010). Integrated treatment approaches the person's current circumstances from diverse viewpoints through using various medical health professionals. The kind of treatment provided is often based on the needs of the person.

The treatment options include inpatient treatment for people who require undergoing a medical detox for alcohol and drugs or those who are suicidal or severely depressed. Group or individual therapy can also be used to address the particular challenges which increase substance abuse and depression. Existing guidelines propose that people with co-occurring disorders get treated for both disorders; nevertheless, the level of unmet needs tends to be great. For instance, in the year 2008, over 2.5 million people were reported to have had co-occurring substance abuse and mental illness disorders (Hunter *et al.*, 2012).

Additionally, studies demonstrate that people treated for substance use often experience challenges accessing mental healthcare services even though they share similar diagnostic and clinical aspects with those being treated in mental health facilities (Havassy, Alvidrez, and Mercile, 2009). Integrated treatment can arise when several treatments are given by different professionals or when a single treatment tackles the two disorders. Based on research, integrated treatment is considered more effective in treating co-occurring disorders due to some of its unique features which include

> **comprehensiveness**—individuals with co-occurring disorders generally have various needs. Integrated treatment has programs which help such individuals. These programs include housing, training in social skills, family psychoeducation, management of the disorder, and pharmacological treatment.

> **integrating services**—when substance use and mental health services are offered by one team or individual, the patient gets a single treatment and relapse plan. The necessity for communication among the various agencies involved is eliminated and this enhances the provision of services.

> **joint decision-making**—this approach which is a part of integrated treatment involves the patient in the treatment process. Patients with co-occurring disorders choose the goals they want to follow and the path the treatment is to follow.

Cognitive Behavioural Therapy in Treating Substance Abuse and Depression

Cognitive behavioural therapy is one of the psychotherapies which are used to treat substance abuse. Cognitive behavioural therapy is an effective treatment in both substance abuse and depression (Gelenberg *et al.*, 2010). Cognitive behavioural therapy helps the affected person to replace negative thoughts with those which enhance positive health (Johnco, Wuthrich, and Rapee, 2014). This kind of psychotherapy allows a person to become involved in his or her recovery. For instance, an individual struggling with substance abuse can read literature concerning the same and also keep the record of the doctor's appointment. Cognitive behavioural therapy helps the individual to apply the lessons learned in their day-to-day life.

Cognitive behavioural therapy allows the patient to develop a relationship with their therapist. During the CBT sessions, the therapist and the client discuss the feelings, moods, and physical health of the patient (Johnco, Wuthrich, and Rapee, 2014). Additionally in these sessions, the therapist frequently questions the patient regarding his or her most pressing issues.

A CBT therapist assists clients to evaluate the correctness and effectiveness of their worrying thoughts. The client is then taught over time how to change his or her negative thinking pattern (Hunter eta l., 2012). During the cognitive behavioural therapy, a therapist assesses a person's symptoms to establish existing problems and plan goals to rise above them. Feedback is given to the client at the conclusion of each session.

Studies demonstrate that many mental illnesses including depression involve the incapacity to manage fear and negative feelings (Pour, 2014). Through many cognitive behavioural therapies, the activity and volume in the amygdala which controls the emotional behaviour are reduced. Cognitive behavioural therapy helps people with addiction issues by assisting them to identify situations which lead to substance use. Moreover, the person through CBT learns how to get away from the triggering situation. Cognitive behavioural therapy approaches and addresses thoughts and emotions which could lead to substance abuse.

Family Systems Therapy in Treating Substance Abuse and Depression

This kind of therapy provides treatment to the entire family and not just the affected individual. Goals of family systems therapy entail educating close family members regarding addiction and depression, enhancing communication in the family and putting in place reasonable boundaries. Family systems therapy also helps in creating a home environment which sustains sobriety. Treating the two disorders concurrently involves addressing the patient's depressive symptoms such as feelings of hopelessness and lack of motivation and also addictive behaviour. During the initial phases of recovery, if the patient has suicidal ideations, inpatient treatment should be recommended.

In the inpatient setting, patients undergo rehabilitation and detoxification under the supervision of the therapist and clinicians. After the patient is ready to move to the next recovery phase an outpatient program can provide more independence. There are many benefits which arise by treating addiction through family therapy. One of the benefits includes both the affected person and his or her family gain an understanding of the impact substance abuse has on their behaviour. The family receives insight and assessment from the therapist.

Additionally, the therapy provides awareness of family dynamics. Family patterns which are maladaptive and which could have contributed to both the depression and substance abuse are addressed during these sessions. Family systems therapy also improves communication in families. Since substance use often goes together with dishonesty, family members may not trust the affected individual. When communication is enhanced, there can be honest interaction between the affected person and other family members.

The Impact of Environmental Factors on Depression

Causes of depression are often complex, partially unknown, and determined by various factors such as environmental and social (Kessler and Bromet, 2013). Environmental and social factors can be modified, thereby become targets for public health actions. The brain is affected by poor social environments which include unemployment and economic instability and this raises the risk of depression (Holz *et al.*, 2015). Recent studies show that other physical features of the environment such as chemical pollutants and noise can also have a neurobiological effect and enhance the risk of depression, particularly among individuals that are genetically vulnerable (Uchida *et al.*, 2018).

Air Pollution and Depression

Airborne pollutants which include carbon monoxide, sulphur dioxide, diesel emissions, and nitrogen oxides among others are emitted from residential heating, industries, and vehicles. Air pollutants can impact the function of the neurotransmitters such as dopamine and serotonin. Research shows that air pollutants can adversely affect the morphology of the neuron in the hippocampus and inflammatory cytokines; this may lead to oxidative stress (Fonken *et al.*, 2011). Air pollution can also impact neural plasticity thereby affecting the performance of the memory, cognition, and other behavioural outcomes.

Physical health conditions linked to air pollution for example asthma, diabetes, and cardiovascular diseases can, through comorbidity, enhance the prevalence of depression in environments that are air polluted. Additionally, depression has comorbidity with various neuropsychiatric disorders which are linked with air pollution, for instance, Alzheimer and cognitive disturbance (Sram *et al.*, 2017). Furthermore, air pollution can lead to oxygen insufficiency, and this can alter various neural systems which include serotonin production (Brenner *et al.*, 2011).

Studies done of developed countries have shown that air pollution reduces people's mental health increasing their risk of developing depression (Cho *et al.*, 2014). Even though the biological means for this relationship is not fully understood, there are likely pathological pathways. These include the fact that air pollution enhances the risk of developing cardiovascular diseases which increases the risk of depression (Kioumourtzoglou *et al.*, 2017). Air pollution can also adversely affect a person's mental health by affecting the digestive and nervous system (Lim *et al.*, 2012).

Furthermore, air pollution can decrease the amount of sunlight and this can cause stress to the nervous system leading to depression (Zhang *et al.*, 2017). Some studies have reported that air pollution reduces face-to-face contact between neighbours thereby enhancing their risk of depression (Lin *et al.*, 2016).

Some pollen which is produced by plants during flowering can trigger allergies. Pollens are mostly linked to low moods due to fatigue and other physical symptoms that occur from allergic symptoms. This relationship can explain the link between depression and pollen exposure. Noise is another environmental factor which has been associated with depression. Excessive noise can lead to negative emotions such as annoyance which might trigger psychophysiological stress reaction, which is linked to depression (Slavich and Irwin, 2014). Studies have reported that noise can lead to disturbances in sleep and this is associated with depression (Sygna *et al.*, 2014).

Urbanisation has brought with it drastic changes in the environment. Recent studies have reported that living in a city affects the function and structure of some parts of the brains vital for stress, social cognition, and processing of emotion (Haddad *et al.*, 2015). According to some studies, when a person spends the first fifteen years of his or her life in an urban area, the pregenual anterior cingulated cortex activation is increased, and the grey matter quantity in the prefrontal cortex reduces. When these two brain parts are interfered with, then the risk of developing mental disorders such as depression is increased (Rauda *et al.*, 2012). Depression is one of the psychiatric disorders whose incidence is constantly found among people who have lived in urban environments from an early age.

Vitamin D Deficiency and Depression

A lack of vitamin D has also been linked to various mental disorders including depression. Studies have shown that people whose vitamin D levels are normal have a low likelihood of developing depression (Chan *et al.*, 2011). Depression among patients with cancer and heart problems has been linked to a deficiency in vitamin D (Johansson *et al.*, 2016). Additionally, depression in young people has been associated with a deficiency in vitamin D (Kerr *et al.*, 2015). Insufficient vitamin D can influence the beginning and development of depression by working together with other factors (Cui *et al.*, 2015).

Vitamin D can be produced by a sunlit skin or ingested through foods. The human body contains numerous vitamin D receptors. Therefore, there are numerous ways through which vitamin D can affect a person's mood. One of the ways is hormonal because vitamin D assists in regulating the testosterone levels in men. Low testosterone has been linked to the impaired mood in both men and women

The risk of developing depression is decreased in people whose level of vitamin D is high. Studies conducted on people who were diagnosed with depression and other mood disorders reported significant improvement after they were treated with vitamin D (Stokes *et al.*, 2016). Increasing evidence shows that one of the primary roles of vitamin D is to sustain the Ca^{2+} homeostasis. Vitamin D controls the expression of signalling toolkit properties of Ca^{2+} whose function is to preserve low levels of Ca^{2+} cytosolic resting levels. Vitamin D also controls the production of serotonin which is a vital factor in depression.

A study conducted in the northern latitudes demonstrated that a significant association exists between late-life depression and vitamin D deficiency (Stewart and Hirani, 2010). Additionally, older men having insufficient vitamin D were more likely to develop depression compared to men of a similar age whose levels of vitamin D were sufficient. Other studies have linked low vitamin D levels to postpartum depression (Murphy *et al.*, 2010).

People diagnosed with depression can have low vitamin D since most of them rarely participate in outdoor activities. Individuals who are always indoors have little access to sunlight and tend to exercise less; this can be linked to impaired moods. Studies have reported that deficiency in the production of vitamins during the months of winter can cause seasonal affective disorder (Melrose, 2015). It is necessary to note that what exists between insufficient vitamin D levels and depression is correlation, not causation.

Exposure to Heavy Metals and Depression

A person can be exposed to heavy metals through diet, industrial emissions, dust in urban and industrial areas, or diet. Heavy metals can have a neurotoxic effect and may enhance the risk of depression. Some of the heavy metals include cadmium which may negatively affect an individual's mental health condition by altering the release of neurotransmitters and damaging the blood-brain barrier. Lead is another heavy metal which has been linked to many health conditions which include impairing the function of the brain.

Studies have shown that exposure to lead can increase the risk of developing depression (McFarlane AC, *et al.*, 2013). Due to the many issues linked to environmental exposures, it is important to apply precautions. Until evidence of harmlessness is established, an individual should limit his or her exposure to environmental exposures. This will stop the increase in the current alarming depression rate.

REFERENCES

Abbott, R. A., Whear, R., Rodgers, L. R., Bethel, A., Coon, J. T., Kuyken, W., and Dickens, C. (2014) 'Effectiveness of mindfulness-based stress reduction and mindfulness based cognitive therapy in vascular disease: A systematic review and meta-analysis of randomised controlled trials', *Journal of Psychosomatic Research*, *76*(5), pp. 341–351.

Alwan, A. (2011) Global status report on noncommunicable diseases 2010', World Health Organization.

American Psychiatric Association (2013) 'Diagnostic and statistical manual of mental disorders' (5th ed.), Washington, DC: American Psychiatric Association.

Andersen, S. L., and Teicher, M. H. (2008) 'Stress, sensitive periods and maturational events in adolescent depression,' *Trends in Neurosciences*, *31*(4), pp. 183–19.

Andreou, E., Alexopoulos, E. C., Lionis, C., Varvogli, L., Gnardellis, C., Chrousos, G. P., and Darviri, C. (2011) 'Perceived stress scale: reliability and validity study in Greece', *International journal of environmental research and public health*, *8*(8), pp. 3287–3298.

Arden, J. B. (2015) *Brain2Brain: Enacting Client Change Through the Persuasive Power of Neuroscience*, John Wiley and Sons.

Baker, A. L., Thornton, L. K., Hiles, S., Hides, L., and Lubman, D. I. (2012) 'Psychological interventions for alcohol misuse among people with co-occurring depression or anxiety disorders: a systematic review', *Journal of Affective Disorders*, *139*(3), pp. 217–229.

Balaratnasingam, S., and Janca, A. (2011) 'Combining sertraline and naltrexone in the treatment of adults with comorbid depression and alcohol dependence', *Current Psychiatry Reports*, *13*(4), pp. 245–247.

Beaulac, J., Carlson, A., and Boyd, R. J. (2011) 'Counseling on physical activity to promote mental health: Practical guidelines for family physicians', *Canadian Family Physician*, *57*(4), pp. 399–401.

between childhood low-level lead exposure and adult mental health problems: the Port Pirie cohort

Blumenthal, J. A., Babyak, M. A., Doraiswamy, P. M., Watkins, L., Hoffman, B. M., Barbour, K. A., . . . and Hinderliter, A. (2007) 'Exercise and pharmacotherapy in the treatment of major depressive disorder', *Psychosomatic Medicine*, *69*(7), p. 587.

Boden, J. M., and Fergusson, D. M. (2011) 'Alcohol and depression', *Addiction*, *106*(5), pp. 906–914.

Brenner, B., Cheng, D., Clark, S., and Camargo Jr, C. A. (2011) 'Positive association between altitude and suicide in 2584 US counties', *High Altitude Medicine and Biology*, *12*(1), pp. 31–35.

Brewer, J. A., Bowen, S., Smith, J. T., Marlatt, G. A., and Potenza, M. N. (2010) 'Mindfulness-based treatments for co-occurring depression and substance use disorders: what can we learn from the brain?', *Addiction*, *105*(10), pp. 1698–1706.

Brody, A. E. (2009) 'Motivational interviewing with a depressed adolescent', *Journal of Clinical Psychology*, *65*(11), pp. 1168–1179.

Brown, R. A., Ramsey, S. E., Kahler, C. W., Palm, K. M., Monti, P. M., Abrams, D., . . . and Miller, I. W. (2011) 'A randomized controlled trial of cognitive-behavioral treatment for depression versus relaxation training for alcohol-dependent individuals with elevated depressive symptoms', *Journal of Studies on Alcohol and Drugs*, *72*(2), pp. 286–296.

Carney, C. E., Segal, Z. V., Edinger, J. D., and Krystal, A. D. (2007) 'A comparison of rates of residual insomnia symptoms following pharmacotherapy or cognitive-behavioral therapy for major depressive disorder', *The Journal of Clinical Psychiatry*, *68*(2), pp. 254–260.

Chaiton, M. O., Cohen, J. E., O'Loughlin, J., and Rehm, J. (2009) 'A systematic review of longitudinal studies on the association between depression and smoking in adolescents', *BMC Public Health*, *9*(1), p. 356.

Chan, R., Chan, D., Woo, J., Ohlsson, C., Mellström, D., Kwok, T., and Leung, P. (2011) 'Association between serum 25-hydroxyvitamin D and psychological health in older Chinese men in a cohort study', *Journal of Affective Disorders*, *130*(1–2), pp. 251–259.

Chan, Y. F., Dennis, M. L., and Funk, R. R. (2008) 'Prevalence and comorbidity of major internalizing and externalizing problems among adolescents and adults presenting to substance abuse treatment', *Journal of Substance Abuse Treatment*, *34* (1), pp. 14–24.

Cho, J., Choi, Y. J., Suh, M., Sohn, J., Kim, H., Cho, S. K., . . . and Shin, D. C. (2014) 'Air pollution as a risk factor for depressive episode in patients with cardiovascular disease, diabetes mellitus, or asthma', *Journal of Affective Disorders*, *157*, pp. 45–51.

Chokroverty, S. (2010) 'Overview of sleep and sleep disorders', *Indian J Med Res*, *131*(2), pp. 126–140.

Clark, Heddy Kovach, Chris L. Ringwalt, and Stephen R. Shamblen (2011) 'Predicting Adolescent Substance Use: The Effects of Depressed Mood and Positive Expectancies', *Addictive Behaviors* 36, pp. 488–493.

Cui, X., Gooch, H., Groves, N. J., Sah, P., Burne, T. H., Eyles, D. W., and McGrath, J. J. (2015) 'Vitamin D and the brain: key questions for future research', *The Journal of Steroid Biochemistry and Molecular Biology*, *148*, pp. 305–309.

Dankel, S. J., Loenneke, J. P., and Loprinzi, P. D. (2016) 'Mild depressive symptoms among Americans in relation to physical activity, current overweight/obesity, and self-reported history of overweight/obesity', *International Journal of Behavioral Medicine*, *23*(5), pp. 553–560.

DeVido, J. J., and Weiss, R. D. (2012) 'Treatment of the depressed alcoholic patient', *Current Psychiatry Reports*, *14*(6), pp. 610–618.

Diagnostic, D. S. M. V. (2013) *Statistical Manual of Mental Health Disorders: DSM-5.5.*

Dinas, P. C., Koutedakis, Y., and Flouris, A. D. (2011) 'Effects of exercise and physical activity on depression', *Irish Journal of Medical Science*, *180*(2), pp. 319–325.

Fluharty, M., Taylor, A. E., Grabski, M., and Munafò, M. R. (2016) 'The association of cigarette smoking with depression and anxiety: a systematic review', *Nicotine and Tobacco Research*, *19*(1), pp. 3–13.

Fonken, L. K., Xu, X., Weil, Z. M., Chen, G., Sun, Q., Rajagopalan, S., and Nelson, R. J. (2011) 'Air pollution impairs cognition, provokes depressive-like behaviors and alters hippocampal cytokine expression and morphology', *Molecular Psychiatry*, *16*(10), p. 987.

Fraser, A. (2013) *The Healing Power of Meditation: Leading Experts on Buddhism, Psychology, and Medicine Explore the Health Benefit s of Contemplative Practice*, Shambhala Publications.

Gangwisch, J. E., Hale, L., Garcia, L., Malaspina, D., Opler, M. G., Payne, M. E., . . . and Lane, D. (2015) 'High glycemic index diet as a risk factor for depression: analyses from the Women's Health Initiative', *The American Journal of Clinical Nutrition*, *102*(2), pp. 454–463.

Gao, S., Jin, Y., Unverzagt, F. W., Liang, C., Hall, K. S., Cao, J., . . . and Bian, J. (2012) 'Selenium level and depressive symptoms in a rural elderly Chinese cohort', *BMC Psychiatry*, *12*(1), p. 72.

Gelenberg, A. J., Freeman, M. P., Markowitz, J. C., Rosenbaum, J. F., Thase, M. E., Trivedi, M. H., . . . and Schneck, C. D. (2010) 'Practice guideline for the treatment of patients with major depressive disorder', third edition, *The American journal of psychiatry*, *167*(10), p. 1.

Girard, J. M., Cohn, J. F., Mahoor, M. H., Mavadati, S., and Rosenwald, D. P., (2013) 'Social risk and depression: Evidence from manual and automatic facial expression analysis', *In*

2013 10th IEEE International Conference and Workshops on Automatic Face and Gesture Recognition (FG), pp. 1–8, IEEE, 2013 (accessed April 2013).

Goldstein, B. I., and Levitt, A. J. (2008) 'The specific burden of comorbid anxiety disorders and of substance use disorders in bipolar I disorder', *Bipolar Disorders*, *10*(1), pp. 67–78.

Goldstein, B. I., Shamseddeen, W., Spirito, A., Emslie, G., Clarke, G., Wagner, K. D., . . . and Mayes, T. (2009) 'Substance use and the treatment of resistant depression in adolescents', *Journal of the American Academy of Child and Adolescent Psychiatry*, *48*(12), pp. 1182–1192.

Gopinath, B., Hickson, L., Schneider, J., McMahon, C. M., Burlutsky, G., Leeder, S. R., and Mitchell, P. (2012) 'Hearing-impaired adults are at increased risk of experiencing emotional distress and social engagement restrictions five years later', *Age and Ageing*, *41*(5), pp. 618–623.

Goyal, M., Haythornthwaite, J., Levine, D., Becker, D., Vaidya, D., Hill-Briggs, F., and Ford, D. (2010) 'Intensive meditation for refractory pain and symptoms', *The Journal of Alternative and Complementary Medicine*, *16*(6), pp. 627–631.

Haddad, L., Schäfer, A., Streit, F., Lederbogen, F., Grimm, O., Wüst, S., . . . and Meyer-Lindenberg, A. (2014) 'Brain structure correlates of urban upbringing, an environmental risk factor for schizophrenia', *Schizophrenia Bulletin*, *41*(1), pp. 115–122.

Hage, M. P., and Azar, S. T. (2012) 'The link between thyroid function and depression', *Journal of Thyroid Research*.

Havassy, B. E., Alvidrez, J., and Mericle, A. A. (2009) 'Disparities in use of mental health and substance abuse services by persons with co-occurring disorders', *Psychiatric Services*, *60*(2), pp. 217–223.

Hechtman, L. (2018) *Clinical Naturopathic Medicine*, Elsevier Health Sciences.

Herring, M. P., Puetz, T. W., O'Connor, P. J., and Dishman, R. K. (2012) 'Effect of exercise training on depressive symptoms among patients with a chronic illness: a systematic review and meta-analysis of randomized controlled trials', *Archives of Internal Medicine*, *172*(2), pp. 101–111.

Holt-Lunstad, J. (2018) 'Why social relationships are important for physical health: a systems approach to understanding and modifying risk and protection', *Annual Review of Psychology*, *69*, pp. 437–458.

Holz, N. E., Laucht, M., and Meyer-Lindenberg, A. (2015) 'Recent advances in understanding the neurobiology of childhood socioeconomic disadvantage', *Current Opinion in Psychiatry*, *28*(5), pp. 365–370.

Hunter, S. B., Watkins, K. E., Hepner, K. A., Paddock, S. M., Ewing, B. A., Osilla, K. C., and Perry, S. (2012) 'Treating depression and substance use: a randomized controlled trial', *Journal of Substance Abuse Treatment*, *43*(2), pp. 137–151.

Hunter, S. B., Witkiewitz, K., Watkins, K. E., Paddock, S. M., and Hepner, K. A. (2012) 'The moderating effects of group cognitive–behavioral therapy for depression among substance users', *Psychology of Addictive Behaviors*, *26*(4), p. 906.

Jerstad, S. J., Boutelle, K. N., Ness, K. K., and Stice, E. (2010) 'Prospective reciprocal relations between physical activity and depression in female adolescents', *Journal of Consulting and Clinical Psychology*, *78*(2), p. 268.

Johansson, P., Alehagen, U., van der Wal, M. H., Svensson, E., and Jaarsma, T. (2016) 'Vitamin D levels and depressive symptoms in patients with chronic heart failure', *International Journal of Cardiology*, *207*, pp. 185–189.

Johnco, C., Wuthrich, V. M., and Rapee, R. M. (2014)' The influence of cognitive flexibility on treatment outcome and cognitive restructuring skill acquisition during cognitive behavioural treatment for anxiety and depression in older adults: Results of a pilot study', *Behaviour Research and Therapy*, *57*, pp. 55–64.

Katagiri, R., Yuan, X., Kobayashi, S., and Sasaki, S. (2017)' Effect of excess iodine intake on thyroid diseases in different populations: A systematic review and meta-analyses including observational studies'; *PloS one*, *12*(3), e0173722.

Kerr, D. C., Zava, D. T., Piper, W. T., Saturn, S. R., Frei, B., and Gombart, A. F. (2015)'Associations between vitamin D levels and depressive symptoms in healthy young adult women', *Psychiatry Research*, *227*(1), pp. 46–51.

Kessler, R. C., and Bromet, E. J. (2013)' The epidemiology of depression across cultures', *Annual Review of Public Health*, *34*, pp. 119–138.

Kioumourtzoglou, M. A., Power, M. C., Hart, J. E., Okereke, O. I., Coull, B. A., Laden, F., and Weisskopf, M. G. (2017) 'The association between air pollution and onset of depression among middle-aged and older women', *American Journal of Epidemiology*, *185*(9), pp. 801–809.

Kofler, M. J., McCart, M. R., Zajac, K., Ruggiero, K. J., Saunders, B. E., and Kilpatrick, D. G. (2011) 'Depression and delinquency covariation in an accelerated longitudinal sample of adolescents', *Journal of Consulting and Clinical Psychology*, *79*(4), p. 458.

Li, Y., Lv, M. R., Wei, Y. J., Sun, L., Zhang, J. X., Zhang, H. G., and Li, B. (2017) 'Dietary patterns and depression risk: a meta-analysis', *Psychiatry Research*, *253*, p. 373–382.

Lim, Y. H., Kim, H., Kim, J. H., Bae, S., Park, H. Y., and Hong, Y. C. (2012) 'Air pollution and symptoms of depression in elderly adults', *Environmental Health Perspectives*, *120*(7), pp. 1023–1028.

Lin, G. Z., Li, L., Song, Y. F., Zhou, Y. X., Shen, S. Q., and Ou, C. Q. (2016) 'The impact of ambient air pollution on suicide mortality: a case-crossover study in Guangzhou, China', *Environmental Health*, *15*(1), p. 90.

Lydecker, K. P., Tate, S. R., Cummins, K. M., McQuaid, J., Granholm, E., and Brown, S. A. (2010) 'Clinical outcomes of an integrated treatment for depression and substance use disorders', *Psychology of Addictive Behaviors*, *24*(3), p. 453.

Ma, J., and Xiao, L. (2010) 'Obesity and depression in US women: results from the 2005–2006 National Health and Nutritional Examination Survey', *Obesity*, *18*(2), pp. 347–353.

Mafra, D., and Fouque, D. (2014) 'Lower physical activity and depression are associated with hospitalization and shorter survival in CKD', *Clinical Journal of the American Society of Nephrology*, *9*(10), pp. 1669–1670.

McCall, W. V., Blocker, J. N., D'Agostino Jr, R., Kimball, J., Boggs, N., Lasater, B., and Rosenquist, P. B. (2010) 'Insomnia severity is an indicator of suicidal ideation during a depression clinical trial', *Sleep Medicine*, *11*(9), pp. 822–827.

McFarlane AC, Searle AK, Van Hooff M, Baghurst PA, Sawyer MG, *et al.* (2013) 'Prospective associations'.

McManus, F., Surawy, C., Muse, K., Vazquez-Montes, M., and Williams, J. M. G. (2012) 'A randomized clinical trial of mindfulness-based cognitive therapy versus unrestricted services for health anxiety (hypochondriasis)', *Journal of Consulting and Clinical Psychology*, *80*(5), p. 817.

McManus, S., Meltzer, H., and Campion, J. (2010) 'Cigarette smoking and mental health in England: Data from the Adult Psychiatric Morbidity Survey 2007', *London, UK: National Centre for Social Research*.

Mead, G. E., Morley, W., Campbell, P., Greig, C. A., McMurdo, M., and Lawlor, D. A. (2009) 'Exercise for depression', *Cochrane Database of Systematic Reviews*, (3).

Melrose, S. (2015) 'Seasonal affective disorder: an overview of assessment and treatment approaches', *Depression Research and Treatment*, *2015*.

Michalak, J., Heidenreich, T., Meibert, P., and Schulte, D. (2008) 'Mindfulness predicts relapse/recurrence in major depressive disorder after mindfulness-based cognitive therapy', *The Journal of Nervous and Mental Disease*, *196*(8), pp. 630–633.

Miller, P. (2013) *Principles of Addiction*, Amsterdam: Elsevier/AP.

Murphy, P. K., Mueller, M., Hulsey, T. C., Ebeling, M. D., and Wagner, C. L. (2010) 'An exploratory study of postpartum depression and vitamin D', *Journal of the American Psychiatric Nurses Association*, *16*(3), pp. 170–177.

National Institute for Clinical Excellence (2009) 'Depression: the treatment and management of depression in adults', (update) *Clinical Guidelines, CG90.*

Ng, M., Fleming, T., Robinson, M., Thomson, B., Graetz, N., Margono, C., . . . and Abraham, J. P. (2014) 'Global, regional, and national prevalence of overweight and obesity in children and adults during 1980–2013: a systematic analysis for the Global Burden of Disease Study 2013', *The Lancet, 384*(9945), pp. 766–781.

Overall, N. C., and Hammond, M. D. (2013) 'Biased and accurate: Depressive symptoms and daily perceptions within intimate relationships', *Personality and Social Psychology Bulletin, 39*(5), pp. 636–650.

Ozen, L. J., Gibbons, C., and Bédard, M. (2016), 'Mindfulness-Based Cognitive Therapy Improves Depression Symptoms After Traumatic Brain Injury', *In Mindfulness-Based Cognitive Therapy*, Springer, Cham., pp. 31–45.

Patten, S. B. (2009) 'Accumulation of major depressive episodes over time in a prospective study indicates that retrospectively assessed lifetime prevalence estimates are too low', *BMC Psychiatry, 9*(1), p. 19.

Piet, J., and Hougaard, E. (2011) 'The effect of mindfulness-based cognitive therapy for prevention of relapse in recurrent major depressive disorder: a systematic review and meta-analysis', *Clinical Psychology Review, 31*(6), pp. 1032–1040.

Popova, S., Mohapatra, S., Patra, J., Duhig, A., and Rehm, J. (2011) 'A literature review of cost-benefit analyses for the treatment of alcohol dependence', *International Journal of Environmental Research and Public Health, 8*(8), pp. 3351–3364.

Pour, T. H. (2014) 'The effect of cognitive behavioural therapy on anxiety in infertile women', *European Journal of Experimental Biology, 4*(1), pp. 415–419.

Pytliak, M., Vargová, V., Mechírová, V., and Felsöci, M. (2011) 'Serotonin receptors—from molecular biology to clinical applications', *Physiological Research, 60*(1), p. 15.

Radua, J., Borgwardt, S., Crescini, A., Mataix-Cols, D.,

Meyer-Lindenberg, A., McGuire, P. K., and Fusar-Poli, P. (2012) 'Multimodal meta-analysis of structural and functional brain changes in first episode psychosis and the effects of antipsychotic medication', *Neuroscience and Biobehavioral Reviews, 36*(10), pp. 2325–2333.

Rao, T. S., Asha, M. R., Ramesh, B. N., and Rao, K. J. (2008) 'Understanding nutrition, depression and mental illnesses', *Indian Journal of Psychiatry, 50*(2), p. 77.

Rapgay, L., and Bystrisky, A. (2009) 'Classical mindfulness: An introduction to its theory and practice for clinical application', *Annals of the New York Academy of Sciences, 1172*(1), pp. 148–162.

Rhew, I. C., Richardson, L. P., Lymp, J., McTiernan, A., McCauley, E., and Vander Stoep, A. (2008) 'Measurement matters in the association between early adolescent depressive symptoms and body mass index', *General Hospital Psychiatry, 30*(5), pp. 458–466.

Richards, Derek (2015) 'Prevalence and clinical course of depression: a review', *Clinical Psychology Review* 31.7, pp. 1117–1125.

Rodgers, S., Hengartner, M. P., Müller, M., Aleksandrowicz, A. A., Rössler, W., and Ajdacic-Gross, V. (2015) 'Serum testosterone levels and symptom-based depression subtypes in men', *Frontiers in Psychiatry, 6*, p. 61.

Rognmo, K., Torvik, F. A., Røysamb, E., and Tambs, K. (2013) 'Alcohol use and spousal mental distress in a population sample: the nord-trøndelag health study', *BMC Public Health, 13*(1), p. 319.

Sánchez-Villegas, A., Delgado-Rodríguez, M., Alonso, A., Schlatter, J., Lahortiga, F., Serra Majem, L., Martínez-González, M. A. (2009) 'Association of the Mediterranean dietary pattern with the incidence of depression: the Seguimiento Universidad de Navarra/University of Navarra follow-up (SUN) cohort', *Archive of General Psychiatry, 66*, pp. 1090–1098.

Schwartz-Mette, R. A., and Rose, A. J. (2016) 'Depressive symptoms and conversational self-focus in adolescents' friendships', *Journal of Abnormal Child Psychology, 44*(1), 87–100.

Sheikh, M., Hantoushzadeh, S., Shariat, M., Farahani, Z., and Ebrahiminasab, O. (2017) 'The efficacy of early iron supplementation on postpartum depression, a randomized double-blind placebo-controlled trial', *European Journal of Nutrition*, 56(2), pp. 901–908.

Sihvola, E., Rose, R. J., Dick, D. M., Pulkkinen, L., Marttunen, M., and Kaprio, J. (2008) 'Early-onset depressive disorders predict the use of addictive substances in adolescence: a prospective study of adolescent Finnish twins', *Addiction*, 103(12), pp. 2045–2053.

Slavich, G. M., and Irwin, M. R. (2014) 'From stress to inflammation and major depressive disorder: a social signal transduction theory of depression', *Psychological bulletin*, 140(3), p. 774.

Smith, P. H., Mazure, C. M., and McKee, S. A. (2014) 'Smoking and mental illness in the US population', *Tobacco Control*, 23(e2), pp. e147–e153.

Smith, P. H., Mazure, C. M., and McKee, S. A. (2014) 'Smoking and mental illness in the US population', *Tobacco Control*, 23(e2), pp. e147–e153. b

Sram, R. J., Veleminsky, J. M., Veleminsky, S. M., and Stejskalova, J. (2017) 'The impact of air pollution to central nervous system in children and adults', *Neuro Endocrinology Letters*, 38(6), pp. 389–396.

Stewart, R., and Hirani, V. (2010) 'Relationship between vitamin D levels and depressive symptoms in older residents from a national survey population', *Psychosomatic Medicine*, 72(7), pp. 608–612.

Stokes, C. S., Grünhage, F., Baus, C., Volmer, D. A., Wagenpfeil, S., Riemenschneider, M., and Lammert, F. (2016) 'Vitamin D supplementation reduces depressive symptoms in patients with chronic liver disease', *Clinical Nutrition*, 35(4), pp. 950–957.

study. *NeuroToxicology* 39:11–17

Swendsen, J., Conway, K. P., Degenhardt, L., Glantz, M., Jin, R., Merikangas, K. R., . . . and Kessler, R. C. (2010) 'Mental disorders as risk factors for substance use, abuse and dependence: results from the 10-year follow-up of the National Comorbidity Survey', *Addiction*, *105*(6), pp. 1117–1128.

Sygna, K., Aasvang, G. M., Aamodt, G., Oftedal, B., and Krog, N. H. (2014) 'Road traffic noise, sleep and mental health', *Environmental Research*, *131*, pp. 17–24.

Tait, R. J., French, D. J., Burns, R., and Anstey, K. J. (2012) 'Alcohol use and depression from middle age to the oldest old: gender is more important than age', *International Psychogeriatrics*, *24*(8), pp. 1275–1283.

Taylor, D. J., Lichstein, K. L., Weinstock, J., Sanford, S., and Temple, J. R. (2007) 'A pilot study of cognitive-behavioral therapy of insomnia in people with mild depression', *Behavior Therapy*, *38*(1), pp. 49–57.

Taylor, D. J., Pigeon, W. R., Hegel, M., Unützer, J., Fan, M. Y., Sateia, M. J., . . . and Perlis, M. L. (2008) 'Is Insomnia a Perpetuating Factor for Late-Life Depression in the IMPACT Cohort? Commentary', *Sleep*, *31*(4).

Townsend, A. L., Biegel, D. E., Ishler, K. J., Wieder, B., and Rini, A. (2006) 'Families of persons with substance use and mental disorders: A literature review and conceptual framework', *Family Relations*, *55*(4), pp. 473–486.

Uchida, S., Yamagata, H., Seki, T., and Watanabe, Y. (2018) 'Epigenetic mechanisms of major depression: Targeting neuronal plasticity', *Psychiatry and Clinical Neurosciences*, *72*(4), pp. 212–227.

Verderber, K. S., Verderber, R. F., and Sellnow, D. D. (2013) *Communicate!*, Cengage Learning.

Volkow, N. D. (2014) 'America's addiction to opioids: heroin and prescription drug abuse', *Senate Caucus on International Narcotics Control*, *14*.

Wand, G. (2008) 'The influence of stress on the transition from drug use to addiction', *Alcohol Research and Health*, *31*(2), p. 119.

Weinberger, A. H., McKee, S. A., and George, T. P. (2012) 'Smoking cue reactivity in adult smokers with and without depression:

A pilot study', *The American journal on addictions*, *21*(2), pp. 136–144.

Williams, J. M. G., and Kuyken, W. (2012) 'Mindfulness-based cognitive therapy: a promising new approach to preventing depressive relapse', *The British Journal of Psychiatry*, *200*(5), pp. 359–360.

World Health Organization. (2016) 'Obesity and overweight', fact sheet (updated June 2016), *Trouvé le, 13*.

Zhang, X., Zhang, X., and Chen, X. (2017) 'Happiness in the air: how does a dirty sky affect mental health and subjective well-being?', *Journal of Environmental Economics and Management, 85*, pp. 81–94.

CHAPTER 6

Borderline Personality Disorder

A dog is happy to lick up a plastic bag as long as he does not have to move his ass from the shade!

'The masses have never thirsted after truth. They turn aside from evidence that is not to their taste, preferring to deify error, if error seduce them. Whoever can supply them with illusions is easily their master; whoever attempts to destroy their illusions is always their victim. An individual in a crowd is a grain of sand amid other grains of sand, which the wind stirs up at will' (Gustave Le Bon).

'A lie can travel halfway around the world while the truth is putting on its shoes' (Mark Twain). The term borderline personality was first used by a psychoanalyst named Adolph Stern in 1938 in the United States (Douglas and James, 2013). The term was used to describe patients who did not fit either in the psychoneurotic or the psychotic group. Later in 1975, Otto Kernberg introduced the term borderline personality organisation to describe a pattern of behaviour and functioning categorised by instability among those affected. The description given to BPD patients included people that were difficult, unstable in their functioning, needy, at risk of suicide, and emotional. Soon after, a pattern of symptoms arose that could be used to describe people with a borderline personality disorder.

The symptoms included lack of a stable image, frequent

changes between periods of despair and confidence, fear of being abandoned, rapid shift in mood, and suicidal ideations. The features which currently define BPD were described in 1978 by Kolb and Gunderson (Edelstein, Hersen, and Thase, 2013). Later in 1980, borderline personality disorder became officially recognised as a personality disorder in the *Diagnostic and Statistical Manual*-III. Borderline personality disorder (BPD) is a mental illness that affects how a person thinks and feels about himself and other people; this adversely affects the person's daily functionality. BPD is part of the class of mental illnesses referred to as personality disorders.

Similar to other personality disorders, BPD is characterised by a regular pattern of feeling, thinking, and relating with other people that often causes considerable problems to the affectedperson. Furthermore, BPD is characterised by a constant pattern of mood variation, behaviour, and self-image. These symptoms may lead to impulsive behaviour and difficulties in relating toothers (APA, 2013). A person with BPD can experience heightened periods of anxiety, depression, and anger. The affected individuals also may experience challenges in trying tocontrol their emotional responses. Consequently, this may lead to suicidal and self-harming behaviours.

An individual with a borderline personality disorder might experience anxiety, depression, and attacks of anger, which can last for a day or a few hours (APA, 2013). These emotions might be linked to periods where the person engages in alcohol or drug abuse and self-injury, which may include cutting. Cognitive distortions that occur in people with BPD can cause constant changes in career plans, values, long-term goals, friendships, and jobs. At times, the affected individuals regard themselves as being unworthy or inadequate. The person might feel empty, bored, or mistreated. These symptoms are most severe when individuals with the disorder lack social support and feel isolated. Individuals with borderline personality disorder often experience unsteady patterns of social relationships (APA,2013). The person may develop an intense emotional attachment to family and friends. However, these attachments can quickly change from love and admiration to dislike and anger. The individual might become rapidly attached and idealise another person. However, when conflict occurs, the person may switch to the other extreme and blame the other individual for being uncaring. People diagnosed with borderline personality disorder are extremely sensitive to rejection. BPD also leads to feelings of abandonment, which puts the affected person at high risk of suicidal ideations.

Similar to other personality disorders, individuals are often in adulthood or adolescence before being evaluated as meeting the full borderline personality disorder criteria. Historically, BPD was believed to be a group of symptoms which comprised of mood problems and distorted reality. Therefore, the disorder was thought to border between schizophrenia and mood problems. Nonetheless, currently, there is an understanding that although BPD symptoms may include such symptoms; it is more linked to other personality disorders in regard to how it might develop and occur in families. Currently, patients with a borderline personality disorder can be seen in all kinds of clinical settings. Studies have shown that these patients account for 20% of inpatients and 10% of outpatients (Zimmerman, Chelminski, and Young, 2008). In most communities, the prevalence of borderline personality disorder seems to be equal between men and women. However, more women tend to seek professional mental health services than men (Paris, 2010). Causes of BPD remain unclear, but it is believed to be a combination of social stressors, biological predispositions, and the way a person understands the world (Kulacaoglu and Kose, 2018). A large number of individuals with borderline personality disorder tend to have experienced traumatic events, which include adversity, abandonment, and abuse. This shows that social, psychological, and biological factors can enhance the risk of developing borderline personality disorder.

Potential Causes of Borderline Personality Disorder

There is no single known cause that can be linked to the development of borderline personality disorder. However, there are likely risk factors that have been linked to the disorder, and they include, among others:

Biological Factors

Although there are no apparent factors that can be attributed to the development of BPD, there are various biological factors that have been linked to the disorder. People whose family has BPD have a higher likelihood of being diagnosed with the disorder (Lopez-Castroman *et al.*, 2012). Borderline personality disorder is a brain disorder. When genetic factors linked to the disorder are present, the person's brain development is adversely affected, leaving him or her prone to BPD.

The biological factors can vary from early childhood environment and genetic influence on the brain and nervous system development. One of the primary features of BPD is emotional regulation. The abnormal transmitter functioning is one of the factors which makes it difficult for people diagnosed with BPD to regulate their emotions. Emotional regulation entails processing, amplifying, maintaining, and attenuating the emotions produced from external and internal stimuli.

Research has shown that the person's risk of developing BPD is expressed by genetic abnormalities (Torgersen *et al.*, 2012). The defects often affect the proper operation of the brain's circuits or pathways, which are involved in impulse control, which includes reasoning, perception, and information processing. Existing research shows that there is no particular gene that can be entirely attributed to borderline personality disorder. It seems that genes that increase the risk of developing BPD can be passed by someone who has the disorder.

Neurotransmitters, especially serotonin, which regulates affect, aggression, and impulses, have been linked to the development of the disorder. When serotonin is dysfunctional, it often leads to impulsivity, suicidal tendencies, and emotional instability, all of which are common among borderline personality disorder patients (Barlow and Durand, 2012). When the serotonin levels are low, a person might not be able to control any destructive impulses (The British Psychological Society and the Royal College of Psychiatrists, 2009). Several studies have shown that BPD can be inherited, primary areas being on traits linked to mood dysregulation, and impulsive aggression.

According to studies, aggression, which is one of the symptoms of borderline personality, is caused by having an impaired regulation of the neural circuits which control emotions. It is important to note that direct hereditary associated with the disorder is not very common (Livesley, 2008). Current studies show that environmental factors impact the intensity and frequency of the genetic expression of behaviours common with borderline personality disorder (Willensen and Boomsma, 2008).

Studies propose that brain function and structure, genetics, cultural, social, and economic factors can increase the risk of developing the disorder. Individuals who have a close member of his/ her family affected by borderline personality disorder are at a higher risk of the same. Additionally, studies have shown that individuals with BPD may have functional and structural alterations in the brain region, which controls emotions and impulses (Lopez-Castroman *et al.*, 2012). Nonetheless, it remains unclear if these alterations are a risk factor of developing BPD; therefore, there is a need for more research.

Psychological Factors

Traumatic events such as emotional, sexual, and physical abuse experienced during childhood have also been linked to the development of BPD. These traumatic experiences are said to bring about developmental hindrances in children, which can later lead to BPD development. Nevertheless, childhood abuse, on its own, cannot cause BPD. When a child experiences abuse, there is a likelihood that it might disorganize the child's attachment to the abusive family member (Gerull *et al.*, 2008).

Studies have shown evidence that the response of the caregiver to the abuse is more important than the abuse in long-term borderline personality disorder outcomes (Gerull *et al.*, 2008). Failure to give and express sympathy plays a crucial role in childhood development. When a caregiver or parent does not portray empathy after a child has undergone a traumatic event, it can impair the development of the child, which may lead to dysfunction in their personal development. If parents or caregivers cannot validate a child immediately after the traumatic experience, it might alter the secure attachment development leading to emotional dysregulation, which can make the child vulnerable to BPD.

Psychosocial Factors

There are times where the development of BPD is believed to be a result of social factors. Studies have identified several factors that can be linked to the development of BPD. For instance, a family that is unstable and is not nurturing can lead to personality dysfunction, which might lead to emotional dysregulation that is common among BPD patients (The British Psychological Society and the Royal College of Psychiatrists, 2009). When children grow in a family environment that is unstable, they fail to learn how to handle emotional distress. During adulthood, the person may adopt the features of the invalidating environment by quashing his/her emotional experiences and depending on other people for a correct reflection of the outside reality.

Additionally, a history of substance abuse and mood disorders can be linked to the development of BPD. Neglect and lack of involvement by caregivers can make the child experience challenges in socialising and may increase the risk of suicidal ideations. A family environment that inhibits logical dialogue regarding a child's view of the world can hinder effective adjustment after trauma (The British Psychological Society and the Royal College of Psychiatrists, 2009).

Neglect and lack of parental involvement have been viewed as a factor that can lead to the development of BPD. Lack of emotional involvement can make the child to experience challenges in socialisation and increase their risk of suicide (The British Psychological Society and the Royal College of Psychiatrists, 2009). Parents who have experienced traumas which remain unresolved have a greater likelihood of experiencing relationship and attachment challenges with their children (Gerull *et al.*, 2008). If a parent presents their previous trauma in the current situation, children are likely to be traumatised and can lead to the development of BPD later.

BPD Prevalence

Various studies show that borderline personality disorder prevalence rates among the general public in the United States vary from 0.5%–5.9% (Zanarini *et al.*, 2011). Some of the latest reviews of epidemiological evidence hold the view that in clinical settings, the prevalence rates of borderline personality disorder vary from 15%–25%. These rates show that a large number of people with BPD are not diagnosed and might not be receiving any treatment (Gunderson, 20009). Regarding gender, earlier studies showed a considerably higher rate of the disorder in women than men.

The gender disparity has been attributed by some authors to sampling biases since most of the earlier prevalence rates were not drawn from the general population but clinical samples. Additionally, women and men are inclined to advocate for diverse sets of borderline personality disorder symptoms (Zanarini *et al.*, 2011). For instance, men have an enhanced likelihood of engaging in impulsive behaviour that self-harming behaviours. On the contrary, women are likely to portray feelings of affective instability and emptiness.

Why Is Borderline Personality Disorder a Misunderstood Disease?

Among the various mental illnesses or disorders, none is more misunderstood than a borderline personality disorder. The disorder is a disease that has experienced a lot of misunderstanding historically and even currently. Some of the reasons why BPD is misunderstood include the fact that it can present itself in over two hundred ways, and BPD hardly stands on its own.

Borderline personality disorder can co-occur with other disorders such as substance abuse, anxiety disorders, bipolar disorder, depression, and eating disorder (Wang *et al.*, 2012). Due to the co-occurrence, another disorder may be diagnosed, and often BPD diagnosis might be overlooked or missed.

Individuals who have been diagnosed with a borderline personality disorder might be on more than one kind of medication. Currently, there are no specific medications that have been approved in the treatment of BPD; this increases the misunderstanding associated with the disorder. Nevertheless, a mental health practitioner can prescribe drugs that can address some symptoms which those diagnosed with BPD experience. A person with borderline personality disorder who has been diagnosed with co-occurring disorders like post-traumatic stress disorder, depression, or anxiety may be given medications to treat these mental health conditions (Sadock, Sadock, and Levin, 2007).

Additionally, BPD is misunderstood by the general population due to the myths associated with the disorder. Some of the myths include the view that BPD cannot be treated, thereby looking at it as a life sentence (Choi-Kain and Gunderson, 2019). Although this is false, most people who have been diagnosed with the disorder tend to feel helpless, thereby not seeking any form of treatment. However, BPD is treatable through various evidence-based psychological therapies such as dialectical behavioural therapy.

Another myth associated with BPD is that all individuals diagnosed with the disorder must have experienced childhood abuse.

Although childhood abuse is regarded as one of the factors which can cause BPD, it is necessary to note that not everyone with the disorder has undergone childhood trauma. Additionally, people also associate BPD with bipolar disorder. Although the symptoms of the two disorders may look similar, the two are different. For instance, both bipolar disorder and BPD causes intense mood swings (Choi-Kain and Gunderson, 2019).

Nonetheless, the two disorders have differences; for example, unstable personal relationships and fear of being abandoned are common in BPD than in bipolar disorder. Due to the misunderstanding, a person with BPD might be misdiagnosed as having bipolar disorder, which adds to the confusion (Choi-Kain and Gunderson, 2019). It is necessary to note that the medications used to treat bipolar disorder cannot help patients diagnosed with a borderline personality disorder.

Some people also erroneously believe that only women can experience BPD (Chapman and Gratz, 2007). This belief is erroneous since although more women than men are diagnosed with BPD, the disorder is found in both genders. A man with BPD symptoms might be unwilling to seek treatment due to fear of being harshly judged by others. On the contrary, a woman may not be afraid to get an unbiased assessment since people might believe she has BPD due to her gender.

Furthermore, the symptoms which men discuss can mistakenly be linked to other disorders such as depression or post-traumatic disorder. Another popular myth associated with a borderline personality disorder is that people who have been diagnosed with the disorder experience similar symptoms and act in the same way. Another erroneous belief regarding the disorder is the view that it is not possible to diagnose BPD in children or adolescents. It is also widely believed that BPD is a personality defect or flaw. Being diagnosed with BPD does not signify that the personality of a person is flawed (Chapman and Gratz, 2007).

People with BPD are also believed to be manipulative and attention-seekers. Therefore, people around an individual diagnosed with a borderline personality disorder may believe that the person does not have any disease but is only seeking attention (Chapman and Gratz, 2007). These are some of the myths which have led to a misunderstanding regarding borderline personality disorder among the general population and also the healthcare providers.

Borderline Personality Disorder According to **DSM-5**

A borderline personality disorder is a common personality disorder that is predominant in clinical populations. A BPD diagnosis is based on a mental health practitioner's clinical evaluation. An appropriate assessment technique can entail presenting the disorder's criteria to patients and enquiring from them if the features correctly describe their condition (Gunderson, 2011). Active involvement of individuals in their BPD assessment can assist them to be more willing to agree to the diagnosis. At times, some mental health professionals prefer to keep the diagnosis from the patients. These professionals may do this either to protect the patient from the stigma associated with the disorder or because it is not treatable.

However, patients with BPD must be aware of their diagnosis as it may help them to embrace treatment more easily (Gunderson, 2011). Generally, psychological assessment entails asking the patient concerning the commencement and severity of the BPD symptoms. The assessment can also include asking questions regarding the impact of the symptoms on the patient's quality of life. Issues that can be addressed in this evaluation can entail self-harming behaviour and suicidal ideations.

Other tests for borderline personality disorder can entail laboratory tests and physical examinations to eliminate other likely factors that can trigger BPD symptoms like substance abuse. The *Diagnostic and Statistical Manual of Mental Disorders* published by the American Psychiatric Association is viewed as the official basis of diagnostic information concerning mental disorders, which includes borderline personality disorder (APA, 2013). *DSM* gives a list of symptoms and details the number of symptoms required and their severity to justify a particular diagnosis. A person is diagnosed with a borderline personality disorder if he or she meets five of the nine criteria in the *DSM*-5.

DSM-5 has defined borderline personality disorder as a persistent pattern of unsteadiness in a person's self-image, interpersonal relationships, and noticeable impulsivity. The symptoms listed in *DSM*-5 to identify the presence of **BPD** include severe impulsivity, which leads to risky behaviours, repeated suicidal or other self-harming threats or behaviours, and persistent feelings of emptiness (APA, 2013). The other symptoms include intense and inappropriate anger, unstable relationships, self-image, or emotions.

The symptoms specified in *DSM*-5, which can qualify for the diagnosis of borderline personality disorder include having an impaired ability to become attached to other people. The person could also be having dysfunctional behavioural issues linked to separation from those whom the person depends on or even other people. Additionally, based on *DSM*-5, for a person to be diagnosed with a borderline personality disorder, the individual should portray a troubled identity denoted by an evident insecure sense of self or self-image (APA, 2013). Borderline personality disorder, according to *DSM*-5, is also marked by continuous feelings of emptiness (APA, 2013). Additionally, the person may have a pattern of intense and unsteady interpersonal relationships characterised by fluctuations between idealisations (love and fondness) and devaluations (anger and dislike). The person with the disorder might dramatically change from viewing another individual as being perfect to seeing the same individual as being worthless. If the person feels supported or cared for by another individual, he or she may believe that this individual can do no wrong. Nevertheless, when the person feels abandoned or rejected, he or she may devalue the person and believe this individual can never do any right.

Borderline personality disorder based on *DSM*-5 also subjects those affected to mood swings marked by irritability, intense episodes of unhappiness or anxiety that lasts for extended periods (APA, 2013).

The person might also experience difficulties in managing these negative feelings when they occur. The mood swings can be so intense that the individual begins to become overwhelmed by immense emotional waves. This intense emotional response can be triggered by experiences or events that are disappointing to the person or stress-related even when the stresses are negligible or minor. For instance, a person might become extremely sad when a loved one is going on a business trip. An individual with a borderline personality disorder can also experience intense rage and have challenges managing the anger or rage. When under stress, individuals with BPD often become paranoid.

The person can also engage in repeated suicidal behaviours or threats or self-mutilating behaviour. The person could also engage in self-harm to relieve the intense emotions caused by BPD. Another symptom of borderline personality disorder, according to *DSM*-5, can also include impulsive behaviour where the person is involved in acts that are potentially self-damaging (APA, 2013). Impulsivity can make the affected individual act before thinking in self-damaging ways. For instance, the person may become involved in substance abuse, indiscriminate sex, reckless driving, overspending, or binge eating. Recurrent self-harming and suicidal behaviour, threats, or gestures can be another indication of borderline personality disorder. The inability to control anger or experiencing intense outrage can also be an indication of borderline personality disorder. For a person to be diagnosed with BPD, he or she should meet at least five of the nine symptoms specified in *DSM*-5

Controversies in the Diagnosis of the Borderline Personality Disorder

BPD has remained one of the most controversial personality disorder subgroups. The word borderline is often used in describing patients viewed as *difficult* and those who are considered untreatable or bring to mind unpleasant feelings and reactions such as helplessness and anger. Historically, borderline personality disorder was used to signify people who were regarded as emotional, needy, and had suicidal tendencies (Gunderson, 2009). The early borderline personality disorder personality descriptions portrayed the disorder as being unmanageable, leading to a sense of hopelessness among clinicians.

Not every person agrees that BPD is an authentic mental health condition. Despite years of studying BPD, the aetiology of the disorder has remained vague. There is a common agreement that BPD is caused by biological and environmental factors, neglect during childhood, and childhood abuse among others. Nevertheless, there is no clear path on what triggers borderline personality disorder. Although traumatic events are a factor in BPD development, there are people who, despite having undergone such experiences, do not have the disorder. Therefore, traumatic experiences cannot be regarded as a determining factor in BPD (Weniger *et al.*, 2009). Two people who have been diagnosed with BPD at times could have only a single common criterion. Borderline personality disorder has comorbidity and overlaps and with other personality disorders. The comorbidity complicates the accurate diagnosis of the disorder. The credibility of people with personality disorders has always been questioned. Controversy regarding people with BPD has been linked to dissociation or the impact the lack of attachment from physical experiences and emotions has on these individuals. Some people also believe that patients diagnosed with BPD are frequent liars. Lying is, therefore, believed to be a distinguishing trait of people with BPD. This erroneous belief can affect the quality of care individuals with BPD might receive in healthcare and legal systems.

Borderline personality disorder commonly appears clinically in the time of transiting from childhood to adulthood and can interrupt the intricate development tasks linked to this period and achieving the adult functioning role. However, diagnosing BPD, among other personality disorders before a person reaches the age of eighteen years, has remained a controversial issue (Chanen, and McCutcheon, 2013). There has been significant debate regarding the diagnosis of personality disorders among adolescents owing to the considerable developmental changes which occur in teenage years (Miller, Muehlenkamp, and Jacobson, 2008). Adolescence is linked to a high level of moodiness and impulsivity. A majority of adult borderline personality disorder patients state having had emotional challenges dating back to childhood and even adolescence. These reports suggest that there is a likelihood of BPD features being present among some adolescents, in spite of whether the disorder's full criteria are met or not.

Another controversy linked to BPD includes the validity and reliability of its diagnostic criteria.

It remains vague how adequately research or clinical diagnoses identify the experiences of people with people disorders. Studies report that BPD frequently overlaps with other personality disorders; therefore, it is difficult to find a person diagnosed with borderline personality disorder only (Krawitz and Jackson, 2008).

Age is another controversial issue in the borderline personality disorder diagnosis. Although much is known regarding the symptoms of borderline personality disorder in adults, little is known concerning the disorder in adolescents. In spite of the prevailing common agreement that various personality disorders have their origin in adolescence and childhood, the diagnosis of BPD before eighteen years is often faced with controversy (Chanen and McCutcheon, 2013). Most mental health professionals believe that individuals under the age of eighteen years still have their personality developing; therefore, diagnosing them with the disorder can be misleading.

Additionally, although the BPD symptoms listed in *DSM*-5 are similar for both adults and adolescents, some experts argue that the BPD symptoms in teenagers are different (Guilé *et al.*, 2018). Although adolescents with BPD may look for professional help, often a delay occurs between the symptoms' onset, seeking help, and identification of the disorder. Controversy regarding diagnosing borderline personality disorder among adolescents and the stigma associated with the disorder can lead to low rates of detection. Additionally, this stigma may cause clinicians to become reluctant to diagnose BPD in this age group (Miller, Muehlenkamp, and Jacobson, 2008).

Clinicians around the world are also sceptical concerning the diagnosis of BPD among youths and children due to various concerns. One of the concerns is that symptoms of the disorder, such as having a troubled self-image, impulsive behaviour, or instability in interpersonal relationships, are common features of adolescence (Miller, Muehlenkamp, and Jacobson, 2008). Another concern among clinicians is the desire to protect patients from the stigma that is associated with a borderline personality disorder.

When adolescents seek mental health services, rarely are they assessed; this has led to a large number of BPD cases remaining unidentified. Overlooking the likelihood of BPD as medical reality among adolescents can hinder successful clinical treatment (Miller, Muehlenkamp, and Jacobson, 2008). Many of the controversies surrounding borderline personality disorder diagnosis in adolescents focus on whether it is legal to diagnose personality disorders in this age group.

A BPD diagnosis among adolescents has strong simultaneous validity, which means it is linked to a high degree of impaired functioning and current distress. Furthermore, BPD features among adolescents are similar to those of adults (Miller, Muehlenkamp, and Jacobson, 2008). Another controversial issue regarding BPD diagnosis in adolescents is the risk that the diagnosis can haunt the individual even after the symptoms are long gone (Silk, 2008).

Since most mental health practitioners are reluctant to diagnose BPD among adolescents, the detection rates tend to below. Moreover, when adolescents are in contact with mental health professionally, rarely are personality disorders evaluated, leading to most cases of borderline personality disorder remaining unrecognised. Disregarding the likelihood of borderline personality disorder among adolescent can hinder successful clinical treatment (Miller, Muehlenkamp, and Jacobson, 2008). Regrettably, a BPD diagnosis can lead to rejection by the health professionals since clients are viewed as *too difficult*. Therefore, it is necessary to provide mental health professionals with information that can assist them in making clinically applicable BPD diagnoses. Provision of the right knowledge to clinicians will help them to make the correct diagnoses without any fear of stigmatising their patients (Silk, 2008). Failure to diagnose BPD can hinder accurate interventions, and the patient may be at risk of wrong intervention, which can be harmful.

Lack of proper assessment can make adolescents with borderline personality disorder be misdiagnosed or remain with no treatment. Without appropriate interventions, adolescents with BPD can experience constant challenges that can adversely impact their development increasing their sense of hopelessness and despair. Borderline personality disorder can be identified in youths who have presented themselves for clinical treatment and have similar symptoms to adults with BPD (Chanen *et al.*, 2008).

In adolescents, a borderline personality disorder may present itself through substance use, anxiety, and eating disorders among other mental health disorders (Kaess *et al.*, 2012). The psychosocial functioning of adolescents with borderline personality disorder tends to be lower in comparison with those with other psychiatric disorders (Kaess *et al.*, 2012). It is necessary to note that it is possible to identify borderline personality disorder in young adults and adolescents.

DSM-5 allows borderline personality disorder diagnosis in patients below eighteen years if the symptoms have persisted for a period longer than one year. *DSM*-5 does not exclude the diagnosis of personality disorders, including BPD among adolescents. However, a proper diagnosis is frequently hindered by a lack of developmentally accurate personality disorder criteria in adolescents (Chanen, and McCutcheon, 2013).

Studies report that most adolescents rarely maintain their BPD diagnosis for a period of more than one to three years after follow-up (Miller, Muehlenkamp, and Jacobson, 2008). Whether a BPD diagnosis continues into adulthood, borderline personality disorder merits intervention. Studies also show that the diagnosis of borderline personality disorder is as valid and reliable among adolescents as in adults (Winograd, Cohen, and Chen, 2008).

Furthermore, the risk factors for borderline personality disorder in adults are similar to those of adolescents. In reality, most environmental BPD risk factors arise during childhood. For instance, neglect, childhood abuse, parental loss, or separation has been associated with borderline personality disorder in both adolescents and adults. Studies have also demonstrated that children whose parents have been diagnosed with mental health conditions such as antisocial personality disorder, substance abuse, or depression are at a high risk of developing BPD. Therefore, there is a need for early diagnosis of the disorder among adolescents (Guilé *et al.*, 2018).

A borderline personality disorder diagnosis in adolescents can be performed when symptoms last for a period longer than one year. Since the adolescents' nature is still developing, the diagnosis should be made carefully. The clinician should base the evaluation on the history, thinking, coping, and emotional pattern of the adolescent. A diagnosis that is appropriately and carefully conducted based on *DSM*-5 criteria can help the client and his or her family and the clinician to plan suitable interventions. An appropriate diagnosis can also lessen the present and future challenges related to BPD. Since adolescents can break away from the diagnosis, it is necessary to continually re-evaluate them to see whether the diagnosis is still correct (Silk, 2008).

Studies report that when adolescents and other young patients' exhibit symptoms indicative of borderline personality disorder, it is essential to evaluate the possible benefits against the stigmatisation risks. Healthcare professionals must receive training on how to handle the stigma associated with the disorder in young clients (Chanen *et al.*, 20008). It is necessary to exercise caution when making a borderline personality disorder diagnosis to ensure its accuracy. At times clinicians view borderline personality disorder as suitable for patients that are difficult to treat.

Health care professionals should perform appropriate clinical evaluations, especially by avoiding classifying all adolescents who engage in self-harming behaviour as having a borderline personality disorder. Clinicians should also openly discuss the BPD diagnosis and psychoeducation to both the adolescents and their families (Chanen *et al.*, 2009).

Comorbidity and Misdiagnosis of BPD

Either due to its position of bordering other conditions or the conceptual confusion, a borderline personality disorder is frequently comorbid with other mental health disorders (Grant *et al.*, 2008). The comorbidity level is so high that it is rare to find a person diagnosed with only BPD.

The disorder can adversely impact various aspects of an individual's life. A proper diagnosis of the disorder is often faced with various challenges. Various factors impede an appropriate diagnosis of the disorder. Some of the factors include the stigmatising attitudes people have regarding BPD, which makes clinicians reluctant to diagnose the disorder.

Additionally, the high comorbidity of BPD with other kinds of mental health disorders can contribute to its misdiagnosis. A borderline personality disorder is strongly linked to other mental disorders besides personality disorders (Grant *et al.*, 2008). Some of the disorders strongly related to BPD include bipolar disorder, post-traumatic stress disorder, depression, substance dependence, and generalised anxiety disorder. Typically, borderline personality patients meet the criteria for other mental health disorders (Harned, Rizvi, and Linehan, 2010).

A borderline personality disorder is also comorbid with other personality disorders such as dependent, histrionic, and narcissistic personality disorders. Although comorbidity is common in both women and men, studies have identified some gender disparities. For instance, antisocial, narcissistic, and substance-use disorders are common in men who have been diagnosed with BPD. On the contrary, panic disorder, dysthymia, major depressive disorder, social phobias, eating disorders, and post-traumatic stress disorder are common in women with BPD (Grant *et al.*, 2008). It is necessary to note that these results can indicate gender's primary impact instead of interaction between BPD and gender.

Popular beliefs regarding borderline personality disorder can decrease the chance of receiving a proper diagnosis. Additionally, the stigma associated with the disorder can make clinicians reluctant to diagnose the condition. Without the correct diagnosis, individuals with a borderline personality disorder may continue struggling with their symptoms. BPD, just like any other mental illness, can become a challenge to diagnose since there is no blood or medical tests which are available in screening the disorder. At times it becomes difficult to diagnose borderline personality disorder due to the similarity of its symptoms to other mental disorders (Harned, Rizvi, and Linehan, 2010).

One of the challenges encountered in the treatment of borderline personality disorder is that in most cases, the disorder has comorbidities. Most mental illnesses have comorbidities, but for individuals with a borderline personality disorder, they tend to be high. Borderline personality disorder commonly coexists with substance use, depression, and anxiety among other mental disorders (Wang *et al.*, 2012). Symptoms of these mental disorders can cause a clinician to miss the BPD diagnosis.

BPD is a heterogeneous disorder, and its symptoms significantly overlap with identity, impulsive, schizophrenic, depressive disorders (Harned, Rizvi, and Linehan, 2010). This overlap can be associated with comorbidity and in clinical practice, it is challenging at times, to establish if the symptoms presented are for borderline personality disorder or other related comorbid conditions. The main disparity between the symptoms of BPD and other conditions is that the disorder undergoes more inconsistency and fluctuation. For instance, a BPD patient may have intense suicidal thoughts, which may last for a short period only. The person may also experience doubts regarding his or her identity, but this can be short-lived.

Various disorders such as eating disorders, substance-related disorders, attention deficit hyperactive disorder, and personality disorders can be comorbid with BPD (Harned, Rizvi, and Linehan,

2010). Depression is also common among patients diagnosed with a borderline personality disorder. Symptoms of depression can also be a sign of borderline personality disorder. At times it is difficult to differentiate between depression and BPD. However, symptoms such as feelings of emptiness, abandonment, suicidal thoughts are most common in borderline personality disorder.

It is not very clear why individuals with BPD have comorbidities; however, this may be caused by the overlap of the symptoms of different mental disorders. The disorder can also be misdiagnosed since mental health professionals may find it difficult to differentiate it from other mood disorders. Borderline personality disorder has several comorbidities with other disorders, which include bipolar disorder (Harned, Rizvi, and Linehan, 2010). BPD is characterised by extreme changes in manic highs and depressive lows.

The affected individual can experience trouble controlling his or her emotions and often is disposed of risky behaviour. These symptoms can also be witnessed in people with borderline personality disorder; this means that a person with either bipolar or borderline personality disorders might have a difficult time getting the correct diagnosis (Harned, Rizvi, and Linehan, 2010). However, there are differences between the two conditions; individuals with BPD tend to have a fear of being abandoned, have an unstable relationship, and have trust issues. These symptoms are not common with people who have bipolar disorder.

Additionally, depressive symptoms in borderline personality disorder last long and are not periodic like for people with bipolar disorder (Wang et al., 2012). Environmental conditions rarely trigger the moods of people with bipolar disorder; nevertheless, people with BPD have their mood respond to environmental changes. The depressed mood caused by bipolar disorder cannot be lifted through a positive event. However, the depressed mood of a person with a borderline personality disorder can be raised through a positive event. Likewise, an adverse experience can diminish the excitement caused by BPD but cannot change the euphoria whose cause is bipolar disorder (Wang et al., 2012).

Borderline personality disorder is a complex disorder whose symptoms are similar to other mental health disorders (Wang *et al.*, 2012). A lot of mental health practitioners have little education or exposure to BP; therefore, it is easy to misdiagnose the disorder with a different mental health condition. When BPD is misdiagnosed as a bipolar disorder, it can adversely affect a patient who may likely receive the wrong medications. To prevent such a misdiagnosis, the patient should be honest and frank with the mental health professional regarding his or her symptoms.

A major depressive disorder is another common comorbidity of borderline personality disorder.

Studies show that people who have been diagnosed with one of the disorders tend to have the other (Wang *et al.*, 2012). Major depressive disorder and borderline personality disorder share some common symptoms, which include sleep problems, lack of interest in activities previously enjoyed, low moods, and fatigue. The similarity in the symptoms of the two disorders can lead to the misdiagnosis of BPD.

Impulsivity is one of the symptoms of borderline personality disorder; people with a substance use disorder can be impulsive; this makes the disorder comorbid with BPD (APA, 2013).

However, for a person to be diagnosed with BPD, he or she should be impulsive in several areas such as binge eating, spending, reckless driving, or sex. Additionally, an individual with a borderline personality disorder might not have substance use issues. Individuals with BPD might also develop an eating disorder in an attempt to regulate their emotions (Wang *et al.*, 2012).

Borderline personality disorder can also be comorbid with the post-traumatic stress disorder (Wang *et al.*, 2012). The two disorders share similar symptoms, which include mood swings, impulsiveness, past trauma, alienation, instability, and avoidance among others. Nonetheless, the two conditions are distinct; therefore, diagnosis and treatment should be different. Individuals with post-traumatic stress disorder do not experience significant challenges in overcoming their emotions. On the contrary, people with BPD may find it challenging to manage their feelings.

Moreover, by addressing past traumas, the emotional response of individuals with PTSD, which occur when these memories are activated, is reduced. On the other, a person with BPD may find it hard to be calm after experiencing intrusive flashbacks and memories. The extreme reaction may continue, regardless of any therapy provided to the person. It is necessary for mental health professionals always to remember that the interventions which can assist individuals with PTSD can aggravate the symptoms of borderline personality disorder. Therefore, an accurate diagnosis of BPD should be made, distinguishing it from PTSD to ensure those affected receive the right treatment (Cloitre *et al.*, 2014).

Self-Harm in Borderline Personality Disorder

People with borderline personality disorder are a high risk of engaging in self-harming behaviours such as self-mutilation (Oumaya *et al.*, 2008). A distressing and common symptom of borderline personality disorder is self-harm. Individuals with the disorder tend to act in an impulsive manner, such as becoming involved in drug and alcohol abuse, promiscuous behaviour, overspending, and self-harm, among others. Suicidal thoughts and self-injurious actions are common in many people with mental illnesses. People who are not affected by mental health conditions such as borderline personality disorder may view the thought of self-harm as pointless or even bizarre.

Nevertheless, to those affected by BPD, self-harm may seem like an effective way of temporary relief from internal pain. The truth, however, is that self-harm increases and intensifies the existing issues. Regrettably, the desire to manage the immediate physical threat created by self- harming behaviour may divert from complex issues. The self-harming practices are one of the primary factors used to diagnose a borderline personality disorder, according to

DSM-5 (American Psychiatric Association, 2013). However, for individuals struggling with a borderline personality disorder, the risk of such behaviours tends to high. Fifty to eighty per cent of people diagnosed with BPD engage in self-harm, the most common method being cutting (Oumaya *et al.*, 2008). A lot of individuals with borderline personality disorder engage in self-harming acts such as burning, overdosing on drugs, scratching their skin, hitting, and cutting among others. Most of these individuals engage in such behaviours as a way of releasing the extreme emotional turmoil they could be experiencing (Oumaya *et al.*, 2008). The presence of self-harming action is a strong predictor that the person in the future might attempt suicide. Self-harm in people with a borderline personality disorder is often linked to emotional imbalance and a disturbing way of processing pain.

Patients with the disorder who are engaged in self-harming behaviour tend to have high levels of pain as related to emotional stress. It is necessary for family members and other caregivers to understand that these are some of the primary motives of the person engaging in self-injurious acts. Signs that a person is engaged in self-harming behaviour to include bruises, burns, and visible scars (Oumaya *et al.*, 2008). Other indications of self-harm include a person accumulating sharp objects, bloody paper towels, and tissues in the trash, and bloodstains on the person's clothes.

The person might also become excessively secretive, spending extended periods in the bathroom alone. Self-harm tends to follow a cycle; the affected individual might become anxious, and the resulting impulse may be self-harm. The person might try to refuse the impulse, which only creates more tension. To release the tension, the individual may engage in self-harming acts; often shame or scars resulting from the behaviour can lead to more anxiety, creating a never- ending cycle.

Chronic self-harming behaviour can put the individual of suicide in the future. The person can become accustomed to the pain of self-harm, and when this ceases to help as a coping technique, he or she can resort to suicide. Even in circumstances where the self-harming acts are mild, the impact can be disastrous. Self-injury can increase a person's risk of intended or accidental death. Feelings of guilt and failure can torment an individual who is affected by borderline personality disorder and who is experiencing difficulties in relationships. Such a person can decide to punish himself by hurting his own body. At times self-harm can be used as a way of punishing another person. For instance, a person can hurt himself to show the impact of the lack of attention from family members or friends is having on him or her (Bresin, 2014).

Why do Individuals with Borderline Personality Disorder Engage in Self-Harming Behaviours?

People affected by borderline personality disorder may engage in self-harming behaviours for several reasons, as outlined below:

- *Escape or relief from emotional pain*—most people with BPD engage in self-harm to avoid or run away from emotional pain. Individuals who are affected by the disorder are usually very emotional. These people tend to experience extreme emotions, which at times could be unbearable or overwhelming (Chapman and Gratz, 2007). Additionally, these individuals may encounter challenges in controlling their feelings and most of the time do not know how to make themselves feel better when angry. For some of these people, the only way to manage these emotions is through self-harm. Studies have shown that some of these individuals resort to self-harm to feel better. However, it is essential to state that relief is usually short-lived. After the self-harming act such as cutting is over, the person is often plagued by feelings of guilt and shame. Additionally, the behaviour prevents the person from learning effective techniques of feeling better.
- *Self-punishment*—people with a borderline personality disorder may engage in self-harming behaviour as a way of

punishing themselves for some supposed wrongdoing. Anger with oneself can lead to agitation, which might influence the affected individual to look for ways to solve the existing problems without consideration of any adverse consequence. Self-punishment does not solve anything. Rather, it affirms that the person deserved the punishment leading to worse feelings.

- *Generate feelings*—individuals with a borderline personality disorder often report feeling numb, detached, incapable of exerting any influence, and empty. The person may engage in self-harm as a way of generating feelings (Chapman and Gratz, 2007). The person might opt to feel pain rather than empty or numb. In such cases, the person may engage in the self-harming behaviour in secret or hidden parts of the body since their aim is not to attract attention.

- *To become less burdensome to other people*—a person with a borderline personality disorder can feel as if he or she is a burden to their family or friends. The individual can have thoughts that other people would be better off without him. Such thoughts can lead to suicide (Chapman and Gratz, 2007).

- *As a way of influencing or communicating with other people*—individuals who are diagnosed with a borderline personality disorder often experience problems in their interpersonal relationships. These people also lack skills in asking other people what they would want. Due to this, the person might feel compelled to look for different ways of communication, which can include self-harm (Chapman and Gratz, 2007). Therefore, self-harming behaviour in borderline personality disorder can be used to seek support and attention.

Self-harming behaviour can lead to feelings of shame and loneliness since it is frequently performed in secret. The guilt and secrecy can harm the individual's interpersonal relationships. Furthermore, self-harming behaviours, such as cutting, can lead to fatal wounds. The risk of developing other mental health conditions such as alcohol and drug abuse and major depression is also enhanced if the behaviour is not addressed early enough. Self-harming can also become addictive; therefore, the necessary therapeutic approach is essential.

Pathology of Narcissism—the Danger of Misperception

The best word that describes narcissism is misdirection because narcissists are the complete opposite of what they appear to be. Anger is not anger; it is fear, empathy, if any, is actually projective identification and blame is a shame!

Narcissism is a spectrum and narcissist are people, therefore, it is all about the brain pathways and a mindset. Narcissism is not a diagnosis, borderline or narcissistic personality disorders are. What makes narcissism special is the process of reality. In this case, reality is processed in different more egocentric way. When disagreement on perception is present, there is diversity and that often creates unhealthy or toxic relationship. The stronger disagreements are more toxic relationship will be.

The perception of a narcissist is often distorted by their emotions, resulting in paranoia, Delusions, and egocentric behaviour. When narcissists are asked to explain their actions or ideas, they often sound illogical, and for that reason, people around them see them as a seriously mentally ill individuals. The main evidence for the narcissists is their feelings and emotions.

For example, if someone sad something and all of the sudden a narcissist gets hurt, the reality for the narcissist is that others are hurting them. Even others have difficulties to understand why a narcissist is hurt. When asked to explain why they are offended, narcissists will present their feelings as proof of others hurting them purposely, trying to convince others that their feelings have been attacked. Unfortunately, these irrational logic circles are the core evidence and basis for narcissists to determine their reality. Due to distorted perception, narcissists' defensive mechanism caused them to often feel hurt, shame, fear, jealousy, and rejection.

Narcissists have a strong quest for winning in order to validate their thoughts, feelings, and emotions. Everything that is happening around them is usually perceived that is because or for them, therefore, they are never hurt by accident. In narcissists' eyes, this world is made for them only, and without their importance, this world will stop. If narcissists are physically violent and you asked them to leave you home because you do not want to tolerate their behaviour, they will be hurt because you asked them to leave, regardless of their inappropriate behaviour. When a narcissists are caught cheating, they turn responsibility to a partner who checked their phone.

Narcissists are always convinced that they are born special and that they never do things wrong.

Mirroring

In order to function, a narcissist needs a constant evaluation from others due to his distortion of Self-image and self-worth (the same way as babies and little children require it). During the honeymoon stage of the relationship, the narcissist believes that the other person is perfect because the other person holds a strong belief that they are indeed perfect. Unfortunately, that does not last long because of jealousy that narcissist feels. If a narcissist perceives that others are better or superior to them, feelings of helplessness, shame and worthlessness occur.

This is often perceived as an attack by a narcissist and usually results as an emotional rage and a hysterical attack. The main problem is that a narcissist is highly dependent on others. Therefore, the evaluation of their self-worth can be achieved only if others around them are doing things wrong. For example, a narcissist can only win or be right if others lose or others are wrong. Narcissistic life is either black or white, perfect of not, nothing in between. The most difficult thing for narcissists to accept is that they are not perfect.

Splitting

Splitting often happens when a mind creates two different categories or two different images for the same thing. This usually happens in babies and young children. It is a common defence mechanism created by people suffering from personality disorders. Narcissists are always accusing others of abusing them because they don't perceive them as perfect. Splitting is causing a lot of problems for narcissists because it affects their evaluation circle. If a narcissist sees themselves perfect, others are immediately worthless. Therefore, they should be treated that way. This is one way of explaining why narcissists are lacking empathy towards others.

Hoovering

As soon narcissists realise that they went too far and the relationship has been ruined, they will do everything they can to stop others to leave or ignore them. Hoovering is all about the control of the recourses. In this case, it is a relationship, which is undoubtedly important for a narcissist to keep playing his manipulative game. Narcissists have an extreme level of anxiety in an area of being rejected and abandoned by others. Because they depend on others just like children, they must keep their relationships going in order to fulfil their psychological needs. If narcissists are not in a position to keep the relationship, the anxiety level rises enormously, resulting in rage, paranoia, violence, cold silence, or simple social withdrawal because their sense of helplessness is caused by the inability to control and manipulate others.

Survival mode is a daily battle for narcissists, and for that reason, they are struggling to show any empathy due to perceiving the world around them as a threat. Sometimes when narcissists are in deep control of the relationship, they can show some empathy. For example, if during the day a news of an accident breaks through, narcissists can feel sorry for the people involved in the accident as long they have nothing to lose and that accident has nothing to do with their relationships.

Here and Now

Narcissists live for now and they have difficulties to understand that their behaviour will cause problems later. A survival situation causes survival mode. In that state, it is impossible to trust, care, or even show some empathy. Survival mode and fear cancel empathy. The most common behaviour pattern by narcissists is problem-creating. Creating a problem out of nothing is usually caused by chronic anger. Narcissists are often claiming that they are offended and day-to-day living with them is tiring, toxic, unpredictable, and damaging.

How to Leave a Narcissist

To conclude, narcissists are empty, toxic, fake, and very miserable people who only spread anger, Hate, and misery around by creating unnecessary problems and nothing else than abuse. Narcissism is a modern disease of our society which destroys and affects many lives in our communities. My recommendations to everyone who is dealing with a narcissist is very simple. Keep being emotionally stable and constantly repeat these four phrases to a narcissist, 'Your anger is your responsibility, not mine. I guess I have to accept how you feel. I can accept your faulty perception of me and others. I am sorry that you feel that way!' Please do not be scared to call the emergency hotline and local mental health team when a narcissist is experiencing emotional and hysterical attacks, especially in front of children. Nobody deserves to be psychologically or physically abused. Before leaving a narcissist, one must understand that such a relationship is abusive and destructive. Once fully aware of it, one will never make a mistake of returning to the toxic relationship. Dealing with a narcissist is not a marriage, friendship, or communication problem; it is a mental health problem. My idol, the greatest British philosopher Bertrand Russell made an excellent point by saying that one without clarity and exact thinking can only make mistakes without knowing it. I guess the danger of misperception is more than just making mistakes. It causes harm! Once disconnected from their intellect, narcissists' emotions will make them jealous, petty, hateful, angry, sadistic, aggressive, possessive, manipulative, paranoid, etc. To conclude, the best way to live a narcissist-free life is to be boring towards them. Narcissists need drama and attention; they are emotionally driven people and as soon as you stop reacting to their behaviour, they will leave you alone. In psychology, there is a method called a grey rock. Will a grey rock respond to everything that narcissists are doing? Rocks are not responding; therefore, you will never see a narcissist argue with a rock. If you can do the same, I can guaranty to you that you will enjoy a narcissist-free life.

Why Narcissists Won't Let Go

Why narcissist won't let go. The reason is very simple, control. Narcissists want to control everything and everyone in order to overcome their real feelings of not being in control. If this is not working, they will keep trying to re-establish the relationship not because they love and care; it is just to gain control over the relationship.

Why Did Narcissists Get This Way?

Nature versus nurture? Nature can, in short, be described as our genetic predisposition, something that we are born with. On the other hand, nurture is everything external that influences and shapes our behaviour. In the case of narcissism, nature plays the greatest role, up to 70%. Some people are just born soft and nice, others just difficult to deal with. I do believe that the best way to become a narcissist is to be raised by one. Having inherited the genetic predispositions from a caregiver and to be constantly exposed to anger, shame, insecurity, crime, lying, and learn manipulation is the best recipe to become a narcissist.

What We Can Learn from Narcissists

We can get a valuable lesson on how to appreciate love and care. Narcissists will show us what love and peace are not. Once far from a narcissist, one can truly appreciate love and care. In addition, taking responsibility for your emotions is another lesson that can be learned. Due to the lack of emotional control, a narcissist will always play a victim in order to escape the responsibility, often blaming others for their emotional state. Responsibility and control over the emotions and actions are strong attributes to stay well and healthy.

Treating Self-Harming Behaviours

Treating self-harming behaviours involves persuading individuals to give up on the act. Therapy can be used to find out the cause of the emotional condition and help the person to learn different approaches to managing them. Treating self-harming behaviour is complex and entails comprehensive and extended therapy. An established therapeutic approach used to treat people who repetitively engage in self-harming behaviour is dialectical behavioural therapy. However, there are other treatment approaches such as transference-focused psychotherapy and mentalisation-based therapy.

Apart from the professional therapies, there are other coping mechanisms that the affected person can adopt to manage or eradicate the behaviour. Some of the coping mechanisms can include identifying the triggers, looking for alternative coping techniques, or confiding in someone.

Dialectical Behavioural Therapy

This is a therapy structured initially to address issues linked to self-harming behaviour in peoplediagnosed with a borderline personality disorder. DBT as a treatment approach for people diagnosed with BPD emphasises on emotional regulation, mindfulness, tolerance to distress, and interpersonal effectiveness. A standard dialectical behavioural therapy employs cognitive and behavioural approaches. Patients learn adaptive coping skills linked to the principal challenging areas attributed to borderline personality disorder. The problem areas addressed in dialectical behaviour therapy include tolerance to distress, interpersonal effectiveness, regulation of one's emotions, and reducing the confusion regarding identity (Linehan *et al.*, 2015). The overarching DBT goal is to address the affected person's underlying issues with emotion dysregulation and help him. People diagnosed with borderline personality disorder learn to adjust their emotions without having to engage in regulatory behaviours or unproductive compensatory such as self-harming behaviours. Dialectical behavioural therapy involves four stages namely the pre-treatment phase and three distinct treatment phases identity (Linehan *et al.*, 2015).

It is the responsibility of the therapist to remain conscious of the goals of the treatment to ensure the activities are directed towards generating a life worth living for the patient. In the pre-treatment phase, the client is oriented to the structure and philosophy of DBT to commit to following the goals of the therapy. For instance, if the client is currently involved in self- mutilation, he should agree that getting rid of the behaviour is a goal to pursue.

In dialectical behavioural therapy, it is often assumed that most of the problems a patient experiences are as a result of a deficit in their behavioural skills and motivational issues. Owing to this, DBT stresses the need to build skills as a way of facilitating behavioural change. DBT applies acceptance skills modules such as tolerance to distress and mindfulness and the change skills modules, which include interpersonal effectiveness and emotion regulation to assist

BPD patients in accepting their reality. Mindfulness skills train BPD patients to focus their attention on the current moment and also address their sense of self-dysregulation and the feeling of disconnection (Neacsiu *et al.*, 2010). The distress acceptance skills are used to enhance the patient's capacity to accept and go through the crisis without becoming overwhelmed. The interpersonal efficiency assists in enhancing relationships and learn how to manage conflicts while upholding self-respect. Skills taught on emotional regulation in DBT help in reducing the emotional vulnerability of the patient. These skills help BPD patients to gain enhanced behavioural and emotional control, leading to reducing the chance of engaging in self-harming behaviours (Neacsiu *et al.*, 2010). These skills are taught in a group set-up, which assists in sharing individual experiences with people who have undergone similar issues.

The aim of skills training is to educate the patient regarding general skills, which can help in solving life challenges. As a primary component of dialectical behaviour therapy, skills training address directly the cognitive, behavioural, and emotional-dysfunctional patterns that lead to self-harming behaviours. Additionally, patients through these skills can enhance their emotional understanding and observation, thereby reducing their emotional vulnerability which can decrease the self-harming behaviours (Neacsiu *et al.*, 2010) DBT also employs telephone coaching for various reasons, which include overcoming challenges BPD patients have in asking for assistance and often depend on extreme behaviours such as self- harming as a way of asking for help. Borderline personality disorder patients are encouraged to ask for assistance before engaging in a self-harming act to be coached and reminded of how to use the skills they have learned. Telephone coaching is a necessary preventive measure as it focuses on self-harming behaviour evaluation and the employment of a different solution to address the issue (Chalker *et al.*, 2015).

Phone calls are an efficient approach to enhancing the satisfaction of a patient and lessening the likelihood of dropping out of therapy (Chalker *et al.*, 2015). A therapist's availability away from planned personal sessions assists in developing a sense of connectedness and security for the **BPD** patient (Coyle, Shaver, and Linehan, 2018). Dialectical behavioural therapy through telephone coaching indirectly decreases the risk of engaging in self-harming behaviours.

A consultation team is an integral part of **DBT**; for therapy to be effective; adequate attention should be given to both the therapist and patient. Every **DBT** therapist should be part of a consultation team and engage in regular meetings. Therapists usually experience intense feelings when dealing with **BPD** patients, which can lead to high-stress levels. The consultation teams play a significant role in assisting therapists to be aware of their limits to evade a burnout (Walsh, Ryan, and Flynn, 2018). Reports from various randomised, controlled trials show that dialectical behaviour therapy is linked to a decrease in the severity and frequency of self-harming behaviours, suicidal ideations, and suicidal attempts. Furthermore, **DBT** has been linked to reduced treatment attrition rates, and reduced frequency in the emergency room compared to other treatments.

Transference-Focused Psychotherapy

This therapy was developed to help people struggling with self-harming behaviours, especially those diagnosed with **BPD**. Transference-focused psychotherapy is based on the psychoanalytic theory. The goal of the therapy is to assist patients in changing their behavioural reactions to stress, particularly in interpersonal relationships. Compared to other treatments, in TFP, the role of the therapist is significant. During the sessions, the therapist works on his or her relationship with the patient. The primary emphasis is on the patients' feelings regarding their relationship with the therapist.

TFP tries to identify the challenging interpersonal issues in the life of the patient and the ensuing emotional conditions, which can lead to self-harm. The patient's innate interpersonal dynamic occurs during his interaction with the therapist. TFP approach helps patients to obtain a systematic, integrated, and balanced pattern of thinking regarding themselves and others. In most cases, TFP entails individual therapy sessions that occur regularly. Transference-focused psychotherapy has been proven effective in lessening anger, which can lead to self-harming behaviour.

Mentalisation-Based Treatment

Mentalisation refers to the process through which a person imagines the feelings and thoughts of oneself and those of others to understand interpersonal relationships (Bateman and Fonagy, 2016). The process of mentalisation is often difficult for people diagnosed with a borderline personality disorder, especially when they are emotionally aroused. Mentalisation-based treatment holds the view that borderline personality disorder symptoms such as self-harm emerge when the patient ceases to mentalise. Consequently, the patient may begin to operate from a certainty that is irrational regarding other people's motives. The patient also experiences hyper-activated attachment interactions making them unable to cope. The therapy holds the view that borderline personality disorder, which frequently leads to self-harm, arises from the patients' lack of knowledge regarding the link between emotions and thoughts. MBT purposes of stabilising the symptoms of borderline personality disorder by strengthening the ability of the patient to mentalise. During the therapy sessions, the therapist assumes a position of curiosity intending to encourage the patients to evaluate their interpersonal and emotional situation on a flexible and grounded lens.

Patients are also trained on how to focus on their thoughts and the likely thoughts in other individual's minds. Patients further learn on the effect of such thoughts on their emotional responses and challenging behaviours such as self-harm. Mentalisation-based treatment helps patients to learn how to control their behaviours, emotions, and impulses. Often, this enhances their relationships with others (Bateman and Fonagy, 2016).

Schema-Based Therapy

Schema-based therapy focuses on identifying and modifying a particular unhealthy pattern of thinking. The theory behind the therapy assumes that when the basic needs of a child, such as love, acceptance, and safety, are unmet. A person develops an unhealthy way of interacting with other people (referred to as maladaptive early schemas). Schemas are patterns held deeply regarding the view of oneself and that of the world (Arntz and Van Genderen, 2011). When people due to childhood trauma or abuse have developed unhealthy schemas, often they resort to harmful techniques of behaving and thinking in responding to the new circumstance. The theory further proposes that most of the BPD symptoms are as a result of hard childhood experiences like being separated from caregivers at an early age, abuse, or maltreatment. These experiences often cause the development of maladaptive early schemas. The purpose of this therapy in borderline personality disorders is to identify the person's significant schemas and relate them to past experiences and current symptoms (Arntz and Van Genderen, 2011).

Afterwards, the patient and therapist develop techniques of processing emotions linked to the schemas and changing destructive coping mechanisms such as self-harm. For instance, the patient and therapist may perform exercises aimed at breaking unhealthy behavioural patterns such as self-harm or altering unhealthy thinking patterns. Both schema-focused therapy and dialectical behavioural therapy have proven effective in decreasing borderline personality disorder symptoms such as self-harm (Arntz and Van Genderen, 2011).

Confidence in Someone

Although it might be frightening to open up on something that one has tried to hide for an extended period, it is often a relief to eventually share on the struggle of self-harming. When talking about the behaviour, it is appropriate to share on the triggers that lead to it since this can help the other person to understand the problem better.

Identify the Self-Harm Triggers

Recovery can be enhanced when the affected individual understands the triggers to self-harm. Some of the triggers may include anger, emptiness, anxiety, shame, sadness, or loneliness. If it is difficult to identify the triggers, the person may need to work on his or her emotional awareness. This refers to the ability to understand their feeling and the reasons for the emotions. Emotional awareness is also the capacity to express one's feelings moment by moment and to follow the link between emotions and actions. Emotions are necessary for our bodies, but they do not have to lead to self-harming actions such as cutting.

What Is the Prognosis of Borderline Personality Disorder?

BPD was previously believed to be chronic, severe, and a disorder with no cures and had a poor prognosis. In the past, when a person was diagnosed with a borderline personality disorder, he or she had little hope of ever recovering. However, this has changed over time; with appropriate treatment, a person diagnosed with the disorder can learn how to manage the symptoms and enjoy a lasting decrease of the symptoms (Paris, 2008). Although individuals diagnosed with a borderline personality disorder can experience a difficult time recovering, they may enjoy prolonged recovery after experiencing extended periods of remission of symptoms. No two individuals diagnosed with BPD experience similar symptoms; therefore, the prognosis for recovery can only be identified on a case-by-case basis. Although borderline personality disorder is linked to many challenges and a high suicide rate even after patients cease to meet the diagnosis criteria, reports show that BPD has a natural tendency to improve

(Paris, 2008). Improvement in a personality disorder, including borderline personality disorder, is not equal to a cure since symptoms might reduce with time; however, some of them last for a lifetime. Although borderline personality disorder was viewed initially as an unmanageable disorder, a lot of evidence shows considerable rates of remittance over time and hence a better prognosis than previously envisaged (Paris, 2009).

Current treatment interventions of BPD, according to studies, have shown that over 90% of those treated have reported a two-year remission and 86 % a four-year remission (Gunderson *et al.*, 2011). Such findings portray a positive outlook of the BPD prognosis than what was previously witnessed. Although borderline personality disorder is not curable, proper treatment can lead to a prolonged period of remission of the symptoms. With the right treatment, most individuals with a borderline personality disorder can get relief from symptoms that are distressing and also realise remission.

A study conducted on patients with BPD who were hospitalised showed that 86% of them sustained a steady improvement from symptoms (Zanarini *et al.*, 2010). It is necessary to note that the personality of a patient can play a significant role during therapy leading to improved clinical outcomes. Studies have shown that borderline personality therapy patients with a high degree of agreeableness trait undergoing dialectical behavioural therapy demonstrate enhanced clinical outcomes. On the contrary, patients with low levels of agreeableness and are not receiving DBT treatment have worse clinical outcomes (Hirsh, 2012).

Patients with a high degree of agreeableness develop a strong working relationship with their therapist leading to enhanced clinical outcomes (Hfcairsh, 2012). With the right treatment, individuals with BPD realise better psychosocial functioning. It is essential to recognise that due to borderline personality disorder's genetic predisposition, there are no absolute treatments for the disorder. The period when the patient's mental health condition has improved is described as partial remission since not all the symptoms ultimately improve. Additionally, the symptoms may come back to some extent, often as a result of stress. The recurrence and deterioration of the symptoms commonly described as relapse often need short periods of other therapy, supportive measures, and medications.

Frequently it is difficult to achieve full recovery since various factors often influence the rate of recovery. Some of these factors include the severity of the disorder before the treatment commences, the condition of the patient's existing relationships, and whether the person has a history of childhood abuse (Hfcairsh, 2012). Additionally, whether or not the individual gets the right treatment and the duration it takes before the treatment is received can influence the prognosis.

Patients who have other disorders such as depression and other emotional problems are likely to have a relapse of their borderline personality disorder symptoms. On the contrary, individuals who have a stable school or employment status after the symptoms have subsided often experience fewer relapses. The prognosis of BPD can be enhanced by including intermittent psychotherapy (Wedig *et al.*, 2013). Most of the borderline personality disorder specialised treatment tends to be expensive and often lasts for a period of one to three years. Consequently, these treatments become costly. Therefore, intermittent treatment can help patients to address different challenges at various times in their lives. For instance, dialectical behaviour therapy focuses mainly on suicidality and self-harm, which are frequently early symptoms of BPD. As these symptoms reduce with time, older patients might have to deal with feelings such as fear of abandonment and emptiness, which DBT does not address (Wedig *et al.*, 2013). An intermittent approach can assist patients in concentrating on particular issues at specific periods in their lives. Besides treatment, a better prognosis can be achieved by providing support to patients diagnosed with BPD to help them achieve complete recovery. Some of the psychosocial programs can include specialists who may assist patients in developing necessary skills for any kind of work.

Borderline Personality Disorder
Neurobiological Roots

Historically BPD was believed to be caused by childhood trauma. Although many mental illnesses are strongly linked to childhood trauma, neurobiological factors have been recognised in patients diagnosed with BPD. Borderline personality disorder has a neurobiological and genetic component. Studies have demonstrated that some symptoms of BPD, especially problems in making decisions and regulation of emotions, could have neurobiological roots (Leander, Moore, and Chartrand, 2009). According to *DSM-5*, borderline personality disorder patients often have an underlying susceptibility to emotional hyper-arousal conditions. These conditions occur due to defects in the neurobiological system, which controls stress and emotional regulation. These individuals are also vulnerable to interpersonal and social stress owing to the defect in the neurobiological systems moderating social reward, cognition, and attachment. When stressed, borderline personality disorder patients cannot control their emotions and often revert to their previous state. Neurobiological studies have implied that the neuropeptide functions can predispose BPD patients to interpersonal problems (Stanley and Siever, 2009). The dysfunction of the hypothalamic adrenal axis (HPA) can play a significant role in developing a borderline personality disorder. Studies have been conducted on the HPA axis in people who have undergone childhood trauma and have been diagnosed with BPD.

The studies have revealed that the HPA axis of people who have experienced childhood abuse is often dysregulated. The production of cortisol, which is released as a response to stress, is regulated by the HPA axis. People with borderline personality disorder also have high levels of cortisol, which indicates a hyperactive HPA axis (Rausch *et al.*, 2015). As a result, these people have a higher biological stress reaction, which can be linked to their vulnerability to irritability. Additionally, research has shown that BPD patients frequently demonstrate high levels of the stress hormone and a decreased sensitivity to feedback

(Rausch *et al.*, 2015). Enhanced activity of HPA and reduced levels of the peripheral oxytocin combined with childhood abuse can lead to the development of BPD (Bertsch *et al.*, 2013). Neuroimaging research on borderline personality disorder patients has shown that these people have a bilateral decrease in their medial temporal lobe, amygdala, and the hippocampus (Siever *et al.*, 2008). BPD patients, due to a smaller amygdala, that is overactive, tend to experience more intense emotions than the general population. An overactive amygdala can lead to extreme anger and desperate efforts to avoid imaginary or real abandonment. Additionally, a highly activated amygdala can make the brain provide excessive significance to a signal which ultimately causes issues in modulating the management and processing of these signals in the other parts of the brain. Impulsivity is a primary characteristic of borderline personality disorder, and it is linked to the control and reward circuits. The erratic and intense emotions experienced by BPD patients can be connected to the hyperactivity of the amygdala. Research showing a decrease in the amygdala's grey matter quantity in older borderline personality disorder patients has been viewed as revealing a progressive pathology that is reversible (Kimmel *et al.*, 2016). The increase of the grey matter volume has also been linked to exaggerated reactions viewed in the amygdala to emotional stimuli. Furthermore, difficulties in emotional regulation among BPD patients have been linked to the inadequate ability of the prefrontal cortex activity, cognitive processes (Silvers *et al.*, 2016). Insufficient and inefficient prefrontal cortexes can be linked to impulsivity in BPD patients. Various studies comparing borderline personality disorder patients with people who do not have the disorder have reported that those with BPD have reduced volumes of the medial temporal lobes, hippocampus, and amygdala (Soloff *et al.*, 2008). The hippocampus plays a significant role in declarative memory and memory consolidation. Additionally, the hippocampus is often sensitive to the impact of stress. The hippocampus of BPD patients tends to be in constant hyper-arousal. The hippocampus among these individuals is also dysfunctional and uncoordinated, constantly misinterpreting threats, and conveying false messages to the amygdala.

A reduced volume of the hippocampus can cause perceptual distortions, identity instability, and neurocognitive deficits. These symptoms are common in borderline personality disorder patients (Soloff *et al.*, 2008). The interpretation is that borderline personality patients are likely to view the world and the people around them as threatening, whereas this may not be the reality. Studies have also reported that people diagnosed with a borderline personality disorder often show abnormal cortisol levels in their bloodstream. The cortisol chemical is usually released when a person is under stress (Rausch *et al.*, 2015). High cortisol levels translate to experiencing overwhelming stress daily. Due to this, the person's coping and resilience skills may be undermined, which can overwhelm the body chemically. Recent evidence on adults with borderline personality disorder shows a gene-environment correlation and interaction with the development of the disorder. This indicates that people with sensitive genotype are at a higher risk of developing BPD when exposed to the predisposing environment. Additionally, the genes that influence BPD features also enhance the probability of becoming exposed to particular negative life situations. One study reported that stabilising the BPD features between mid to late adolescence is mostly influenced by genetic and environmental factors (Bornovalova *et al.*, 2009).

REFERENCES

American Psychiatric Association (2013) 'Diagnostic and statistical manual of mental disorders', BMC Med, 17, pp. 133–137.

Arntz, A., and Van Genderen, H. (2011) *Schema Therapy for Borderline Personality Disorder*, John Wiley & Sons.

Bateman, A., and Fonagy, P. (2016) *Mentalization-Based Treatment for Personality Disorders: A Practical Guide*, Oxford University Press.

Bertsch, K., Schmidinger, I., Neumann, I. D., and Herpertz, S. C. (2013) 'Reduced plasma oxytocin levels in female patients with a borderline personality disorder', *Hormones and Behavior*, *63*(3), pp. 424–429.

Bornovalova, M. A., Hicks, B. M., Iacono, W. G., and McGue, M. (2009) 'Stability, change, and heritability of borderline personality disorder traits from adolescence to adulthood: A longitudinal twin study', *Development and Psychopathology*, *21*(4), pp. 1335–1353.

Bresin, K. (2014) 'Five indices of emotion regulation in participants with a history of non suicidal self-injury: A daily diary study', *Behavior Therapy*, *45*(1), pp. 56–66.

Brunner, R., Henze, R., Richter, J., and Kaess, M. (2015) 'Neurobiological findings in youth with a borderline personality disorder', *Scandinavian Journal of Child and Adolescent Psychiatry and Psychology*, *3*(1), pp. 22–30.

Chalker, S. A., Carmel, A., Atkins, D. C., Landes, S. J., Kerbrat, A. H., and Comtois, K. A. (2015) 'Examining challenging behaviors of clients with a borderline personality Disorder', *Behavior Research and Therapy*, *75*, pp. 11–19.

Chanen, A. M., and McCutcheon, L. (2013) 'Prevention and early intervention for borderline personality disorder: current status and recent evidence', *The British Journal of Psychiatry*, *202*(s54), pp. s24–s29.

Chanen, A. M., Jovev, M., Djaja, D., McDougall, E., Yuen, H. P., Rawlings, D., and Jackson, H. J. (2008) 'Screening for borderline personality disorder in outpatient youth', *Journal of personality disorders*, *22*(4), pp. 353–364.

Chanen, A. M., Jovev, M., McCutcheon, L. K., Jackson, H. J., and McGorry, P. D. (2008) 'Borderline personality disorder in young people and the prospects for prevention and early intervention', *Current Psychiatry Reviews*, *4*(1), pp. 48–57.

Chanen, A. M., McCutcheon, L. K., Germano, D., Nistico, H., Jackson, H. J., and McGorry, P. D. (2009) 'The HYPE Clinic: an early intervention service for borderline personality Disorder', *Journal of Psychiatric Practice*, *15*(3), pp. 163–172.

Chapman, A., and Gratz, K. (2007) *The Borderline Personality Disorder Survival Guide: Everything You Need to Know About Living With BPD*, New Harbinger Publications.

Choi-Kain, L. W., and Gunderson, J. G. (eds.) (2019) *Applications of Good Psychiatric Management for Borderline Personality Disorder: A Practical Guide*, American Psychiatric Pub.

Cloitre, M., Garvert, D. W., Weiss, B., Carlson, E. B., and Bryant, R. A. (2014) 'Distinguishing PTSD, complex PTSD, and borderline personality disorder: A latent class analysis', *European Journal of Psychotraumatology*, *5*(1), p. 25097.

Coyle, T. N., Shaver, J. A., and Linehan, M. M. (2018) 'On the potential for iatrogenic effects of psychiatric crisis services: the example of dialectical behavior therapy for adult women with a borderline personality disorder', *Journal of Consulting and Clinical Psychology*, *86*(2), p. 116.

Crowell, S. E., and Kaufman, E. A. (2016) 'Development of self-inflicted injury: Comorbidities and continuities with borderline and antisocial personality traits', *Development and Psychopathology*, *28*(4pt1), pp.1071–1088.

Douglas, B., and James, P. (2013) *Common Presenting Issues in Psychotherapeutic Practice*, Sage.

Durand, V. M., and Barlow, D. H. (2012) *Essentials of Abnormal Psychology*, Cengage Learning.

Edelstein, B. A., Hersen, M., and Thase, M. E. (eds.) (2013) *Handbook of Outpatient Treatment of Adults: Nonpsychotic Mental Disorders*, Springer Science+Business Media.

Gerull, F., Meares, R., Stevenson, J., Korner, A., and Newman, L. (2008) 'The beneficial effect on family life in treating borderline personality', *Psychiatry*, *71*(1), pp. 59–70.

Gerull, F., Meares, R., Stevenson, J., Korner, A., and Newman, L. (2008). The beneficial effect on family life in treating borderline personality. *Psychiatry*, *71*(1), 59-70.

Guilé, J. M., Boissel, L., Alaux-Cantin, S., and de La Rivière, S. G. (2018) 'Borderline personality disorder in adolescents: prevalence, diagnosis, and treatment strategies', *Adolescent Health, Medicine, and Therapeutics*, *9*, p. 199.

Gunderson, J. G. (2009) 'Borderline personality disorder: ontogeny of a diagnosis', *American Journal of Psychiatry*, *166*(5), pp. 530–539.

Gunderson, J. G. (2011) 'Borderline personality disorder', *New England Journal of Medicine*, *364*(21), pp. 2037–2042.

Gunderson, J. G., Stout, R. L., McGlashan, T. H., Shea, M. T., Morey, L. C., Grilo, C. M., . . . and Ansell, E. (2011) 'The ten-year course of borderline personality disorder: psychopathology and function from the Collaborative Longitudinal Personality Disorders Study', *Archives of general psychiatry*, *68*(8), pp. 827–837.

Gunderson, John G. (2009) 'Borderline personality disorder: ontogeny of a diagnosis', *American Journal of Psychiatry* 166.5, pp. 530–539.

Harned, M. S., Rizvi, S. L., and Linehan, M. M. (2010) 'Impact of co-occurring posttraumatic stress disorder on suicidal women with a borderline personality disorder', *American Journal of Psychiatry*, *167*(10), pp. 1210–1217.

Hirsh, J. B., Quilty, L. C., Bagby, R. M., and McMain, S. F. (2012) 'The relationship between agreeableness and the development of the working alliance in patients with a borderline personality disorder', *Journal of Personality Disorders*, *26*(4), pp. 616–627.

Kaess, M., von Ceumern-Lindenstjerna, I. A., Parzer, P., Chanen, A., Mundt, C., Resch, F., and Brunner, R. (2013) 'Axis I and II comorbidity and psychosocial functioning in female adolescents with a borderline personality disorder', *Psychopathology*, *46*(1), pp. 55–62.

Kimmel, C. L., Alhassoon, O. M., Wollman, S. C., Stern, M. J., Perez-Figueroa, A., Hall, M. G., . . . and Radua, J. (2016) 'Age-related parieto-occipital and other gray matter changes in borderline personality disorder: a meta-analysis of cortical and subcortical structures', *Psychiatry Research: Neuroimaging*, *251*, pp 15–25.

Krawitz, R., and Jackson, W. (2008) 'Borderline Personality Disorder (BPD): In the Midst of Vulnerability, Chaos, and Awe', *Brain Sciences*, *18*(1), pp. 20–23.

Kulacaoglu, F., and Kose, S. (2018) 'Borderline Personality Disorder (BPD): In the Midst of Vulnerability, Chaos, and Awe', *Brain Sciences*, *8*(11), pp. 201–202.

Leander, N. P., Moore, S. G., and Chartrand, T. L. (2009) *Mystery Moods: Their Origins and Consequences*, Na.

Linehan, M. M., Korslund, K. E., Harned, M. S., Gallop, R. J., Lungu, A., Neacsiu, A. D., . . . and Murray-Gregory, A. M. (2015) 'Dialectical behavior therapy for high suicide risk in individuals with borderline personality disorder: a randomized clinical trial and component analysis', *JAMA Psychiatry*, *72*(5), pp. 475–482.

Livesley, J. (2008), 'Toward a genetically-informed model of borderline personality Disorder', *Journal of Personality Disorders*, *22*(1), pp. 42–71.

Lopez-Castroman, J., Galfalvy, H., Currier, D., Stanley, B., Blasco-Fontecilla, H., Baca-Garcia, E., . . . and Oquendo, M. A. (2012) 'Personality disorder assessments in acute depressive episodes: stability at follow-up', *The Journal of Nervous and Mental Disease, 200*(6), p. 526.

Miller, A. L., Muehlenkamp, J. J., and Jacobson, C. M. (2008) 'Fact or fiction: Diagnosing borderline personality disorder in adolescents', *Clinical Psychology Review, 28*(6), pp. 969–981.

Moffitt, T. E., in alphabetical order, Arseneault, L., Jaffee, S. R., Kim-Cohen, J., Koenen, K. C., . . . and Viding, E. (2008) 'Research review: *DSM*-V conduct disorder: Research needs for an evidence base', *Journal of Child Psychology and Psychiatry, 49*(1), pp. 3–33.

Neacsiu, A. D., Rizvi, S. L., and Linehan, M. M. (2010) 'Dialectical behavior therapy skills use as a mediator and outcome of treatment for borderline personality disorder', *Behavior Research and Therapy, 48*(9), pp. 832–839.

Oumaya, M., Friedman, S., Pham, A., Abou, T. A., Guelfi, J. D., and Rouillon, F. (2008) 'Borderline personality disorder, self-mutilation, and suicide: a literature review', *L'Encephale, 34*(5), pp. 452–458.

Paris, J. (2008) 'Clinical trials of treatment for personality disorders', *Psychiatric Clinics of North America, 31*(3), pp. 517–526.

Paris, J. (2009) 'The treatment of borderline personality disorder: implications of research on diagnosis, etiology, and outcome', *Annual Review of Clinical Psychology, 5*, pp. 277–290.

Paris, J. (2010) 'Estimating the prevalence of personality disorders in the community', *Journal of Personality Disorders, 24*(4), pp. 405–411.

Rausch, J., Gäbel, A., Nagy, K., Kleindienst, N., Herpertz, S. C., and Bertsch, K. (2015) 'Increased testosterone levels and cortisol awakening responses in patients with borderline personality disorder: gender and trait aggressiveness matter. Psychoneuroendocrinology', *Borderline personality disorder. 55*, Oxford University Press., pp. 116–127.

Sadock, B. J., Sadock, V. A., and Levin, Z. E. (eds.) (2007) *Kaplan and Sadock's Study Guide and Self-Examination Review in Psychiatry*, Lippincott Williams and Wilkins.

Shaffer, D., and Jacobson, C. (2009) 'Proposal to the *DSM*-V childhood disorder and mood disorder work groups to include non-suicidal self-injury (NSSI) as a *DSM*-V disorder', *American Psychiatric Association*, pp. 1–21.

Siever, L. J. (2008) 'Neurobiology of aggression and violence', *American Journal of Psychiatry*, *165*(4), pp. 429–442.

Silk, K. R. (2008) 'Personality disorder in adolescence: The diagnosis that dare not speak its Name'.

Silvers, J. A., Hubbard, A. D., Biggs, E., Shu, J., Fertuck, E., Chaudhury, S., . . . and Brodsky, B. S. (2016) 'Affective lability and difficulties with regulation are differentially associated with the amygdala and prefrontal response in women with Borderline Personality Disorder', *Psychiatry Research: Neuroimaging*, *254*, pp. 74–82.

Skodol, A. E., Gunderson, J. G., Shea, M. T., McGlashan, T. H., Morey, L. C., Sanislow, C. A., . . . and Pagano, M. E. (2005) 'The collaborative longitudinal personality disorders study (CLPS): Overview and implications', *Journal of Personality Disorders*, *19*(5), pp. 487–504.

Soloff, P., Nutche, J., Goradia, D., and Diwadkar, V. (2008) 'Structural brain abnormalities in borderline personality disorder: a voxel-based morphometry study', *Psychiatry Research: Neuroimaging*, *164*(3), pp. 223–236.

Stanley, B., and Siever, L. J. (2009) 'The interpersonal dimension of borderline personality disorder: toward a neuropeptide model', *American Journal of Psychiatry*, *167*(1), pp. 24–39.

Torgersen, S., Myers, J., Reichborn-Kjennerud, T., Røysamb, E., Kubarych, T. S., and Kendler, K. S. (2012) 'The heritability of Cluster B personality disorders assessed both by personal interview and questionnaire', *Journal of Personality Disorders*, *26*(6), pp. 848–866.

Walsh, C., Ryan, P., and Flynn, D. (2018) 'Exploring dialectical behaviour therapy clinicians' experiences of team consultation meetings', *Borderline Personality Disorder and Emotion Dysregulation*, *5*(1), p. 3.

Wang, L., Ross, C. A., Zhang, T., Dai, Y., Zhang, H., Tao, M., . . . and Xiao, Z. (2012) 'Frequency of borderline personality disorder among psychiatric outpatients in Shanghai', *Journal of Personality Disorders*, *26*(3), pp. 393–401.

Wedig, M. M., Frankenburg, F. R., Reich, D. B., Fitzmaurice, G., and Zanarini, M. C. (2013) 'Predictors of suicide threats in patients with borderline personality disorder over 16 years of prospective follow-up', *Psychiatry Research*, *208*(3), pp. 252–256.

Weniger, G., Lange, C., Sachsse, U., and Irle, E. (2009) 'Reduced amygdala and hippocampus size in trauma-exposed women with borderline personality disorder and without posttraumatic stress disorder', *Journal of Psychiatry and Neuroscience*, 34, pp. 383–388.

Winograd, G., Cohen, P., and Chen, H. (2008) 'Adolescent borderline symptoms in the community: prognosis for functioning over 20 years', *Journal of Child Psychology and Psychiatry*, *49*(9), pp. 933–941.

Zanarini, M. C., Frankenburg, F. R., Reich, D. B., and Fitzmaurice, G. (2010) 'Time to the attainment of recovery from borderline personality disorder and stability of recovery: A 10-year prospective follow-up study', *American Journal of Psychiatry*, *167*(6), pp. 663–667.

Zanarini, M. C., Horwood, J., Wolke, D., Waylen, A., Fitzmaurice, G., and Grant, B. F. (2011) 'Prevalence of *DSM*-IV borderline personality disorder in two community samples: 6,330 English 11-year-olds and 34,653 American adults', *Journal of Personality Disorders 25*(5), pp. 607–619.

Zimmerman, M., Chelminski, I., and Young, D. (2008) 'The frequency of personality disorders in psychiatric patients', *Psychiatric Clinics of North America*, *31*(3), pp. 405–420.

CHAPTER 7

BPD and Brain Anatomy

The brain consists of many structures that are involved in processing events, memories, emotions, and information. Various studies have related emotional issues experienced by borderline personality disorder patients to the brain. BPD is, in reality, a brain disorder.

Individuals with a borderline personality disorder often have abnormal activities in the brain region that regulate fear and emotion. Additionally, these individuals often have unusual activity in regions of the brain that regulate fear and emotion. People diagnosed with BPD studies have shown that they have less grey matter in the front parts of their brains. As a result, their emotions tend to be inhibited, making these individuals have an emotional response to situations that others would consider trivial. The brains of people diagnosed with BPD tend to work differently from individuals without the disorder. For instance, the brain of a healthy individual usually senses when one should become uncomfortable in a particular situation. However, the brain of people with BPD does not function correctly, making them interpret people and situations inaccurately.

Differences in the brain between people diagnosed with borderline personality disorder and their healthy counterparts can be attributed to stress, drug abuse, genes, or exposure to unhealthy situations among others involved (Wingfield *et al.*, 2010). Various studies have looked at the potential factors and causes, which can lead to the development of borderline personality disorder. However, there has been no conclusive evidence regarding a single cause that can be solely linked to the development of BPD. Research has also demonstrated that the executive system of people with BPD also does not function properly. As a result, these individuals are prone to make impulsive decisions. Bearing in mind the heterogeneity of BPD, it is likely that a combination of various factors is involved (Wingfield *et al.*, 2010). Some of the factors attributed to borderline personality disorder development include traumatic events early in life such as maternal separation or childhood abuse. Other factors associated with BPD include genetics, psychosocial or environmental stressors, or neurobiological alterations among others (Steele and Siever, 2010).

Over the years, neurobiological abnormalities have begun to be associated with the development of borderline personality disorder (Foti *et al.*, 2010). Studies have reported that individuals with borderline personality disorders have a higher probability of having brain anatomy that is altered than their healthy counterparts. The alteration may include a smaller hippocampus and amygdala (Nunes *et al.*, 2009). People with BPD can also have sluggish serotonin systems; this is linked to impulsivity, anger, depression, irritability, and low mood.

Prefrontal Dysfunctions in Borderline Personality Disorder

The prefrontal cortex is responsible for decision-making, rationality, and reason. Individuals diagnosed with borderline personality disorder have a prefrontal cortex that is inefficient and inactive. Studies have demonstrated that impaired prefrontal cortex can lead to impulsivity, which is one of the symptoms of BPD. Various studies performed using functional MRI (fMRI) have evaluated the neural networks underlying borderline personality disorder stimulus interference. The studies have revealed that people diagnosed with

BPD have little activation in the prefrontal area (Wingefield *et al.*, 2009). Studies have also demonstrated that prefrontal cortex activities influence various functions in the limbic system, including the amygdala. The prefrontal cortex activity balances the functions of the amygdala. Research has shown that when patients with borderline personality disorder patients are exposed to stressful memories, they tend to experience reduced activity in some regions of the prefrontal cortex. The lowered activity of the prefrontal cortex hinders the function of the amygdala (Nunes *et al.*, 2009). Consequently, when people diagnosed with BPD encounter stressful situations, their emotions often get out of control. The involvement of the prefrontal cortex in regulating emotions has been demonstrated in various neuroimaging studies. The studies revealed that the prefrontal structures during emotional processing by borderline personality disorder patients are reduced (Smoski *et al.*, 2011). Additionally, reduced activation of the PFC was reported to be higher when a BPD patient was responding to adverse stimuli in comparison to neutral stimuli (Schulze *et al.*, 2016).

Brain scans on aggressive individuals have shown that they have the activity of their prefrontal cortex tends to be low. Studies have also demonstrated that the PFC functioning of individuals diagnosed with borderline personality disorder is often disordered, especially if the person has post-traumatic stress disorder (Kaplan *et al.*, 2016). Additionally, patients with BPD have reduced activation in the anterior cingulate cortex. Studies have also demonstrated that when these patients are compared to healthy individuals, they have reduced activation in the fronto-limbic area, including the dorsal anterior cingulate cortex and the medial frontal gyrus. The dorsal region of ACC is often linked to cognitive functions like complex motor control, executive functions, and attention modulations.

The rostral ACC, on the other hand, has been associated with the regulation of emotions. The medial prefrontal gyrus is responsible for the regulation of stress and emotion (Wingefield *et al.*, 2009). Research has shown that patients diagnosed with borderline personality disorder have an overactive dorsal and subgenual ACC, and this has been linked to negative emotions (Ruocco *et al.*, 2013).

The Amygdala and Insula in Borderline Personality Disorder

Amygdala, a small almond-shaped structure's primary function is to process emotions and store emotional memories. The amygdala is a section of the brain structures that are highly interconnected and complex (Porr, 2010). It is part of the limbic system, and that influences the mood dysregulation in borderline personality disorder. The amygdala is that region of the brain that processes adverse emotions like fear and also pleasure reactions.

The amygdala can be considered as the alarm system of the brain where the fight-or-flight reactions occur. The body, through the thalamus, transmits sensory input to the amygdala, which further transmits signals to other regions such as the face, activating facial responses. Studies have reported that the amygdala is dysfunctional in patients diagnosed with phobias, anxiety disorders, post-traumatic stress disorders, BPD, and autism. The amygdala is also linked to other parts of the brain involved in the sense of smell (Porr, 2010).

The amygdala is often associated with the responsibility of allocating significance to signals transmitted from the somatosensory system, particularly the adverse emotional stimuli. The amygdala can be viewed as the centre of processing emotions while the prefrontal cortex is regarded as the amygdala's brake pedal. Additionally, the amygdala modulates structures that assist in interpreting these signals and make the body to respond to them. Various studies have demonstrated that there is a link between an enhanced activation in the left amygdala and borderline personality disorder (Schulze *et al.*, 2016).

An overactive amygdala can predispose borderline personality disorder patients to hypervigilance. Consequently, these patients become more reactive to other people's expressions, mainly when they are vague. Furthermore, studies have shown that borderline personality disorder patients, when exposed to happy, sad, fearful, and neutral faces, have increased activity of the left amygdala (Widiger, 2012).

The hyper reaction can cause other people to be apprehensive when interacting with individuals diagnosed with BPD. Consequently, borderline personality disorder patients may confirm their view that these people had hidden motives. The perceived adverse signals can further provoke an over activation of the amygdala, leading to the fight-or-flight system (Porr, 2010). As a result, the person may engage in frantic efforts as a way of escaping imaginary or real abandonment. An overactive amygdala causes the brain to provide too much significance to a particular signal.

This further leads to challenges in modulating how these signals are managed and processed in other parts of the brain. According to studies, borderline personality disorder patients often have been found to have a smaller amygdala compared to their healthy counterparts (Nunes *et al.*, 2009). As a result, people diagnosed with BPD often experience emotions more intensely compared to the general population. Additionally, the person may take longer to *cool down* from the emotions he or she is experiencing. The cause of a smaller volume of the amygdala remains unknown. However, environmental factors like stress early in a person's life and genetic may lead to a smaller amygdala.

Studies based on functional MRI have also reported that when emotional responses are triggered, the amygdala often seems to work overtime (Porr, 2010). In individuals diagnosed with borderline personality disorder, the amygdala appears always to be working overtime.

Studies have also reported an overactive insula in borderline personality disorder patients. The overactive insula is frequently associated with the challenges these individuals experience while processing their emotions. In many studies on healthy people, the insula has been linked to the awareness of one's physical experiences, pain perception, and perceived social exclusion (Menon and Uddin., 2010).

In most research, the study is on the activity of the amygdala in borderline personality disorder patients after exposing them to a stimulus that induces fear. The results of these studies report enhanced amygdala activity to specific kinds of stimuli, such as unresolved life circumstances, adverse and positive emotional pictures (Hazlett *et al.*, 2012).

The Hypothalamic-Pituitary-Adrenal Axis

The hypothalamic-pituitary-adrenal axis is another region of the brain associated with a borderline personality disorder. The hypothalamic-pituitary-adrenal comprises the pituitary gland and the hypothalamus. Both these regions control how the body responds to stress. When the HPA is overactive, there is an increased concentration in the body of the stress hormone referred to as cortisol. Borderline personality disorder patients often overreact to life stresses, which other people in similar circumstances would consider to be minor (Chapman and Gratz, 2007).

Since trauma and early life stresses are key risk reasons in the development of various mental disorders, including BPD, various studies have looked into the HPA axis function due to its role in regulating stress responses. The HPA axis comprises the anterior pituitary gland, the adrenal cortex, and the hypothalamus. These two parts of the brain influence the response of the brain to stress (Chapman and Gratz, 2007).

Exposing the body to stress causes the hypothalamus to release peptides such as the corticotrophin-releasing factor (CRF) and the arginine vasopressin. HPA axis can, therefore, be regarded as a significant factor in the stress response. The hypothalamus produces the corticotrophin-releasing hormone (CRH), which is transported through the blood to the anterior pituitary. CRH activates the production of the adrenocorticotropic hormone (ACTH). After

ACTH reaches the receptors in the adrenal cortex, cortisol is then released (Widiger, 2012).

Cortisol slows down additional production of CRH from the hypothalamus through the negative feedback loop (Widiger, 2012). A normal stress response leads to the production of cortisol that controls metabolism, enhances the immune repose, and assists memory. However, constant exposure to cortisol can have adverse impacts on the brain, which can include damaging the hippocampus and memory deficiency (Zimmerman and Choi-Kain, 2009). Studies have reported that borderline personality disorder patients that have been exposed to extended childhood abuse often have high levels of cortisol and ACTH. As a result, their HPA axis response tends to be enhanced due to the increased sensitivity of the CRH receptors located in the pituitary gland (Widiger, 2012).

If the HPA axis is overactive, it leads to higher volumes of the cortisol hormone. Therefore, an overactive HPA axis translates to a hyperactive biological stress reaction (Chapman and Gratz, 2007). Studies have reported that individuals diagnosed with borderline personality disorder demonstrate exaggerated stress responses in comparison to people without the condition. Other studies have shown that an overactive HPA axis can lead to suicidal ideation and completion. The hippocampus has primary responsibility for regulating the HPA axis reaction to stress. Studies have demonstrated that patients diagnosed with a borderline personality disorder often have a dysregulated HPA axis. The reason for the dysregulation has been linked to genetic vulnerability and stress in early life (Tottenham and Sheridan, 2010). The function of the HPA is primarily to sustain homeostasis when a person's body is exposed to life stressors. However, in people that have a history of child abuse, studies have shown that the HPA axis is often dysregulated. Since traumatic events may increase the HPA axis activity production, this can be used to explain how childhood abuse is common in people diagnosed with a borderline personality disorder.

Hippocampus in BPD

The hippocampus is a pair of tubes that have the shape of a horseshoe; it is located in the right and left brain hemisphere. The hippocampus is linked to the short and long-term memory, emotional response, and spatial-orientation in the data processor of the body. When a situation is communicated through the visual cortex, the hippocampus chooses the right emotional response, fight or flight. In people diagnosed with a borderline personality disorder, their hippocampus tends to be continuously aroused (Nunes *et al.*, 2009). The hippocampus among borderline personality disorder patients constantly misconstrues threats and communicates erroneous messages to the amygdala. Consequently, these individuals are likely to view circumstances and people around them as being threatening. In reality, this might not be the reality or intention of these people. The volume of the hippocampus in BPD patients is often small (Nunes *et al.*, 2009). Early life stress has been linked to the hippocampus damage in BPD patients.

Corpus Callosum

A borderline personality disorder is characterised by primary symptoms of disturbed cognition, dysregulation, and impulsivity. In the human brain, the corpus callosum is the biggest white matter tract; it links the two parts in the brain hemisphere. The corpus callosum is the primary commissure connecting the cerebral hemispheres (Naidich *et al.*, 2012).

The millions of fibres in the corpus callosum consists are coarsely structured in a topographical manner. The corpus callosum is linked to the integration of information that is inter-hemispheric, which is necessary for the efficient coordination of behaviour, cognition, and emotion. Any structural changes of the corpus callosum can impair communication in the inter-hemisphere; this can lead to various behavioural, emotional, and cognitive issues.

Inter-hemispheric communication is involved in various perceptual and cognitive functions, which include visuospatial processing, memory, speech, and language. In borderline personality disorder, these functions are commonly impaired. Studies have shown that when communication in the inter-hemisphere is damaged, it can lead to suicidal behaviour (Cyprian *et al.*, 2011). Consequently, structural changes of the corpus callosum are more common in mental disorders characterised by deficits in impulse control and emotion regulation (Emsell *et al.*, 2013).

Deficits in impulse control and emotional regulation can lead to suicidal and self-injurious behaviours in borderline personality disorder (Boisseau *et al.*, 2013). Studies have shown that the structure of the corpus callosum of patients diagnosed with a borderline personality disorder is different from that of their health counterparts (Gan *et al.*, 2016). Structural alterations are more common in parts of the corpus callosum that are linked with the tempo-parietal and prefrontal parts of the brain.

Structural and functional changes in the tempo-parietal and prefrontal parts of the brain are significantly involved in impulse control and emotion regulation. This has been exhibited continuously in borderline personality disorder (Kraus Utz *et al.*, 2014). Therefore, it is likely that structural changes in the genu and splenium of the corpus callosum can cause alterations in the amygdala (Niedtfeld *et al.*, 2013). Corpus callosum develops from childhood to adolescence, mainly in the posterior regions. The development of the corpus callosum occurs concurrently with the development of the mental and cognitive function.

Adverse circumstances in early childhood have been connected to abnormalities in the corpus callosum (Carrion *et al.*, 2009). Studies have shown that sexual abuse during childhood, which is common among borderline personality disorder patients, is linked to the smaller corpus callosum. For instance, studies on female survivors of sexual abuse have shown a smaller corpus callosum. Therefore, it is possible to presume that abnormalities in the corpus callosum arising from childhood abuse can mediate odd personality development.

Studies have also demonstrated that children and teenagers with post-traumatic stress disorder have smaller corpus callosum.

Closely observing these facts, I took some time do to my own research and I have investigated further what corpus callosum involvement has on speech. In the study called 'Corpus Callosum and speech impairment in people diagnosed with BDP and Schizophrenia', I also pinpointed how individuals who have deficits in the corpus callosum are affected in their thought patterns and speech. The role that corpus callosum plays in mediating information transference from one hemisphere to another will also be studied. What other researchers have done in regard to this study will also be looked at and recommendations given on the way forward in regard to this research.

REFERENCES

Abraham, P. F., and Calabrese, J. R. (2008) 'Evidenced-based pharmacologic treatment OF borderline personality disorder: A shift from SSRIs to anticonvulsants and atypical antipsychotics?', *Journal of Affective Disorders*, *111*(1), pp. 21–30.

American Psychiatric Association (2013) 'Diagnostic and statistical manual of mental disorders', *BMC Med*, *17*, pp. 133–137.

Arntz, A., and Van Genderen, H. (2011) *Schema Therapy for Borderline Personality Disorder*, John Wiley & Sons.

Bateman, A. W. (2012) 'Treating borderline personality disorder in clinical practice'.

Bateman, A. W., and Fonagy, P. E. (2012) *Handbook of Mentalizing In Mental Health Practice*, American Psychiatric Publishing, Inc.

Bateman, A., and Fonagy, P. (2010) 'Mentalization based treatment for borderline personality Disorder', *World Psychiatry*, *9*(1), p. 11.

Bateman, A., and Fonagy, P. (2016) *Mentalization-Based Treatment for Personality Disorders: A Practical Guide*, Oxford University Press.

Bateman, A. W., and Krawitz, R. (2013) *Borderline Personality Disorder: An Evidence-Based Guide for Generalist Mental Health Professionals*, Oxford University Press.

Bellino, S., Paradiso, E., and Bogetto, F. (2008) 'Efficacy and tolerability of pharmacotherapies for borderline personality disorder', *CNS Drugs*, *22*(8), pp. 671–692.

Bertsch, K., Schmidinger, I., Neumann, I. D., and Herpertz, S. C. (2013) 'Reduced plasma oxytocin levels in female patients with a borderline personality disorder', *Hormones and Behavior*, *63*(3), pp. 424–429.

Blum, N., St. John, D., Pfohl, B., Stuart, S., McCormick, B., Allen, J., . . . and Black, D. W. (2008) 'Systems Training for Emotional Predictability and Problem Solving (STEPPS) for outpatients with borderline personality disorder: a randomized controlled trial and 1-year follow-up', *American Journal of Psychiatry, 165*(4), pp. 468–478, *Borderline Personality Disorder,* Oxford University Press.

Bornovalova, M. A., Hicks, B. M., Iacono, W. G., and McGue, M. (2009) 'Stability, change, and heritability of borderline personality disorder traits from adolescence to adulthood: A longitudinal twin study', *Development and Psychopathology, 21*(4), pp. 1335–1353.

Boisseau, C. L., Yen, S., Markowitz, J. C., Grilo, C. M., Sanislow, C. A., Shea, M. T., . . . and McGlashan, T. H. (2013) 'Individuals with single versus multiple suicide attempts over 10 years of prospective follow-up', *Comprehensive Psychiatry, 54*(3), pp. 238–242.

Bresin, K. (2014) 'Five indices of emotion regulation in participants with a history of nonsuicidal self-injury: A daily diary study', *Behavior Therapy, 45*(1), pp. 56–66.

Bridler, R., Häberle, A., Müller, S. T., Cattapan, K., Grohmann, R., Toto, S., . . . and Greil, W. (2015) 'Psychopharmacological treatment of 2195 in-patients with borderline personality disorder: a comparison with other psychiatric disorders', *European Neuropsychopharmacology, 25*(6), pp. 763–772.

Brown, J., Blum, N., and Black, D. W. (2013) 'Systems Training for Emotional Predictability and Problem Solving: An Advanced Understanding', *Journal of Law Enforcement, 3*(4).

Brüne, M., Dimaggio, G., and Edel, M. A. (2013) 'Mentalization-Based Group Therapy for Inpatients with Borderline Personality Disorder: Preliminary Findings', *Clinical Neuropsychiatry, 10*(5).

Brunner, R., Henze, R., Richter, J., and Kaess, M. (2015) 'Neurobiological findings in youth with a borderline personality disorder', *Scandinavian Journal of Child and Adolescent Psychiatry and Psychology, 3*(1), pp. 22–30.

Carlstedt, R. A. (2009) *Handbook Of Integrative Clinical Psychology, Psychiatry, and Behavioral Medicine: Perspectives, Practices, and Research*, Springer Publishing Company.

Carrion, V. G., Weems, C. F., Watson, C., Eliez, S., Menon, V., and Reiss, A. L. (2009)

'Converging evidence for abnormalities of the prefrontal cortex and evaluation of midsagittal structures in pediatric posttraumatic stress disorder: an MRI study', *Psychiatry Research: Neuroimaging, 172*(3), pp. 226–234.

Chalker, S. A., Carmel, A., Atkins, D. C., Landes, S. J., Kerbrat, A. H., and Comtois, K. A. (2015) 'Examining challenging behaviors of clients with a borderline personality disorder', *Behavior Research and Therapy, 75*, pp. 11–19.

Chanen, A. M., and McCutcheon, L. (2013) 'Prevention and early intervention for borderline personality disorder: current status and recent evidence', *The British Journal of Psychiatry, 202*(s54), pp. s24–s29.

Chanen, A. M., Jovev, M., Djaja, D., McDougall, E., Yuen, H. P., Rawlings, D., and Jackson, H. J. (2008) 'Screening for borderline personality disorder in outpatient youth', *Journal of Personality Disorders, 22*(4), pp. 353–364.

Chanen, A. M., Jovev, M., McCutcheon, L. K., Jackson, H. J., and McGorry, P. D. (2008) 'Borderline personality disorder in young people and the prospects for prevention and early intervention', *Current Psychiatry Reviews, 4*(1), pp. 48–57.

Chanen, A. M., Mccutcheon, L. K., Germano, D., Nistico, H., Jackson, H. J., and Mcgorry, P. D. (2009) 'The HYPE Clinic: an early intervention service for borderline personality Disorder', *Journal of Psychiatric Practice, 15*(3), pp. 163–172.

Chanen, A. M., Jackson, H. J., McCutcheon, L. K., Jovev, M., Dudgeon, P., Yuen, H. P., . . . and

Clarkson, V. (2009) 'Early intervention for adolescents with borderline personality disorder: quasi-experimental comparison with treatment as usual', *Australian and New Zealand Journal of Psychiatry, 43*(5), pp. 397–408.

Chapman, A., and Gratz, K. (2007) *The Borderline Personality Disorder Survival Guide: Everything You Need to Know About Living with BPD*, New Harbinger Publications.

Choi-Kain, L. W., and Gunderson, J. G. (eds.) (2019) *Applications of Good Psychiatric Management for Borderline Personality Disorder: A Practical Guide*, American Psychiatric Pub.

Choi-Kain, L. W., Albert, E. B., and Gunderson, J. G. (2016) 'Evidence-based treatments for borderline personality disorder: implementation, integration, and stepped care', *Harvard Review of Psychiatry*, *24*(5), pp. 342–356.

Clarkin, J. F., Levy, K. N., Lenzenweger, M. F., and Kernberg, O. F. (2013) 'Evaluating three treatments for borderline personality disorder: A multiwave study', *Focus*, *11*(2), pp. 269–276.

Cloitre, M., Garvert, D. W., Weiss, B., Carlson, E. B., and Bryant, R. A. (2014) 'Distinguishing PTSD, complex PTSD, and borderline personality disorder: A latent class analysis', *European Journal of Psychotraumatology*, *5*(1), p. 25097.

Coyle, T. N., Shaver, J. A., and Linehan, M. M. (2018) 'On the potential for iatrogenic effects of psychiatric crisis services: the example of dialectical behavioral therapy for adult women with a borderline personality disorder', *Journal of Consulting and Clinical Psychology*, *86*(2), p. 116.

Cyprien, F., Courtet, P., Malafosse, A., Maller, J., Meslin, C., Bonafé, A., . . . and Artero, S. (2011) 'Suicidal behavior is associated with reduced corpus callosum area', *Biological psychiatry*, *70*(4), pp. 320–326.

Crowell, S. E., and Kaufman, E. A. (2016) 'Development of self-inflicted injury: Comorbidities and continuities with borderline and antisocial personality traits', *Development and Psychopathology*, *28*(4pt1), pp. 1071–1088.

Das, P., Calhoun, V., and Malhi, G. S. (2014) 'Bipolar and borderline patients display differential patterns of functional connectivity among resting state networks', *Neuroimage*, *98*, pp. 73–81.

Dimeff, L. A., and Koerner, K. E. (2007) *Dialectical Behavior Therapy in*

Clinical Practice: Applications Across Disorders and Settings, Guilford Press.

Douglas, B., and James, P. (2013) *Common Presenting Issues in Psychotherapeutic Practice*, Sage.

Durand, V. M., and Barlow, D. H. (2012) *Essentials of Abnormal Psychology*, Cengage Learning.

Ducasse, D., Lopez-Castroman, J., Dassa, D., Brand-Arpon, V., Dupuy-Maurin, K., Lacourt, L., . . . and Olié, E. (2019) 'Exploring the boundaries between borderline personality disorder and suicidal behavior disorder', *European Archives of Psychiatry and Clinical Neuroscience*, pp. 1–9.

Edelstein, B. A., Hersen, M., and Thase, M. E. (eds.) (2013) *Handbook of Outpatient Treatment of Adults: Nonpsychotic Mental Disorders*, Springer Science+Business Media.

Emsell, L., Leemans, A., Langan, C., Van Hecke, W., Barker, G. J., McCarthy, P., . . . and McDonald, C. (2013) 'Limbic and callosal white matter changes in euthymic bipolar I disorder: an advanced diffusion magnetic resonance imaging tractography study', *Biological Psychiatry*, *73*(2), pp. 194–201.

Gan, J., Yi, J., Zhong, M., Cao, X., Jin, X., Liu, W., and Zhu, X. (2016) 'Abnormal white matter structural connectivity in treatment-naïve young adults with borderline personality disorder', *Acta Psychiatrica Scandinavica*, *134*(6), pp. 494–503.

Gerull, F., Meares, R., Stevenson, J., Korner, A., and Newman, L. (2008) 'The beneficial effect on family life in treating borderline personality', *Psychiatry*, *71*(1), pp. 59–70.

Guilé, J. M., Boissel, L., Alaux-Cantin, S., and de La Rivière, S. G. (2018) 'Borderline personality disorder in adolescents: prevalence, diagnosis, and treatment strategies', *Adolescent Health, Medicine, and Therapeutics*, *9*, p. 199.

Gunderson, J. G. (2009) 'Borderline personality disorder: ontogeny of a diagnosis', *American Journal of Psychiatry*, *166*(5), pp. 530–539.

Gunderson, J. G. (2011) 'Borderline personality disorder', *New England Journal of Medicine*, *364*(21), pp. 2037–2042. Gunderson, J. G. (2016) 'The emergence of a generalist model to meet public health needs for patients with borderline personality disorder', *American Journal of Psychiatry*, *173*(5), pp. 452–458.

Gunderson, J. G., Stout, R. L., McGlashan, T. H., Shea, M. T., Morey, L. C., Grilo, C. M., . . . and Ansell, E. (2011) 'The ten-year course of borderline personality disorder: psychopathology and function from the Collaborative Longitudinal Personality Disorders Study', *Archives of General Psychiatry*, *68*(8), pp. 827–837.

Gunderson, J. G., Stout, R. L., Shea, M. T., Grilo, C. M., Markowitz, J. C., Morey, L. C., . . . and McGlashan, T. H. (2014) 'Interactions of borderline personality disorder and mood disorders over ten years' *Journal of Clinical Psychiatry*, *75*(8), p. 829.

Gunderson, John G. (2009) 'Borderline personality disorder: ontogeny of a diagnosis', *American Journal of Psychiatry,* 166.5, pp. 530–539.

Gunderson, J. G., Weinberg, I., and Choi-Kain, L. (2013) 'Borderline personality disorder', *Focus*, *11*(2), pp. 129–145.

Hancock-Johnson, E., Griffiths, C., and Picchioni, M. (2017) 'A focused systematic review of pharmacological treatment for borderline personality disorder', *CNS Drugs*, *31*(5), pp. 345–356.

Harned, M. S., Rizvi, S. L., and Linehan, M. M. (2010) 'Impact of co-occurring posttraumatic stress disorder on suicidal women with a borderline personality disorder', *American Journal of Psychiatry*, *167*(10), pp. 1210–1217.

Herpertz, S. C., Zanarini, M., Schulz, C. S., Siever, L., Lieb, K., and Möller, H. J. (2007) 'Treatment of personality disorders: World Federation of Societies of Biological Psychiatry (WFSBP) Guidelines for Biological Treatment of Personality Disorders', *World Journal of Biological Psychiatry*, *8*(4), pp. 212–244.

Hirsh, J. B., Quilty, L. C., Bagby, R. M., and McMain, S. F. (2012) 'The relationship between agreeableness and the development of the working alliance in patients with a borderline personality disorder', *Journal of Personality Disorders*, *26*(4), pp. 616–627.

Horvath, A. O., Del Re, A. C., Flückiger, C., and Symonds, D. (2011) 'Alliance in individual Psychotherapy', *Psychotherapy*, *48*(1), p. 9.

Hopwood, C. J., Swenson, C., Bateman, A., Yeomans, F. E., and Gunderson, J. G. (2014) 'Approaches to psychotherapy for borderline personality: Demonstrations by four master Clinicians', *Personality Disorders: Theory, Research, and Treatment*, *5*(1), p. 108.

Kaess, M., von Ceumern-Lindenstjerna, I. A., Parzer, P., Chanen, A., Mundt, C., Resch, F., and Brunner, R. (2013) 'Axis I and II comorbidity and psychosocial functioning in female adolescents with a borderline personality disorder', *Psychopathology*, *46*(1), pp. 55–62.

Kaplan, C., Tarlow, N., Stewart, J. G., Aguirre, B., Galen, G., and Auerbach, R. P. (2016) 'Borderline personality disorder in youth: The prospective impact of child abuse on non- suicidal self-injury and suicidality', *Comprehensive psychiatry*, *71*, pp. 86–94.

Kimmel, C. L., Alhassoon, O. M., Wollman, S. C., Stern, M. J., Perez-Figueroa, A., Hall, M. G., . . . and Radua, J. (2016) 'Age-related parieto-occipital and other gray matter changes in borderline personality disorder: a meta-analysis of cortical and subcortical structures', *Psychiatry Research: Neuroimaging*, *251*, pp. 15–25.

Kulacaoglu, F., and Kose, S. (2018). Borderline Personality Disorder (BPD): In the Midst of Vulnerability, Chaos, and Awe. *Brain sciences*, *8*(11), 201.

Laurenssen, E. M., Hutsebaut, J., Feenstra, D. J., Bales, D. L., Noom, M. J., Busschbach, J. J., . . . and Luyten, P. (2014) 'Feasibility of mentalization-based treatment for adolescents with borderline symptoms: A pilot study', *Psychotherapy*, *51*(1), p. 159.

Leander, N. P., Moore, S. G., and Chartrand, T. L. (2009) *Mystery Moods: Their Origins and Consequences*, Na.

Lieb, K., Völlm, B., Rücker, G., Timmer, A., and Stoffers, J. M.

(2010) 'Pharmacotherapy for borderline personality disorder: Cochrane systematic review of randomised trials', *The British Journal of Psychiatry*, *196*(1), pp. 4–12.

Linehan, M. M. (2018) *Cognitive-Behavioral Treatment of Borderline Personality Disorder*, Guilford Publications.

Leiberich, P., Nickel, M. K., Tritt, K., and Gil, F. P. (2008) 'Lamotrigine treatment of aggression in female borderline patients, Part II: an 18-month follow-up', *Journal of Psychopharmacology*, *22*(7), pp. 805–808.

Linehan, M. M., Korslund, K. E., Harned, M. S., Gallop, R. J., Lungu, A., Neacsiu, A. D., . . . and Murray-Gregory, A. M. (2015) 'Dialectical behavior therapy for high suicide risk in individuals with borderline personality disorder: a randomized clinical trial and component analysis', *JAMA Psychiatry*, *72*(5), pp. 475–482.

Livesley, J. (2008) 'Toward a genetically-informed model of borderline personality disorder', *Journal of Personality Disorders*, *22*(1), pp. 42–71.

Lopez-Castroman, J., Galfalvy, H., Currier, D., Stanley, B., Blasco-Fontecilla, H., Baca-Garcia, E., . . . and Oquendo, M. A. (2012) 'Personality disorder assessments in acute depressive episodes: stability at follow-up', *The Journal of Nervous and Mental Disease*, *200*(6), p. 526.

May, J. M., Richardi, T. M., and Barth, K. S. (2016) 'Dialectical behavior therapy as treatment for borderline personality disorder', *Mental Health Clinician*, *6*(2), pp. 62–67. 'Borderline personality disorder in adolescents', *Clinical Psychology Review*, *28*(6), pp. 969–981.

McMain, S. F., Links, P. S., Gnam, W. H., Guimond, T., Cardish, R. J., Korman, L., and Streiner, D. L. (2009) 'A randomized trial of dialectical behavior therapy versus general psychiatric management for borderline personality disorder', *American Journal of Psychiatry*, *166*(12), pp. 1365–1374.

Mercer, D., Douglass, A. B., and Links, P. S. (2009) 'Meta-analyses of mood stabilizers, antidepressants and antipsychotics in the treatment of borderline personality disorder: effectiveness for depression and anger symptoms', *Journal of Personality Disorders*, *23*(2), pp. 156–174.

Miller, A. L., Muehlenkamp, J. J., and Jacobson, C. M. (2008) 'Fact or fiction: Diagnosing'.

Moffitt, T. E., in alphabetical order, Arseneault, L., Jaffee, S. R., Kim-Cohen, J., Koenen, K. C., . . . and Viding, E. (2008) 'Research review: *DSM*-V conduct disorder: Research needs for an evidence base', *Journal of Child Psychology and Psychiatry*, *49*(1), pp. 3–33.

Naidich, T. P., Castillo, M., Cha, S., and Smirniotopoulos, J. G. (2012) *Imaging of the Brain: Expert Radiology Series*, Elsevier Health Sciences.

Neacsiu, A. D., Rizvi, S. L., and Linehan, M. M. (2010) 'Dialectical behavior therapy skills use as a mediator and outcome of treatment for borderline personality disorder', *Behavior Research and Therapy*, *48*(9), pp. 832–839.

Niedtfeld, I., Schulze, L., Krause-Utz, A., Demirakca, T., Bohus, M., and Schmahl, C. (2013) 'Voxel-based morphometry in women with borderline personality disorder with and without comorbid posttraumatic stress disorder', *PloS One*, *8*(6).

Oumaya, M., Friedman, S., Pham, A., Abou, T. A., Guelfi, J. D., and Rouillon, F. (2008) 'Borderline personality disorder, self-mutilation, and suicide: a literature review', *L'Encephale*, *34*(5), pp. 452–458.

Paris, J. (2008) 'Clinical trials of treatment for personality disorders', *Psychiatric Clinics of North America*, *31*(3), pp. 517–526.

Paris, J. (2009) 'The treatment of borderline personality disorder: implications of research on diagnosis, etiology, and outcome', *Annual Review of Clinical Psychology*, *5*, pp. 277–290.

Paris, J. (2010) 'Estimating the prevalence of personality disorders in the community', *Journal of Personality Disorders*, *24*(4), pp. 405–411.

Paris, J. (2019) *Treatment of Borderline Personality Disorder: A Guide to Evidence-Based Practice*, Guilford Publications.

Parker, G. (2011) 'Clinical differentiation of bipolar II disorder from personality-based "emotional dysregulation" conditions', *Journal of Affective Disorders*, *133*(1–2), pp. 16–21.

Parry, G. D., Crawford, M. J., and Duggan, C. (2016) 'Iatrogenic harm from psychological therapies–time to move on', *The British Journal of Psychiatry*, *208*(3), pp. 210–212.

Paton, C., Crawford, M. J., Bhatti, S. F., Patel, M. X., and Barnes, T. R. (2015) 'The use of psychotropic medication in patients with emotionally unstable personality disorder under the care of UK mental health services', *The Journal of Clinical Psychiatry*, *76*(4), pp. 512–518.

Porr, V. (2010) *Overcoming Borderline Personality Disorder: A Family Guide for Healing and Change*, Oxford University Press.

Rausch, J., Gäbel, A., Nagy, K., Kleindienst, N., Herpertz, S. C., and Bertsch, K. (2015) 'Increased testosterone levels and cortisol awakening responses in patients with borderline personality disorder: gender and trait aggressiveness matter', *Psychoneuroendocrinology*, *55*, pp. 116–127.

Reddy, M. S., and Vijay, M. S. (2017) 'Empirical reality of dialectical behavioral therapy in borderline personality', *Indian Journal of Psychological Medicine*, *39*(2), p. 105.

Ripoll, L. H. (2012) 'Clinical psychopharmacology of borderline personality disorder: an update on the available evidence in light of the Diagnostic and Statistical Manual of Mental Disorders–5', *Current Opinion in Psychiatry*, *25*(1), pp. 52–58.

Ripoll, L. H. (2013) 'Psychopharmacologic treatment of borderline personality Disorder', *Dialogues in Clinical Neuroscience*, *15*(2), p. 213.

Rogers, B., and Acton, T. (2012) '"I think we're all guinea pigs really": a qualitative study of medication and borderline personality disorder', *Journal of Psychiatric and Mental Health Nursing*, *19*(4), pp. 341–347.

Ruocco, A. C., Amirthavasagam, S., Choi-Kain, L. W., and McMain, S. F. (2013) 'Neural correlates of negative emotionality in borderline personality disorder: an activation-likelihood-estimation meta-analysis', *Biological Psychiatry*, *73*(2), pp. 153–160.

Sadock, B. J., Sadock, V. A., and Levin, Z. E. (eds.) (2007) *Kaplan and Sadock's Study Guide and Self-Examination Review in Psychiatry*, Lippincott Williams and Wilkins.

Schulze, L., Schmahl, C., and Niedtfeld, I. (2016) 'Neural correlates of disturbed emotion processing in borderline personality disorder: a multimodal meta-analysis', *Biological Psychiatry*, *79*(2), pp. 97–106.

Shaffer, D., and Jacobson, C. (2009) 'Proposal to the *DSM*-V childhood disorder and mood disorder work groups to include non-suicidal self-injury (NSSI) as a *DSM*-V disorder', *American Psychiatric Association*, pp. 1–21.

Siever, L. J. (2008) 'Neurobiology of aggression and violence', *American Journal of Psychiatry*, *165*(4), pp. 429–442.

Silk, K. R. (2008) 'Personality disorder in adolescence: The diagnosis that dare not speak its Name'.

Silvers, J. A., Hubbard, A. D., Biggs, E., Shu, J., Fertuck, E., Chaudhury, S., . . . and Brodsky, B. S. (2016) 'Affective lability and difficulties with regulation are differentially associated with the amygdala and prefrontal response in women with Borderline Personality Disorder', *Psychiatry Research: Neuroimaging*, *254*, pp. 74–82.

Skodol, A. E., Gunderson, J. G., Shea, M. T., McGlashan, T. H., Morey, L. C., Sanislow, C. A., . . . and Pagano, M. E. (2005) 'The collaborative longitudinal personality disorders study (CLPS): Overview and implications', *Journal of Personality Disorders*, *19*(5), pp. 487–504.

Soloff, P., Nutche, J., Goradia, D., and Diwadkar, V. (2008) 'Structural brain abnormalities in borderline personality disorder: a voxel-based morphometry study', *Psychiatry Research: Neuroimaging*, *164*(3), pp. 223–236.

Stanley, B., and New, A. (eds.) (2017) *Borderline Personality Disorder*, Oxford University Press.

Stanley, B., and Siever, L. J. (2009) 'The interpersonal dimension of borderline personality disorder: toward a neuropeptide model', *American Journal of Psychiatry*, *167*(1), pp. 24–39.

Starcevic, V., and Janca, A. (2018) 'Pharmacotherapy of borderline personality disorder: replacing confusion with prudent pragmatism', *Current Opinion in Psychiatry*, *31*(1), pp. 69–73.

Steele, H., and Siever, L. (2010) 'An attachment perspective on borderline personality disorder: Advances in gene-environment considerations', *Current Psychiatry Reports*, *12*(1), pp. 61–67.

Stoffers-Winterling, J. M., Völlm, B. A., Rücker, G., Timmer, A., Huband, N., and Lieb, K. (2012) 'Psychological therapies for people with borderline personality disorder', *Cochrane Database of Systematic Reviews*, (8).

Smoski, M. J., Salsman, N., Wang, L., Smith, V., Lynch, T. R., Dager, S. R., . . . and Linehan, M. M. (2011) 'Functional imaging of emotion reactivity in opiate-dependent borderline personality disorder', *Personality Disorders: Theory, Research, and Treatment*, *2*(3), p. 230.

Torgersen, S., Myers, J., Reichborn-Kjennerud, T., Røysamb, E., Kubarych, T. S., and Kendler, K. S. (2012) 'The heritability of Cluster B personality disorders assessed both by personal interview and questionnaire', *Journal of Personality Disorders*, *26*(6), pp. 848–866.

Tottenham, N., Hare, T. A., Quinn, B. T., McCarry, T. W., Nurse, M., Gilhooly, T., . . . and

Thomas, K. M. (2010) 'Prolonged institutional rearing is associated with atypically large amygdala volume and difficulties in emotion regulation', *Developmental Science*, *13*(1), pp. 46–61.

Trull, T. J., Jahng, S., Tomko, R. L., Wood, P. K., and Sher, K. J. (2010) 'Revised NESARC personality disorder diagnoses: gender, prevalence, and comorbidity with substance dependence disorders', *Journal of Personality Disorders*, *24*(4), pp. 412–426.

Walsh, C., Ryan, P., and Flynn, D. (2018) 'Exploring dialectical behaviour therapy clinicians' experiences of team consultation meetings', *Borderline Personality Disorder and Emotion Dysregulation*, 5(1), p. 3.

Wang, L., Ross, C. A., Zhang, T., Dai, Y., Zhang, H., Tao, M., . . . and Xiao, Z. (2012) 'Frequency of borderline personality disorder among psychiatric outpatients in Shanghai', *Journal of Personality Disorders*, 26(3), pp. 393–401.

Wedig, M. M., Frankenburg, F. R., Reich, D. B., Fitzmaurice, G., and Zanarini, M. C. (2013) 'Predictors of suicide threats in patients with borderline personality disorder over 16 years of prospective follow-up', *Psychiatry Research*, 208(3), pp. 252–256.

Weniger, G., Lange, C., Sachsse, U., and Irle, E. (2009) 'Reduced amygdala and hippocampus size in trauma-exposed women with borderline personality disorder and without posttraumatic stress disorder', *Journal of Psychiatry and Neuroscience*, 34, pp. 383–388

Widiger, T. A. (ed.) (2012) *The Oxford Handbook of Personality Disorders*, Oxford University Press.

Wingenfeld, K., Spitzer, C., Rullkötter, N., and Löwe, B. (2010) 'Borderline personality disorder: hypothalamus pituitary adrenal axis and findings from neuroimaging studies', *Psychoneuroendocrinology*, 35(1), pp. 154–170.

Winograd, G., Cohen, P., and Chen, H. (2008) 'Adolescent borderline symptoms in the community: prognosis for functioning over 20 years', *Journal of Child Psychology and Psychiatry*, 49(9), pp. 933–941.

Völlm, B. A., Chadwick, K., Abdelrazek, T., and Smith, J. (2012) 'Prescribing of psychotropic medication for personality disordered patients in secure forensic settings', *The Journal of Forensic Psychiatry and Psychology*, 23(2), pp. 200–216.

Zanarini, M. C., Frankenburg, F. R., Reich, D. B., and Fitzmaurice, G. (2010) 'Time to the attainment of recovery from borderline personality disorder and stability of recovery: A 10-year prospective follow-up study', *American Journal of Psychiatry*, 167(6), pp. 663–667.

Zanarini, M. C., Frankenburg, F. R., Reich, D. B., Harned, A.

L., and Fitzmaurice, G. M. (2015) 'Rates of psychotropic medication use reported by borderline patients and axis II comparison subjects over 16 years of prospective follow-up', *Journal of Clinical Psychopharmacology*, *35*(1), p. 63. 'English 11-year-olds and 34,653 American adults', *Journal of Personality Disorders*, *25*(5), pp. 607–619.

Zanarini, M. C., Frankenburg, F. R., Reich, D. B., Harned, A. L., and Fitzmaurice, G. M. (2015) 'Rates of psychotropic medication use reported by borderline patients and axis II comparison subjects over 16 years of prospective follow-up', *Journal of Clinical Psychopharmacology*, *35*(1), p. 63.

Zanarini, M. C., Horwood, J., Wolke, D., Waylen, A., Fitzmaurice, G., and Grant, B. F. (2011) 'Prevalence of *DSM*-IV borderline personality disorder in two community samples: 6,330'.

Zimmerman, M., Chelminski, I., and Young, D. (2008) 'The frequency of personality disorders in psychiatric patients', *Psychiatric Clinics of North America*, *31*(3), pp. 405–420.

Corpus Callosum and speech impairment in people diagnosed with BDP and schizophrenia.

Abstract

The study seeks to investigate the correlation that exists between corpus callosum and speech impairment in patients suffering from schizophrenia and borderline personality disorder and understanding of expressive language disturbance. The objectives are to find out what are the causes of schizophrenia and borderline personality disorder, also what the symptoms of disorders are. The study also seeks to find out what causes language impairment among those people who suffer from schizophrenia and borderline personality disorder. In this regard theories which causes abnormalities in speech will be discussed, and various researchers who have conducted research in this area be identified. The study also aims at studying what corpus callosum is and also the involvement that it has on speech, also how individuals who have deficits in the corpus callosum are affected in their thought patterns and speech. The role that corpus callosum plays in mediating information transference from one hemisphere to another will also be studied. What other researchers have done in regard to this study will also be looked at and recommendations given on the way forward in regard to this research.

A Bridge Too Far: Could Corpus Callosum Dysfunction under Scope Language Impairments in Borderline Personality Disorder and Schizophrenia?

Schizophrenia is a long-term mental disorder that causes an abnormality in the thoughts, feelings, and behaviour of the individual affected. In this regard, the persons suffering from this condition are depicted as having lost touch with the real events of the world. The individual may have difficulty expressing normal emotions while in a social setting. According to the *DSM*-5 criteria, there are a number of symptoms that one can use to identify the presence of the disease. The disease is not associated with a particular laboratory result but rather by the experience of at least two of the following symptoms:

disorganised speech, hallucinations, delusions, negative symptoms, and catatonic behaviour. Either of the initial three must be one of the symptoms evident in the patient (Mohapatra, Panda, Sahoo, Dey, and Rath, 2015). Additionally, it is essential that the signs presented to the suffering individual must prevail for at least six months. At this time, the patient should have experienced at least a month of active symptoms that show significant social or occupational deterioration (Subramaniam et al, 2017). In identifying the mental disorder, it is important that the symptoms do not occur as a result of another disorder.

There are three distinct symptoms presented in the patient including the cognitive, negative, and positive symptoms. The positive symptoms are those depicted as psychotic such as hallucinations that are mainly auditory, delusions, and speech or behaviour that is disorganised (Innocenti, Ansermet, and Parnas, 2003; Cassidy et al., 2014). The negative symptoms manifest in the form of a decreased emotional range, loss of interest, poor speech, and tremendous inertia. Finally, the cognitive symptoms may demonstrate significant neurocognitive deficit such as the poor working memory, attention, and executive function. These individuals may find it difficult to understand the nuances of relating to others (Li et al., 2015; Jamadar et al., 2014; Palaniyappan et al., 2013). Persons suffering from this mental disorder may experience symptoms associated with mood changes where their happiness or sadness may be a result of depression.

Despite a lack of clarity on the cause of the mental disorder, there are a number of assumptions made to describe its occurrence. There is the hereditary factor, the biological aspect of impaired brain chemistry or structure, and the immune disorders along with viral infections (Müller, Weidinger, Leitner, and Schwarz, 2015; Thoresen et al, 2014). It may, therefore, be difficult to clearly identify what causes the disease. The individual suffering from this disease is more likely to be unable to function appropriately at work, school or in relationships (Covington et al., 2005). The biological anomaly is presented in two instances either as an imbalance of the brain chemicals or neurotransmitters or the improper development of connections of the brain during growth in the womb leading to the mental condition (Pouget *et al.*, 2016). Due to an imbalance of neurotransmitters, schizophrenic individuals will react differently to stimuli such as bright lights or loud music when compared to a healthy person.

Corpus callosum, also identified as CC, is the largest band of nerve tissue connecting the two hemispheres of the brain or commissure. This part of the brain is integral to the appropriate communication between these two hemispheres (Vissers, Cohen, and Geurts, 2012; Cui *et al.*, 2011). It is evident that the CC connects to the contralateral hemisphere of the brain whereby various functions of the brain are performed including motor, cognitive, and sensory activities. An image of the corpus callosum is included in appendix A. There are cases where this important part of the brain may be defective particularly beginning from birth. In this regard, this occurrence is known as agenesis of the corpus callosum (ACC), an uncommon congenital deficiency causing about 200 million axons to be either partially or completely absent (Mohapatra, Panda, Sahoo, Dey, and Rath, 2015) and (Jalili *et al*, 2010). This developmental abnormality may occur in isolation or as a combination of other central nervous system deformities. The widespread use of magnetic resonance imaging (MRI) has increased the ability to find the condition. The following research will argue for the possibility of ACC or CC dysfunction in underscoring language impairments in individuals suffering from schizophrenia.

The term borderline personality was first used by a psychoanalyst named Adolph Stern in 1938 in the United States (Douglas and James. 2013). The term was used to describe patients who did not fit either in the psychoneurotic or the psychotic group. Later in 1975, Otto Kernberg introduced the term borderline personality organisation to describe a pattern of behaviour and functioning categorized by instability among those affected. The description given to BPD patients included people that were difficult, unstable in their functioning, needy, at risk of suicide, and emotional. Soon after, a pattern of symptoms arose that could be used to describe people with a borderline personality disorder.

The symptoms included lack of a stable image, frequent changes between periods of despair and confidence, fear of being abandoned, rapid shift in mood, and suicidal ideations. The features which currently define BPD were described in 1978 by Kolb and Gunderson (Edelstein, Hersen, and Thase, 2013). Later in 1980, borderline personality disorder became officially recognised as a personality disorder in the Diagnostic and Statistical Manual-111. Borderline personality disorder (BPD) is a mental illness that affects how a person thinks and feels about himself and other people; this adversely affects the person's daily functionality. BPD is part of the class of mental illnesses referred to as personality disorders. Similar to other personality disorders, BPD is characterised by a regular pattern of feeling, thinking, and relating with other people that often causes considerable problems to the affected person. Furthermore, BPD is characterised by a constant pattern of mood variation, behaviour, and self-image. These symptoms may lead to impulsive behaviour and difficulties in relating to others (APA, 2013). A person with BPD can experience heightened periods of anxiety, depression, and anger. The affected individuals also may experience challenges in trying to control their emotional responses. Consequently, this may lead to suicidal and self-harming behaviours.

An individual with a borderline personality disorder might experience anxiety, depression, and attacks of anger, which can last for a day or a few hours (APA, 2013). These emotions might be linked to periods where the person engages in alcohol or drug abuse and self-injury, which may include cutting. Cognitive distortions that occur in people with BPD can cause constant changes in career plans, values, long-term goals, friendships, and jobs. At times, the affected individuals regard themselves as being unworthy or inadequate. The person might feel empty, bored, or mistreated. These symptoms are most severe when individuals with the disorder lack social support and feel isolated. Individuals with a borderline personality disorder often experience unsteady patterns of social relationships (APA,

2013). The person may develop an intense emotional attachment to family and friends. However, these attachments can quickly change from love and admiration to dislike and anger. The individual might become rapidly attached and idealize another person. However, when conflict occurs, the person may switch to the other extreme and blame the other individual for being uncaring. People diagnosed with borderline personality disorder are extremely sensitive to rejection. BPD also leads to feelings of abandonment, which puts the affected person at high risk of suicidal ideations.

Similar to other personality disorders, individuals are often in adulthood or adolescence before being evaluated as meeting the full borderline personality disorder criteria. Historically, BPD was believed to be a group of symptoms which comprised of mood problems and distorted reality. Therefore, the disorder was thought to border between schizophrenia and mood problems. In support, physically and psychologically abused children demonstrate deficits in producing questions, descriptive utterances and discourse skills (Coster, Gestern, Beeghly, and Cicchetti, 1989) in other words, expressive language is impaired while perceptive language appears intact. The fact links a psychological and physical abuse in early childhood with expressive language disturbance in people diagnosed with borderline personality disorder (Beeghly, and Cicchetti, 1994).

Linguistic/Language Impairments in Schizophrenia and Borderline Personality Disorder

Language is depicted as a vehicle for effective communication whereby the individual has pre-existing thoughts that provide content. The person speaking should have an appropriate understanding of the social environment in an effort to construct intelligent information. As a result, when an individual presents delusional thoughts, such as being a superhero, this is depicted as a case of thought disturbance and not that of language (Binz, and Brüne, 2010). The language in itself is only a reflection of the underlying problem (Hinzen and

Rossello, 2015). The mental disorder is characterised by instances where individuals experience significant distortion in terms of thought and speech. According to Kuperberg and Caplan (2003), the abnormalities of language are a primary trait found in psychosis that significantly manifests in the schizophrenic syndrome. It is evident that there is a number of ways in which this impairment may be presented for easy identification including thought disorder and difference from other psychoses.

Psychopathologists have taken the traditional viewpoint that disturbances of speech evident in schizophrenia reflect the underlying problem in the individual and not the primary disorder. In this regard, the patient is likely to experience derailed and incoherent train of thought bringing about unintelligent speech (Stephane, Pellizzer, Fletcher, and McClannahan, 2007). Despite a clear distinction between language and thought as it affects schizophrenic persons, there is a problem identifying the occurrence. There are researchers who recognise thought disorder as a term referring to the subjective changes affecting the patient (Huang *et al.*, 2015). Others distinguish the various language anomalies in writing and speech as thought disorders. On that note, differentiating the problem and the various processes involved becomes confusing. The terminology is now used purely to describe the various phenomena resulting in the impairment of verbal communication as per language output of the patient. According to Kuperberg (2010), it has little to do with the assumption of underlying causes, but on the way the phenomena cause social and vocational dysfunction.

There are two broad and distinct manifestations of the thought disorders including the negative and positive. The negative-thought disorder usually occurs more frequently along with other negative non-linguistic symptoms. It is portrayed by poor speech also known as alogia (Manschreck, Merrill, Jabbar, Chun, and Delisi, 2012; Zhou et al, 2015). On the other hand, there is the positive-thought disorder where there is the development of a discourse that is disorganised and difficult to follow in meaning. This condition occurs more frequently along with other positive symptoms. The latter disorder may be portrayed as derailment whereby the patient's train of thought slips off from the main point, and the presented ideas may be indirectly or completely unrelated. Tangentiality is another common trait where the response provided by the individual is irrelevant to the question (Keperberg, 2010). In this case, the patient may include words in a sentence that are unrelated to the general context of discourse. At the single-word level, abnormalities may be noted where patients produce neologisms or use common words in a bizarre manner such as *time vessel* in reference to a watch (Keperberg, 2010).

There are also instances where the positive-thought disorder is presented as unintelligible speech, where both the single words and sentences constructed do not have a discernible meaning. The phenomena of thought disorder have been gathered by researchers in the discipline to develop scales on the severity of the condition as presented by individual patients (Bleich-Cohen et al, 2012). Statistical processes of speech and written language produced by a patient would demonstrate that it is easier to predict omitted words in the transcript of a healthy individual than that of the former. There are cases where the language impairment presented is in comprehension (Okada et al, 2016). However, these abnormalities are more subtle and less documented than instances of language production. For instance, schizophrenia and BPD patients are more likely to perform poorly in tasks that use verbal materials than those with non-verbal materials. Kuperberg (2010) also shows that the patients experience problems in interpreting sentences that are long and grammatically complex. Past schizophrenia and BPD studies have demonstrated the relationship between language impairment, syntactic simplification, reduced idea density, and lexical irregularities (Covington, *et al.*, 2005; DeLisi, 2001; Kemper, *et al.*, 2001; Snowdon, *et al.*, 1996; Thomas, *et al.*, 1996).

Reasons for the Impairment

Experts in schizophrenia and BPD and their significant impairments of language have provided two distinct explanations of the reasons for the abnormalities encountered. The first theory asserts that language anomalies occur due to the unusual automatic spread of activation in the structure and function within the semantic memory. This theory identifies the problem as one that arises from a faster and automatic activation of words to build sentences and meaning (Kuperberg, 2010). The assumed model is presented as a network of words and concepts that are connected as per the co-occurrence. Using this assumption, it is evident that the brain is unable to effectively draw out the words and concepts that are closely associated with each other such that a meaningful sentence is formed. The theory appropriately provides an explanation for the derailment and tangentiality characteristics that bring about the *loosening of associations* (Kuperberg, 2010). In this case, words produced are semantically related but when stringing them together they do not form a coherent sentence due to its comprehension (Okada et al, 2016).

The process of spread activation is recognised as the moment when a node becomes active in the brain, the activation begins to spread through the links between them until it brings out the most appropriate answer for a given question. Each node represents a particular concept or word that has a particular set of properties and a link to another node with similar characteristics (Kuperberg, 2010). For the case of individuals with schizophrenia, this automatic mechanism is faster and even more seamless than it is required. The process of linking these concepts and words according to the degree of association is jumbled such that an individual is unable to retrieve meaning, facts, and ideas of the general world. This occurrence provides clear evidence that the corpus callosum commissure is dysfunctional (Randanovic, de Sousa, Valiengo, Gattaz, and Forlenza, 2012). It fails to provide the individual with the ability to appropriately interact with the social environment such that general word knowledge is stored appropriately with an effective linking system for future retrieval. As a result, patients string together words that do not apply to the discourse. For instance, identifying family members as, 'father, mother, son, and Holy Ghost' is a case of loosening associations (Kuperberg, 2010).

Another theory that describes the reasons for language dysfunction is evident when the build-up and context used are also abnormal. In this case, the context of sentences produced is impaired due to deficiencies of the working memory and the executive functioning. The theory highlights that within the multiple domains of cognitive function, significant deficits creating a poor production of speech in auditory or written form (Ho, Moonis, Ginat, and Eisenberg, 2013). Numerous studies have shown that schizophrenic patients have the tendency to perform poorly on various executive functions as is the case for in their working memory. The research incorporates neuropsychological measures as a means of examining the relationship between working memory or executive functioning and language impairment (Randanovic et al, 2012). These measures are appropriate in highlighting the severity of the positive-thought disorder recognising its presence as the reflecting factor of the neurodevelopmental aetiology (Sun et al, 2015). The inability of some parts of the brain to function appropriately influences the occurrence of the clinical condition.

The working memory is an important part of the cognitive system that is responsible for immediate conscious perception and processing of language. A healthy individual is capable of interacting with the social environment and understanding the appropriate words to express ideas and feelings (Stephane, Pellizer, Fletcher, and McClannahan, 2007) and (Sun et al, 2016). However, for the schizophrenic patient, this task may be difficult due to numerous factors such as overwhelming stimuli in the surrounding. Referential communication makes it almost impossible to perform accordingly. The executive function is a part of mental skills enabling the brain to act on information received. Some of the tasks include planning, organisation, prioritization, attention, and remembering (Stephane,

Pellizer, Fletcher, and McClannahan, 2007). The deficit of the corpus callosum makes it difficult for the patient to perform such activities. The organisation of words into a meaningful sentence that relates to the context of the social setting is undertaken by the executive function (Kuperberg, 2010). However, when the two hemispheres of the brain cannot communicate to receive the stimuli from the environment and react in relation to the same, a positive-thought disorder is presented.

The Wernicke's and Broca's areas are two significant areas of the cerebral cortex associated with the speech production and comprehension respectively. An image of both areas is included as appendix B. Broca's area is associated with language processing such that lesions to this part may cause a grammatical speech production. Its specific location is in the frontal gyrus on the left inferior part. The Broca's anterior part helps understand semantics and the posterior part for phonetics. Dysfunction of this area creates the Broca's or expressive aphasia where speech includes important content words, but function words are eliminated or left out. For instance, a patient may say, 'Mom, drive, store' when meaning 'My mom drives me to the store.' It is the act of leaving these functional words that it is referred to as *telegraphic speech*. This part takes control of motor functions associated with speech production such as how to appropriately pronounce words and facial neuron control.

On the other hand, Wernicke's area is responsible for language development as it ensures comprehension of speech. The Wernicke's area is found in the left posterior superior part of the temporal gyrus. Carl Wernicke, who discovered this region of the brain, identified that damage of the Wernicke's area makes it difficult to produce and comprehend written and spoken the language. The condition is referred to as Wernicke's aphasia or fluent, sensory or receptive aphasia. Speech produced in this case sounds normal and may be grammatically correct but does not make sense. Usually, irrelevant and non-existent words may be included in the produced sentences. In this regard, the Wernicke's area is important for comprehension, language recognition, semantic processing, and interpretation of language. Effective language comprehension and production work through the combined effort of these two areas through nerve fibres that connect them. Damage to these fibres results in a condition referred to as conduction aphasia where patients are unable to repeat words or phrases appropriately but comprehend and speak coherently (Li et al, 2014).

Description of Corpus Callosum

As mentioned earlier, the largest white matter in the placental mammals that connects the two hemispheres of the brain is called the corpus callosum. This part of the brain contains hundreds of millions of intra- and inter-hemispheric axonal projections used in creating the connection between the different parts of the brain (Schipul, Keller, and Just, 2011). Despite previous beliefs that the corpus callosum is of no use to the central nervous system, studies on callosal lesions and the numerous corpus callosotomies have shown otherwise. The latter procedures have shown that the white matter structure is indeed important for effective treatment of uncontrollable epilepsy that prevents spreading seizures to the rest of the brain. The very first procedure did not seem to portray a significant effect on the functional or cognitive deficits on the individual despite successful treatment of epilepsy (Baldeweg, and Hirsch, 2015). However, continued behavioural research shows that severing it prevents complete blocking of communication between the two hemispheres. As a result, this dissociation between the left and right makes it difficult to transfer learned information (Karlsgodt, 2016).

This research looks into the condition of schizophrenia and the subsequent development of language dysfunction. In the past, callosotomy procedures involved complete splitting of the brain including some very important commissures. However, in modern times patients of these procedures severed the corpus callosum but have kept the commissures intact (Halgren et al, 2012). The continued uncertainty of schizophrenia and BPD and their negative effects on the social and cognitive life of the individuals it affects have brought about the need to investigate this procedure further. The empirical research is essential to identify the communication between the two hemispheres and functional roles of the corpus callosum (Docherty, Berenbaum, and Kerns, 2011). The question posed in this thesis seeks to identify whether the callosal dysfunction could lead to increased risk of language impairment among individuals who suffer from schizophrenia and BPD along with those who are at great risk (Carter, 2011). In this regard, it is important to identify how and when direct communication takes place between the left and right hemispheres.

Explore in the more details, the anatomical composition of the brain and the way it functions provide a broader outlook on the effect of callosal dysfunction and the altered morphology. Communication in the brain takes place intra-hemispheric and inter-hemispheric (Cassidy et al, 2014). In the former practice, the white matter structure creates a connection among various cortices of the occipital, parietal, temporal and frontal lobes through cortico-cortical pathways (Kuperberg, 2010). The information present in this region is also made available for transfer between the two hemispheres. The latter process involves communication through brain commissures that are three in major ones: anterior, hippocampal, and corpus callosum commissures. The final one is the largest and most connected of them all though only present in placental mammals.

The corpus callosum (CC) is heavily involved in information processing and contributes to brain function lateralisation through selection pressure. This process involves the tendency for particular neural functions to be more dominant in a single cerebral hemisphere (Xu et al, 2014). Through the exchange of information between the right and the left and specialisation of brain functions, the CC saves the cortical space. For instance, language and speech are predominantly functions of the left hemisphere. Further investigation of the brain structure's role in information communication provides clarity to the role played by CC in this mediation.

Involvement of the Corpus Callosum

There are approximately 200 million axons that connect the corpus callosum to the two cerebral hemispheres. Each of these fibres is fixed at birth though, the myelination process continues through to puberty (Knyazeva, 2013). This process is important as myelin, allows for faster transmission of information, and enables the brain to conduct more complex functions. Though there are no clear anatomical subdivisions of the CC, there are distinct sub-regions that in accordance with the topographical organisation of the cortical areas: the genu, truncus, and splenium (Knyazeva, 2013). The width and size of the corpus callosum are depicted to vary among individuals and across the different genders. Controversial studies have identified that women have a larger white matter than men while other research experiments do not distinctly point out a significant difference (Radanovic, Sousa, Valiengo, Gattaz, and Forlenza, 2013). These contradictions could merely be because of corrections as men have larger brains, varied patient groups, and differing technological measurements.

Partial callosotomy and lesion studies provide important information on functional specificity. The differing types of callosal lesions give essential knowledge on the specific function of a given sub-region (van Meer et al, 2016). An intact splenium and the posterior callosal body in partial callosotomy patients compared to complete callosotomy patients and a control group provided evidence that tactile stimuli travelled through the posterior callosal body (Kuperberg, 2010). As a result, the patients who only received a partial procedure performed better off than those who did a complete operation. Further studies show that the size of fibre and its composition varies along the topography of the cortex (Xu *et al.*, 2014). The genu which is also the anterior part has the highest density of myelinated axons that are thin in size and attach to the higher-order sensory areas and the prefrontal cortex (Kuperberg, 2010). The fibres reduce in density towards the truncus as they attach to the parietal and temporal lobes.

The truncus is also referred to as the mid-body region of the CC. While the middle portion affixes to the primary and secondary somatosensory and motor areas, thick axons are present in the posterior mid-body that attach to the primary and secondary auditory areas (Pouget et al, 2016). This information shows that the mid-region is significantly responsible for build-up and production of speech. As the CC extends to the posterior regions, splenium, the density of axons increases once again as it connects to the occipital lobe associated with visual senses (Yalınçetin et al, 2016). There is a thinned area connecting the truncus and the splenium known as the isthmus that affixes to the somatosensory, motor, and primary auditory areas (Ribolsi, Daskalakis, Siracusano, and Koch, 2014). This anatomical composition provides a clear indicator of the importance of the white matter structure in brain functions. However, it is important to note that the brain can process the information on a single hemisphere of inter-hemispheric transfer is recognised as hazardous to one's health.

Sectioning of the corpus callosum presented significant behavioural and functional changes in the animals with the desired response slowly learned. According to results on the subject patients and healthy group, change of behavioural response from the use of one hand to another had little interference in the former group transition period. This demonstrates the proper functioning of the two hemispheres and does not heavily influence lateralisation (Pietrasanta, Restani, and Caleo, 2012; Pietrasanta et al, 2014; Caspers et al, 2015). The human studies would be used to identify the impact of higher cognitive functions. This procedure does not lead to the complete lateralisation of motor control as processing is conducted in both hemispheres (Najjar, S., and Pearlman, 2015). However, language and speech are affected. Callosotomised patients were noted to only effectively name objects placed in the right hand. They could recognise the object on the left and select it from a list. This result demonstrates the restriction of language processing to the left hemisphere. The superiority of the right hemisphere is evident in the episodic grouping, perceptual memory, complex auditory processing, and mental rotation among others (Docherty,

Berenbaum, and Kerns, 2011). The left is specialised for intelligence, cognitive functioning, language and speech, and semantic memory.

Literature Review

Recent studies suggest that through significant morphology of the corpus callosum, the individual is more likely to experience dysfunction in language and speech (Walterfang, 2010; Peters, and Karlsgodt, 2015). The white matter structure of the brain forms nearly 50% of the entire organ hence showing its importance in the performance of the various functions. The abnormal connectivity between the two cerebral hemispheres is depicted to have a significant effect on the onset of the schizophrenia disease (Fogelson, Litvak, Peled, Fernandez-del-Olmo, and Friston, 2014). Callosotomy is depicted as a proposed treatment option for individuals who experience uncontrollable epilepsy seizures (Del Re et al, 2016). This procedure is undertaken only when the quality of health of the affected individual is at high risk. Research shows that the partial procedure on the corpus callosum could ensure continued proper functioning of the brain. Each hemisphere will experience specialisation and lateralisation of its particular functions (Ditman, Goff, and Kuperberg, 2011). However, a complete callosotomy may cause dysfunction in the cognitive processes. Instances of thought disorder may begin to affect the individual creating inability to interact in the social environment.

Agenesis of corpus callosum shows that disorder affecting individuals from birth. In this case, the white matter is depicted to have failed to develop normally particularly during pregnancy (Sass et al, 2014). The fibres which would otherwise form axons that extend from one hemisphere to another usually become longitudinally oriented in each to create Probst bundles. This abnormal growth restricts the co-dependent relationship between the two cerebral hemispheres (Pietrasanta, Restani, and Caleo, 2012; Isobe *et al.*, 2016). The language level, in this case, is severely affected as the patient cannot effectively coordinate between the stimuli received from the social environment and the processed information in either of the hemispheres. Language impairment may be impaired from the phonetics through to phonology. According to a study by Mohapatra, Panda, Sahoo, Dey, and Rath (2015), corpus callosum dysfunction may manifest along with other anomalies of commissures including hippocampal and anterior commissures. Such a disorder may worsen the language problem for the individual making it almost impossible to communicate an idea, feelings and perform normal cognitive tasks (Docherty, Berenbaum, and Kerns, 2011).

The deficits of the corpus callosum in reference to language impairment are manifested into two distinct disorders: thought disorder and schizophasia. The research by Colle *et al.* (2013) indicates that the most impaired language level in patients with schizophrenia and BPD is pragmatics. In this regard, individuals suffering from these illnesses are unable to use language convey meaning within a given context (Bucca, 2012). Even in cases where syntax and semantic components of language are depicted to be intact, the person cannot effectively engage in discourse. The research conducted by Van der Knaap (2010) shows that the lack of effective interaction between the two hemispheres creates a stumbling barrier in the sharing of information. It is important to note that communication is not just the uttering of words, sentences, and paragraphs of meaning but involves much more such as interpreting facial expressions, agency, intention, social salience, and interpreting tone of voice (Niznikiewicz, Kubicki, Mulert, and Condray, 2013; Cui *et al.*, 2011). Due to the separation of sensory areas like motor, auditory, and tactile areas, the individual is unable to participate in social activities as their behaviour is incoherent with the context of the setting.

Future Research Recommendations

From the above research, it is evident that the experts in this field have not reached a consensus on the nature of the role played by the corpus callosum in mediating relocating of information between the hemispheres. The study by Van der Knaap (2010) presents both inhibitory and excitatory nature probably as a means of giving the reader the opportunity to choose either of the two. On the other hand, Bhatia, Saha, and Doval (2015) assert that the white matter plays an inhibitory role. In this case, understanding the mediator function of the corpus callosum is an important factor of better understanding the resulting language impairments that affect patients of BPD and schizophrenia (Thoresen et al., 2014). Despite immense evidence available to support each theory, it is a study of healthy and aged individuals usually presents an excitatory model. This perspective identifies the increased interconnection between the two hemispheres minimising instances of lateralisation of a single side in particular functions. Instead, it purports for greater co-dependence between the two (Hinzen, and Rosselló, 2015; Barrera, McKenna, and Berrios, 2008). The conclusion is not definite and still calls for future research to underline a common understanding.

Morphology studies are another cause for variation between experts and researchers in the corpus callosum. The cause for the distinction is the type of measurements, post-mortem studies, correction for brain volume, MRI and faulty head positioning and head tilt has brought about varied opinions (Balevich et al., 2015; Kazi, Joshi, Kelkar, Mahajan, and Ghawate, 2013). It is evident that the most appropriate measure of measuring the connectivity of the corpus callosum is the size. However, research has shown that men have bigger sizes compared to women whereas individuals with a pre-existing condition such as ADHD have a smaller volume. The conflict of views on the morphology of the white matter structure has delayed developments for the appropriate measures of diagnosis and interventions to curb the effect on language impairment (Collinson et al., 2014; Mohammadi, Zhand, Moghadam, and Golalipour, 2011). Future research should seek to provide unanimous measures of measuring connectivity between the two cerebral hemispheres such that appropriate assistance is made available for individuals with callosal dysfunctions at an early stage.

Future research should also focus on the impact of deficits of the white brain matter in reference to the pragmatic components of language along with other communicative techniques such as non-verbal components. Majority of the literature on language impairments in BPD and schizophrenia present instances of production of written and auditory language. Very few seek to identify other numerous disorders. For instance, the schizophasia disorder has received little attention on the ways such individuals with unintelligent discourse, clanging, and neologism are affected by the lack of connectivity between the cerebral hemispheres (Niznikiewicz, Kubicki, Mulert, and Condray, 2013; Binz, and Brüne, 2010).

Conclusion

Callosal lesions among other disorders affecting the white matter tracts in the brain clearly have an effect on the emphasis of language impairment among schizophrenic individuals. The corpus callosum is depicted as one of the most important commissures of the brain. The structure that forms nearly 50% of the brain is involved in the intra- and inter-hemispheric transfer of information received from the surrounding social environment. Research has shown that improper functioning of this structure or prevailing deficits results in impaired functioning of the brain. The two hemispheres may attempt to specialise or lateralise particular activities. This occurrence is however nearly impossible as depicted in the research only results in the presentation of abnormal behaviour. In the case of a schizophrenic patient, the lack of connectivity for the corpus callosum causes unintelligent discourse in the build-up and production of the speech. Lesion studies have shown the need for coordination in the brain due to each cortical area having a particular role to play in the performance of cognitive, semantic, and executive functions.

References

Baldeweg, T., and Hirsch, S. R. (2015) 'Mismatch negativity indexes illness-specific impairments of cortical plasticity in schizophrenia: a comparison with bipolar disorder and Alzheimer's disease', *International Journal of Psychophysiology, 95(2), pp. 138–141*.

Balevich, E. C., Haznedar, M. M., Wang, E., Newmark, R. E., Bloom, R., Schneiderman, J. S., . . . and Buchsbaum, M. S. (2015) 'Corpus callosum size and diffusion tensor anisotropy in adolescents and adults with schizophrenia', *Psychiatry Research: Neuroimaging, 231*(3), pp. 207–215.

Barrera, A., McKenna, P. J., and Berrios, G. E. (2008) 'Two new scales of formal thought disorder in schizophrenia', *Psychiatry Research, 157*(1), pp. 119–125.

Beeghly, M., and Cicchetti, D., (1994) 'Child maltreatment, attachment, and the self system: emergence of an internal state lexicon in toddlers at high social risk', *Development and Psychopathology, 6*(1), pp. 5–30.

Bhatia, M. S., Saha, R., and Doval, N. (2016) 'Delusional Disorder in a Patient with Corpus Callosum Agenesis', *Journal of Clinical and Diagnostic Research: JCDR, 10*(12), VD01.

Binz, B., and Brüne, B. (2010) 'Pragmatic language abilities, mentalizing skills and executive functioning in schizophrenia spectrum disorders', *Clinical Neuropsychiatry, 7*(3), pp. 76–84.

Bleich-Cohen, M., Sharon, H., Weizman, R., Poyurovsky, M., Faragian, S., and Hendler, T. (2012) 'Diminished language lateralization in schizophrenia corresponds to impaired inter-hemispheric functional connectivity', *Schizophrenia Research, 134*(2), pp. 131–136.

Bucca, A. (2012) 'The shared ideation of the paranoic delusion. Implications of empathy, theory of mind and language', *Journal of Psychopathology, 18*(4), pp. 235–240.

Carter, C. J. (2011) 'Schizophrenia: a pathogenetic autoimmune disease caused by viruses and pathogens and dependent on genes', *Journal of Pathogens*, pp. 9–28.

Caspers, S., Axer, M., Caspers, J., Jockwitz, C., Jütten, K., Reckfort, J., . . . and Zilles, K. (2015) 'Target sites for transcallosal fibers in human visual cortex–a combined diffusion and polarized light imaging study', *Cortex, 72*, pp. 38–47.

Cassidy, C., Buchy, L., Bodnar, M., Dell'Elce, J., Choudhry, Z., Fathalli, F., . . . and Iyer, S. (2014) 'Association of a risk allele of ANK3 with cognitive performance and cortical thickness in patients with first-episode psychosis', *Journal of Psychiatry and Neuroscience: JPN, 39*(1), p. 29.

Colle, L., Angeleri, R., Vallana, M., Sacco, K., Bara, B. G., and Bosco, F. M. (2013) 'Understanding the communicative impairments in schizophrenia: a preliminary study', *Journal of Communication Disorders, 46*(3), pp. 188–212.

Collinson, S. L., Gan, S. C., San Woon, P., Kuswanto, C., Sum, M. Y., Yang, G. L., . . . and Sim, K. (2014) 'Corpus callosum morphology in first-episode and chronic schizophrenia: combined magnetic resonance and diffusion tensor imaging study of Chinese Singaporean patients', *The British Journal of Psychiatry, 204*(1), pp. 42–57.

Covington, M. A., He, C., Brown, C., Naçi, L., McClain, J. T., Fjordbak, B. S., . . . and Brown, J. (2005) 'Schizophrenia and the structure of language: the linguist's view', *Schizophrenia Research, 77*(1), pp. 76–87.

Covington, M., Riedel, W., Brown, C., He, C., Morris, E., Weinstein, S., *et al.* (2007) 'Does ketamine mimic aspects of schizophrenia speech?', *Journal of Psychopharmacology, 21*(3), pp. 338–346.

Coster, W., Gersten, M., Beeghly, M., and Cicchetti, D. (1989)

'Communicative functioning in maltreated toddlers', *Developmental Psychology, 25*(6), pp. 1020–1029.

Cui, L., Chen, Z., Deng, W., Huang, X., Li, M., Ma, X., . . . and Collier, D. A. (2011) 'Assessment of white matter abnormalities in paranoid schizophrenia and bipolar mania patients', *Psychiatry Research: Neuroimaging, 194*(3), pp. 347–353.

Del Re, E. C., Konishi, J., Bouix, S., Blokland, G. A., Mesholam-Gately, R. I., Goldstein, J., . . . and Petryshen, T. (2016) 'Enlarged lateral ventricles inversely correlate with reduced corpus callosum central volume in first episode schizophrenia: association with functional measures', *Brain Imaging and Behavior*, 10(4), pp. 1264–1273.

Ditman, T., Goff, D., and Kuperberg, G. R. (2011) 'Slow and steady: sustained effects of lexico-semantic associations can mediate referential impairments in schizophrenia', *Cognitive, Affective, and Behavioral Neuroscience*, 11(2), pp. 245–258.

Docherty, A. R., Berenbaum, H., and Kerns, J. G. (2011) 'Alogia and formal thought disorder: Differential patterns of verbal fluency task performance', *Journal of Psychiatric Research*, 45(10), pp. 1352–1357.

Fogelson, N., Litvak, V., Peled, A., Fernandez-del-Olmo, M., and Friston, K. (2014) 'The functional anatomy of schizophrenia: a dynamic causal modeling study of predictive coding', *Schizophrenia Research*, 158(1), pp. 204–212.

Halgren, C., Kjaergaard, S., Bak, M., Hansen, C., El-Schich, Z., Anderson, C. M., . . . and Nielsen, M. (2012) 'Corpus callosum abnormalities, intellectual disability, speech impairment, and autism in patients with haploinsufficiency of ARID1B', *Clinical Genetics*, 82(3), pp. 248–255.

Hinzen, W., and Rosselló, J. (2015) 'The linguistics of schizophrenia: thought disturbance as language pathology across positive symptoms', *Frontiers in Psychology*, 6(971), pp. 1–17.

Ho, M. L., Moonis, G., Ginat, D. T., and Eisenberg, R. L. (2013) 'Lesions of the corpus callosum', *American Journal of Roentgenology*, 200(1), W1–W16.

Huang, X., Du, X., Song, H., Zhang, Q., Jia, J., Xiao, T., and Wu, J. (2015) 'Cognitive impairments associated with corpus callosum infarction: a ten cases study', *International Journal of Clinical and Experimental Medicine*, 8(11), p. 21991.

Innocenti, G. M., Ansermet, F., and Parnas, J. (2003) 'Schizophrenia, neurodevelopment and corpus callosum', *Molecular Psychiatry*, 8(3), pp. 184–199.

Isobe, M., Miyata, J., Hazama, M., Fukuyama, H., Murai, T., and Takahashi, H. (2016) 'Multimodal neuroimaging as a window into the pathological physiology of schizophrenia: current trends and issues', *Neuroscience Research*, 102, pp. 18–29.

Jalili, M., Meuli, R., Do, K. Q., Hasler, M., Crow, T. J., and Knyazeva, M. G. (2010) 'Attenuated asymmetry of functional connectivity in schizophrenia: A high-resolution EEG study', *Psychophysiology*, 47(4), pp. 689–698.

Jamadar, S., O'Neil, K. M., Pearlson, G. D., Ansari, M., Gill, A., Jagannathan, K., and Assaf, M. (2013) 'Impairment in semantic retrieval is associated with symptoms of schizophrenia but not bipolar disorder', *Biological Psychiatry*, 73(6), pp. 491–516.

Karlsgodt, K. H. (2016) 'Diffusion imaging of white matter in schizophrenia: Progress and future directions', *Biological Psychiatry: Cognitive Neuroscience and Neuroimaging*, 1(3), pp. 209–217.

Kazi, A. Z., Joshi, P. C., Kelkar, A. B., Mahajan, M. S., and Ghawate, A. S. (2013) 'MRI evaluation of pathologies affecting the corpus callosum: A pictorial essay', *The Indian Journal of Radiology and Imaging*, 23(4), p. 282.

Knyazeva, M. G. (2013) 'Splenium of corpus callosum: patterns of interhemispheric interaction in children and adults', *Neural Plasticity*, p. 3–22.

Kuperberg, G. R. and Caplan, D. (2003) chapter 19, *Language Dysfunction in Schizophrenia*, pp. 444–466, http://www.nmr.mgh.harvard.edu/kuperberglab/publications/chapters/Kuperberg%26Caplan_Neuropsych_2003.pdf, (accessed 17 March 2003).

Kuperberg, G. R. (2010) 'Language in Schizophrenia Part 1: An Introduction', *Language and Linguistics Compass*, 4(8), pp. 439–471.

Li, J., Edmiston, E. K., Chen, K., Tang, Y., Ouyang, X., Jiang, Y., ... and Jiang, W. (2014) 'A comparative diffusion tensor imaging study of corpus callosum sub region integrity in bipolar disorder and schizophrenia', *Psychiatry Research: Neuroimaging*, 221(1), pp. 58–62.

Manschreck, T. C., Merrill, A. M., Jabbar, G., Chun, J., and Delisi, L. E. (2012) 'Frequency of normative word associations in the speech of individuals at familial high-risk for schizophrenia', *Schizophrenia Research*, 140(1), pp. 99–103.

Mohammadi, M. R., Zhand, P., Moghadam, B. M., and Golalipour, M. J. (2011) 'Measurement of the corpus callosum using magnetic resonance imaging in the North of Iran', *Iranian Journal of Radiology*, 8(4), pp. 218–23.

Mohapatra, S., Panda, U., Sahoo, A., Dey, S., and Rath, N. (2015) 'Neuropsychiatric manifestations in a child with agenesis of the corpus callosum', *Journal of Neurosciences in Rural Practice*, 6(3), pp. 456–457.

Müller, N., Weidinger, E., Leitner, B., and Schwarz, M. J. (2015) 'The role of inflammation in schizophrenia', *Frontiers in Neuroscience*, 9(372), pp. 1–9.

Najjar, S., and Pearlman, D. M. (2015) 'Neuroinflammation and white matter pathology in schizophrenia: systematic review', *Schizophrenia Research*, 161(1), pp. 84–98.

Niznikiewicz, M. A., Kubicki, M., Mulert, C., and Condray, R. (2013) 'Schizophrenia as a Disorder of Communication,' *Schizophrenia Research and Treatment*, pp. 1–4.

Okada, N., Fukunaga, M., Yamashita, F., Koshiyama, D., Yamamori, H., Ohi, K., ... and Nemoto, K. (2016) 'Abnormal asymmetries in subcortical brain volume in schizophrenia', *Molecular Psychiatry*, 21(10), p. 1460.

Palaniyappan, L., Mahmood, J., Balain, V., Mougin, O., Gowland, P. A., and Liddle, P. F. (2015) 'Structural correlates of formal thought disorder in schizophrenia: an ultra-high field multivariate morphometry study', *Schizophrenia Research*, 168(1), pp. 305–312.

Peters, B. D., and Karlsgodt, K. H. (2015) 'White matter development in the early stages of psychosis', *Schizophrenia Research*, 161(1), pp. 52–59.

Pietrasanta, M., Restani, L., and Caleo, M. (2012) 'The corpus callosum and the visual cortex: plasticity is a game for two', *Neural Plasticity*, pp. 7–22.

Pietrasanta, M., Restani, L., Cerri, C., Olcese, U., Medini, P., and Caleo, M. (2014) 'A switch from inter-ocular to inter-hemispheric suppression following monocular deprivation in the rat visual cortex', *European Journal of Neuroscience*, 40(1), pp. 2283–2292.

Pouget, J. G., Han, B., Mignot, E., Ollila, H. M., Barker, J., Spain, S., . . . and Bossini-Castillo, L. (2016) 'Polygenic analysis of schizophrenia and 19 immune diseases reveals modest pleiotropy,' *bioRxiv*, 068684, http://www.biorxiv.org/content/biorxiv/early/2016/08/09/068684.full.pdf (accessed in 2016).

Radanovic, M., Sousa, R. T. D., Valiengo, L., Gattaz, W. F., and Forlenza, O. V. (2013) 'Formal Thought Disorder and language impairment in schizophrenia', *Arquivos de neuro-psiquiatria*, 71(1), pp. 68–81.

Ribolsi, M., Daskalakis, Z. J., Siracusano, A., and Koch, G. (2014) 'Abnormal asymmetry of brain connectivity in schizophrenia', *Frontiers in Human Neuroscience*, p. 8.

Sass, K., Heim, S., Sachs, O., Straube, B., Schneider, F., Habel, U., and Kircher, T. (2014) 'Neural correlates of semantic associations in patients with schizophrenia', *European Archives of Psychiatry and Clinical Neuroscience*, 264(2), pp. 78–95.

Schipul, S. E., Keller, T. A., and Just, M. A. (2011) 'Inter-regional brain communication and its disturbance in autism', *Frontiers in Systems Neuroscience*, 5(10), pp. 1–10.

Stephane, M., Pellizzer, G., Fletcher, C. R., and McClannahan, K. (2007) 'Empirical evaluation of language disorder in schizophrenia', *Journal of Psychiatry and Neuroscience*, 32(4), pp. 239–261.

Subramaniam, K., Gill, J., Fisher, M., Mukherjee, P., Nagarajan, S., and Vinogradov, S. (2017) 'White matter microstructure predicts cognitive training-induced improvements in attention and executive functioning in schizophrenia', *Schizophrenia Research*, https://doi.org/10.1016/j.schres.2017.06.062.

Sun, H., Lui, S., Yao, L., Deng, W., Xiao, Y., Zhang, W., . . . and Sweeney, J. A. (2015) 'Two patterns of white matter abnormalities in medication-naive patients with first-episode schizophrenia revealed by diffusion tensor imaging and cluster analysis', *JAMA Psychiatry*, 72(7), pp. 554–572.

Sun, Y., Chen, Y., Lee, R., Bezerianos, A., Collinson, S. L., and Sim, K. (2016) 'Disruption of brain anatomical networks in schizophrenia: a longitudinal, diffusion tensor imaging based study', *Schizophrenia Research*, 171(1), pp. 149–157.

Thoresen, C., Endestad, T., Sigvartsen, N. P. B., Server, A., Bolstad, I., Johansson, M., . . . and Jensen, J. (2014) 'Frontotemporal hypoactivity during a reality monitoring paradigm is associated with delusions in patients with schizophrenia spectrum disorders', *Cognitive Neuropsychiatry*, 19(2), pp. 65–81.

Van der Knaap, L. J. (2010) *The Corpus Callosum and Brain Hemisphere Communication; How does the corpus callosum mediate interhemispheric transfer*, master's thesis, Utrecht University.

Van Meer, N., Houtman, A. C., Van Schuerbeek, P., Vanderhasselt, T., Milleret, C., and Tusscher, M. P. (2016) 'Interhemispheric Connections between the Primary Visual Cortical Areas via the Anterior Commissure in Human Callosal Agenesis', *Frontiers in Systems Neuroscience*, p. 10.

Vissers, M. E., Cohen, M. X., and Geurts, H. M. (2012) 'Brain connectivity and high functioning autism: a promising path of research that needs refined models, methodological convergence, and stronger behavioral links', *Neuroscience and Biobehavioral Reviews*, 36(1), pp. 519–589.

Walterfang, M., (2010) *The Specificity of Morphological Changes of the Corpus*

Callosum in Schizophrenia and Related Major Mental Disorders, doctoral dissertation, University of Melbourne, Department of Psychiatry, https://minerva-access.unimelb.edu.au/bitstream/handle/11343/35752/265523_Walterfang_thesis.pdf?sequence=1.

Xu, J. Q., Hui, C. L. M., Longenecker, J., Lee, E. H. M., Chang, W. C., Chan, S. K. W., and Chen, E. Y. H. (2014) 'Executive function as predictors of persistent thought disorder in first-episode schizophrenia: a one-year follow-up study', *Schizophrenia Research*, 159(2), pp. 319–358.

Yalınçetin, B., Ulaş, H., Var, L., Binbay, T., Akdede, B. B., and Alptekin, K. (2016) 'Relation of formal thought disorder to symptomatic remission and social functioning in schizophrenia', *Comprehensive Psychiatry*, 70, pp. 98–104.

Zhou, Y., Ma, X., Wang, D., Qin, W., Zhu, J., Zhuo, C., and Yu, C. (2015) 'The selective impairment of resting-state functional connectivity of the lateral sub region of the frontal pole in schizophrenia', *PloS one*, 10(3), e0119176.

CHAPTER 8

Why the Current BPD Treatments Are Not Successful

In the 1970s, psychoanalytic psychotherapy was practically the only therapy used to treat borderline personality disorder. The disorder was believed to need extended period, individual, and comprehensive treatment to reconstruct the personality and eradicate the problematic personality disorder symptoms (Gunderson, Weinberg, and Choi-Kain, 2013). Minimal success was witnessed in the treatment of BPD with psychoanalytic psychotherapy. The failure was credited to the pathologic motivations among borderline personality disorder patients (Gunderson, 2009). Improvements of BPD symptoms through psychoanalytic psychotherapy were sporadic.

In most BPD patients, the psychoanalytic psychotherapy worsened their symptoms due to the unplanned toxic relationship between the BPD core psychopathology and the approach used by the therapist (Gunderson, 2014). The neutrality of the therapist increased the patient's fear of abandonment and projection. Additionally, the passivity of the therapist enhanced the patient's fear of being neglected. The patients viewed the approach used by the therapist to interpret negative emotions as being invalidating and blaming. In the 1980s psychoanalytic psychotherapy started to be slowly replaced by biologic psychiatry. Although helpful therapeutic approaches were still lacking, clinicians were more informed on what to avoid when dealing with BPD patients. Support and empathy became more appreciated as a necessary part of therapy. By the 1990s, dialectical behavioural therapy was developed to specifically treat borderline personality disorder patients (Dimeff and Koerner, 2007). Soon after, other therapies such as the transference-focused psychotherapy, schema-focused therapy, and mentalisation-based therapy were developed for the treatment of BPD. The treatment approaches of borderline personality disorder have evolved significantly over the years. Currently, psychotherapy has remained to be the preferred borderline personality disorder treatment.

Studies have reported that around 75% of individuals with borderline personality disorder seek mental healthcare services from healthcare practitioners compared to people diagnosed with other personality disorders (Tomko, 2014). In most cases, these BPD patients will be provided with psychological interventions and often for extended periods (Zanarini, 2015). Over the last few decades, the treatment of borderline personality disorder has grown.

Treatments for BPD can be divided into pharmacotherapy and psychotherapy since few studies have been conducted on other kinds of treatments such as electroconvulsive therapy. There are various challenges in the provision of adequate care for borderline personality disorder patients. One of the challenges is the different views held by the various guidelines. For instance, the American Psychiatric Association of the Borderline Personality Disorder Treatment has not been updated for several years. However, this guideline gives complex pharmacotherapy data that focuses on diverse BPD symptoms and also psychotherapy (Herpetz *et al.*, 2007).

On the contrary, NICE guidelines state that medicines should not be used specifically to treat borderline personality disorder or any symptoms linked to the disorder. The World Federation of Societies of Biological Psychiatry, on the other hand, developed guidelines that address the pharmacotherapy of borderline personality disorder. The guidelines recommend that some drugs can assist in enhancing some BPD symptoms. However, these guidelines state there is no single drug that can ultimately enhance borderline personality disorder psychopathology (Herpetz *et al.*, 2007). The different views in these guidelines leave mental health professionals with more questions than answers regarding the treatments of borderline personality disorder.

Generally, the treatment of borderline personality disorder includes a combination of psychotherapies and medication. Some of the commonly used psychotherapies in the BPD treatment include dialectical behavioural therapy, mentalisation-based therapy, schema-focused therapy, and the transference-focused psychotherapy (Dimeff and Koerner, 2007). The psychotherapies can be based on conventional psychotherapeutic schools like cognitive behavioural therapy or psychodynamic psychotherapy. The psychological intervention can also be client-centred. Medications used in treating BPD include antidepressants, antipsychotics, mood stabilisers, and anxiolytics. These treatments, although commonly applied in treating BPD, are not quite effective and in most cases, very costly (Zanarini *et al.*, 2015). At times, these treatments can also lead to damaging side effects and have a minimal positive outcome. In this chapter, we will address some of these treatments, both psychotherapies and pharmacotherapies and identify their limitation in treating borderline personality disorder.

Psychotherapies for Borderline Personality Disorder

Until recently, the treatment of borderline personality disorder focused on evidence-based psychotherapies like transference-based therapy, mentalisation-based therapy, dialectical behavioural therapy, and schema-focused therapy. These therapies are intensive in both their clinical resource time and training requirements (Choi-Kain eta l., 2016). Most of these approaches are expensive and rarely assimilate medication. Additionally, the psychotherapies are not adequately available and seldom attend to the public health needs of borderline personality disorder patients. Based on these findings, there is increasing evidence that more readily learned and less intensive treatment approaches can be more effective in treating **BPD** patients (Bateman, 2012). Similar to other interventions, psychotherapy should and maybe scientifically evaluate to identify its efficacy. In the first part of this chapter, we will look at the four commonly used evidence-based psychotherapies, namely the dialectical behavioural therapy, mentalisation-based therapy, schema-focused therapy, and the transference-focused psychotherapy. We will also look to see if they are effective in eliminating borderline personality disorder symptoms.

Dialectical Behavioural Therapy

Marsha Linehan developed dialectical behavioural therapy, a cognitive behaviour treatment for the treatment of individuals that were chronically suicidal (Dimeff and Koerner, 2007). The therapy was first tested on women that were diagnosed with borderline personality disorder and exhibited suicidal tendencies. Linehan suggested that the primary feature of borderline personality disorder is emotional deregulation. She further held the view that emotional dysregulation can either be inherent or caused by environmental factors. A borderline personality disorder patient is often irritable and often takes a long time to become calm down. Emotional dysregulation is associated with interpersonal turmoil and impulsivity; these are common symptoms in people diagnosed with **BPD**. DBT is based on the theory that people develop borderline personality disorder from genetic vulnerability to emotional dysregulation and an environment that invalidates their experiences. As a result, a pattern of unsuccessful relationships between a child and the caregiver is developed. Such interactions often invalidate or minimise the child's experience, thereby escalating other dysfunctional coping techniques.

Dialectical behavioural therapy entails individual therapy sessions that are conducted every week (Stanley and New, 2017). The weekly individual sessions focus primarily on the treatment of self-harming and life-threatening behaviours. The organisation of the skills training sessions is similar to that of a classroom. In these sessions, two therapists are usually involved. The therapists primarily focus on four areas namely mindfulness, emotion regulation, distress tolerance, and acceptance of stressful situations. DBT recommends that borderline personality disorder patients can learn how to manage their interactions and sensitivities with others by acquiring skills that improve mindfulness.

These skills assist them in handling distress, controlling their emotions, and managing relationships. The methods applied in DBT emphasise the acceptance of perspectives that seem contradictory between validation and change. Dialectical behavioural therapy is designed for clinicians to work in teams and is regarded as one of the most times rigorous for clinicians and patients. Although the dialectical behavioural therapy has been effective in most patients, like any other therapy, it has its own limitation. For instance, DBT is often very demanding. Attending group and therapy sessions every week can be challenging for a person, especially one that has been diagnosed with mental illnesses such as BPD (Reddy and Vijay, 2017).

DBT is not only demanding for the patient but for the therapist, who in most instances, has to be available twenty-four hours seven days a week. The therapist is expected to provide behavioural coaching whenever the patients require it (Reddy and Vijay, 2017). Patients that have been diagnosed with BPD engage in challenging behaviour which may interfere with the therapy. For instance, a patient can call the therapist at odd hours which are outside the therapy sessions (Linehan eta l., 2015). Patients may also not be fully cooperative during therapy, argue with the therapist, or even quit the therapy (Oumaya *et al.*, 2010). DBT also places significant demands on the therapist's emotional resources, particularly when dealing with borderline patients that have suicidal tendencies. In such circumstances, the therapist may become emotionally drained, therefore unable to successfully help the patient. Borderline personality disorder patients can be so demanding, which often makes the therapist burn out more quickly (Reddy and Vijay, 2017).

Therapists have limits regarding what they are willing to do for their patients.

Patients' behaviours that are above what a therapist is prepared to put up with can interfere with the therapy. An example is where a borderline personality disorder patient refuses to accept or engage in therapeutic approaches which a therapist believes are necessary. Consequently, this issue might become the focus of the therapy, thereby limiting the effectiveness of DBT. Other behaviours from a BPD patient that can push the limits of a therapist include constantly phoning the therapist (Linehan, 2018). A borderline personality disorder patient can also insist on regular interaction with the family members of the therapist, demand solution beyond the therapist's solution, or demand more sessions than the therapist can offer (Linehan, 2018). DBT therapists are trained to ensure strong and clear boundaries are maintained. People diagnosed with borderline personality disorder rarely maintain boundaries. Consequently, when boundaries are kept, these patients may run away from them. Most DBT therapists seldom differentiate between natural and artificial boundaries.

Additionally, dialectical behavioural therapy also applies the black and white approach; this means that is the patients feel their feelings are not validated. Frequently they isolate themselves, thereby limiting the success of the therapy. A borderline personality disorder patient might also have challenges in maintaining a relationship (Linehan, 2018). For DBT to be effective, there has to be a working patient-therapist relationship. BPD patients might also be reluctant to expose their feelings and fears to the therapist. Therefore, despite the many DBT sessions the patient may attend, he or she may come out the same. At times, people diagnosed with BPD are afraid to share their painful histories or traumatic experiences; this further limits the success of DBT. A significant part to the success of the dialectical behavioural therapy depends on the patient accepting that he or she has a borderline personality disorder. Additionally, the patient must be willing to participate in DBT therapy. It is often difficult for individuals who have both BPD and narcissistic personality disorder to acknowledge that they have a problem; this further complicates the effectiveness of DBT.

The various sessions required in DBT often translate to high cost, which becomes a barrier to most people as they might not afford (Stanley and New, 2017). At times a person may have an insurance that covers dialectical behavioural therapy; however, the co-payments might become a significant burden on the individual. Additionally, in most circumstances, there are continuous battles during reimbursement by insurance companies. Most of these companies hardly recognise the total DBT modality as a treatment that is billable. The companies might just cover the personal sessions and at a lower rate.

Consequently, the service provider might become reluctant to provide DBT to those who require it for fear of not being reimbursed by the insurance companies. In most situations, patients are required to pay from their pocket; this becomes difficult for those who are from low-income households. Generally, borderline personality disorder accounts for considerably higher health costs compared to other personality disorders. The reasons for the high medical expenses involved in treating BPD can be attributed to frequent hospitalisations and greater use of outpatient services (May, Richardi, and Barth,2016). The many sessions involved in DBT may necessitate that patients have to get time off from their work. Consequently, the person may be declared redundant, thereby losing his or her job. This leads to a vicious cycle, where BPD patients can no longer afford the DBT sessions, and this further worsens their mental health condition. Despite the time and costs involved in DBT, the therapy does not cure borderline personality disorder but only provide patients with life skills which can assist them in managing their symptoms (Stanley and New, 2017). Dialectical behavioural therapy primarily focuses on suicidal and self-harming behaviours, but there is no evidence regarding how it addresses other BPD symptoms. The success of DBT in the treatment of borderline personality disorder is dependent on the cooperation and willingness of the patient. When a patient is forced into the therapy, studies show that the treatment is rarely effective. Therefore, the therapy is limited since, at times, patients due to some of the symptoms of BPD may not be in a position to agree to DBT (Porr, 2010). In dialectical behavioural therapy, the patient is expected to avoid medications and hospitals as a way of managing emotional stress. This approach is not right since psychotherapeutic approaches are not effective in obtaining considerable improvement regarding some BPD symptoms.

Moreover, by avoiding medications and hospitals, dialectical behavioural therapy may take longer to have any significant on borderline personality disorder symptoms. Based on studies, when dialectical behavioural therapy was used to other general psychiatric management approaches in BPD, it did not show any significant differences (McMain et al., 2009). Therefore, despite the high cost and extended periods, borderline personality disorder patients do not benefit more by using DBT compared to other psychiatric management techniques. To become a trained DBT therapist may take several years. The therapy is usually designed to be conducted in a team setting which requires several therapists. Setting up a dialectical behavioural therapy team entails several therapists who have enough amount of time to be trained. These trainings are mostly available in few centres. Therefore, since the number of DBT trained therapists is minimal, its effectiveness is thereby minimised. Dialectical behavioural therapy also excludes BPD patients with comorbid issues such as eating disorders, substance and alcohol abuse. People with comorbidities account for a large number of those diagnosed with personality disorders such as borderline personality disorder. Therefore, excluding this group from DBT limits the effectiveness of the therapy.

Schema-Focused Therapy

A psychologist developed this therapy at the Columbia University, Dr Jeffrey Young. This therapy is based on the basis that borderline personality disorder patients have four world views originating in childhood (maladaptive schemas). Schema-focused therapy's initial purpose was to provide treatment for various personality disorders such as **BPD**. The purpose of schema-focused therapy is to assist borderline personality disorder patients to do away with these schemas and acquire a new pattern of behaviour.

Schema-focused therapy incorporates approaches and ideas from cognitive behavioural therapy and attachment theory. The aim of using various approaches in schema therapy is to enhance the patients' self-image, thereby lessening self-harming behaviours and improve interpersonal relationships. Similar to dialectical behavioural therapy, schema-focused therapy emphasises strongly on the therapeutic connection. The theory behind this therapy assumes that when basic childhood needs like love, acceptance, and safety are not fully met, there is a risk of developing harmful ways of interacting with the world.

The wrong interaction is referred to as maladaptive early schemas. Schemas are expansive and pervasive thinking and behaving patterns. They are patterns that are held deeply and are strongly linked to one's world view and sense of self. The schema theory holds that the schemas are activated when events occurring in a person's current life look like those from his past that were linked to the schema's formation. If an individual, due to a challenging childhood experience developed harmful schemas, it is possible to resort to damaging ways of behaving and thinking, which will influence his or her response to the present situation. The schema theory suggests that most borderline personality disorder symptoms are as a result of childhood traumatic experiences. Examples of maladaptive schemas entail shame among individuals who believe that they cannot be loved, therefore wrecking their relationships for fear of abandonment. Another example of a maladaptive schema includes emotional deprivation where a person believes other people are unwilling to fulfil their needs. Consequently, the person might find himself in relationships with individuals that are emotionally distant. Social isolation is another example of a maladaptive schema when a person feels the world does not accept him or her.

Schema therapy proposes that there are three main styles of coping individuals use to deal with the wrong beliefs or maladaptive schemas. One of the coping techniques used is surrender, where individuals take part in behaviours that support their existing beliefs. Avoidance is another coping style used by individuals to avoid situations that elicit vulnerability or fear. People can also overcompensate by participating in behaviours that oppose their beliefs; at times, they do this to an extreme level. The focus of the therapist is to develop a therapeutic relationship and utilise approaches such as assertiveness training, role-playing and guiding. These techniques are used to assist the patient face previous traumatic experiences and daily events.

Schema-focused therapy often takes years for it to be effective, and this can be both costly and time-consuming for the patient. Additionally, there is little evidence to show that re-evaluating past experiences which are an approach used in schema-focused therapy completely eradicates the symptoms of borderline personality disorder. An approach often used in this therapy is to encourage patients to communicate with situations or individuals from their past. Some patients may be afraid or unwilling to do this; therefore, the success of schema-focused therapy is limited.

Mentalisation-Based Therapy

Two psychologists developed the mentalisation-based therapy at the University of London, namely Drs Anthony Bateman and Peter Fonagy. Mentalisation refers to the capacity to recognise feelings and behaviour and how they are linked to particular mental states both in an individual and in other people (Bateman and Fonagy, 2012). Many mental health conditions make the affected person experience challenges with mentalisation. The mentalisation theory is founded on attachment theory and was developed from the psychodynamic theory (Laurenssen *et al.*, 2014). The purpose of the mentalisation-based theory is to assist patients to develop mentalising skills.

It is believed that borderline personality disorder is linked to a disorganised attachment which leads to problems in self-control and attention. It is also believed that **BPD** patients have minimal ability to mentalise due to issues that may have happened in their childhood relationships. The lack of mentalisation is regarded as one that adversely affects future psychiatric impact and is believed to be significant in the borderline personality disorder aetiology (Bateman and Fonagy, 2012). The purpose of the mentalisation-based therapy, therefore, is to address what is regarded as essential deficit among **BPD** patients (Bateman and Fonagy, 2010).

It is presumed that childhood experiences impact on the quality of a person's future relationships (Brüne, Dimaggio, and Edel, 2013). The treatment of borderline personality disorder through mentalisation-based therapy focuses on enhancing the sense of self and assisting the person. The purpose of this therapy is to build up a therapeutic approach where the patients' thoughts and those of others turn out to be the primary focus of the treatment. The goal is to assist patients to recognise how they feel about themselves and other people and their impact on their responses.

Mentalisation holds the view that the ability to mentalise is developed during early childhood during a child's interaction with his or her caregiver (Bateman and Fonagy, 2012). In circumstances where the relationship between a child and a caregiver is interrupted, mentalisation development is disrupted. This view is supported by the fact that childhood abuse or an early loss of a caregiver is often related to a high risk of developing a borderline personality disorder. In most cases, mentalisation-based therapy is conducted weekly for not less than eighteen months.

The long period may be associated with increased costs which some patients might not afford leading some to drop out of the therapy. Additionally, there are other causes of BPD besides attachment such as functional and structural alterations in the brain region which controls emotions and impulses (Lopez-Castroman *et al.*, 2012). Other causes of borderline personality disorder such as genetic and biological factors disorder are rarely considered or addressed in the mentalisation-based therapy (Lopez-Castroman *et al.*, 2012). Therefore, mentalisation-based therapy, which is based on attachment issues as the primary cause of BPD, cannot provide adequate treatment to patients. Furthermore, there is no scientific evidence regarding the efficacy of mentalisation-based therapy in borderline personality disorder patients.

Systems Training for Emotional Predictability and Problem-Solving (STEPPS)

System training for emotional predictability and problem-solving is a group therapy that merges skills training and cognitive behaviour elements with a systems factor for people with whom the patient has regular interaction. This therapy is quickly learned and applied by therapists of diverse professional and educational backgrounds. The therapy adds and does not substitute the patients' current treatment. It is necessary to note that individual therapy is not part of the STEPPS program. The program has three primary components which include psychoeducation regarding borderline personality disorder (Blum *et al.*, 2008). The other component of this program is training the patient on emotional management. The third component of the STEPPS program is training on behaviour management skills (Blum *et al.*, 2008). In the first component, the patient learns how to substitute misconceptions regarding BPD with the consciousness of the behaviours, feelings, and thoughts that describe it and spot it and the schemas that influence their behaviours (Blum *et al.*, 2008). BPD is viewed as an emotional intensity disorder; this becomes more preferable to the patients than a borderline personality disorder.

In the second component, the patient is taught skills such as communication and problem management. These skills help the patient to manage the emotional and cognitive impacts of borderline personality disorder. In the third component of the STEPPS program, the patient is taught behavioural skills such as health monitoring, healthy eating habits, avoidance of self-harm, leisure activities, regular exercise, sleep hygiene, and goal setting (Blum *et al.*, 2008).

In most instances, the STEPPS therapy sessions are carried out in twenty-week group sessions.

Studies have demonstrated that borderline personality disorder patients who have had self-harming behaviours and suicidal ideations experience no significant changes by attending the STEPPS program (Blum *et al.*, 2008). These outcomes may be an indication that shorter therapies can also be more useful for borderline personality disorder. Systems training for emotional predictability and problem-solving therapy are used as an addition to other forms of BPD treatment. STEPPS is both labour-intensive and time-consuming. Furthermore, this therapy requires considerable training of the therapists, which in most cases, lacks. There is no evidence that STEPPS alone has been effective in treating borderline personality disorder. In situations where BPD symptoms have improved, the use of other medications and psychotherapies could likely have been the cause (Blum *et al.*, 2008). Additionally, a borderline personality disorder can experience an improvement in their symptoms due to the social support encountered in the STEPPS program and not through the therapy itself. Therefore, there is no evidence to support the effectiveness of the STEPPS program in the treatment of borderline personality disorder (Brown, Blum, and Black, 2013).

Transference-Focused Psychotherapy

The transference-focused therapy is founded on the theory initially proposed by a psychiatrist by the name Dr Otto Kernberg. The psychiatrist held the view that borderline personality disorder develops from an individual's incapacity to incorporate positive and adverse images of oneself and others. Kernberg holds the view that extreme early violent behaviour can lead young children to split their positive or adverse images of themselves or their caregiver. The extreme aggression can have been inherent or caused be actual frustrations. Viewing people and situations as either being all good or all bad has its roots in one's childhood which are carried to adulthood.

Consequently, such a situation creates internal turmoil leading to the development of borderline personality disorder symptoms. The primary purpose of transference-focused psychotherapy is to decrease self-harming behaviour and BPD symptoms by modifying self-representations and those of others. The approaches often used in TFP include transference interpretations, confrontations, and clarifications. In the treatment of borderline personality disorder, TFP centres on applying the interaction with a therapist to amend how patients relate to the people around them. Transference refers to the process through which emotions are conveyed between people. In the transference- focused psychotherapy, it is assumed that feelings regarding significant individuals in a person's life like siblings and parents are transferred to the therapist. The borderline personality disorder patients respond to the therapist as they would to significant people in their lives.

Through approaches developed from psychoanalytic psychotherapy, the patient and clinician work jointly to comprehend the dynamics of previous interactions and associated feelings. Both the clinician and patient look at how past interactions and their associated emotions impact the current functioning of the patient. It is believed that through TFP, the therapist can recognise how the patients interact with other individuals. The therapist can then apply the information received to assist patients in developing better interpersonal relationships. TFP holds the view that the primary cause of borderline personality disorder is linked to the impaired relationships a person has during childhood.

Consequently, the person continues to experience dysfunctional relationships in his/her adolescence and adulthood. TFP is based on the theory that the interactions individuals have with their caregivers during childhood help them to developmental depictions of other people and also a sense of self. Whenever something wrong occurs at this stage, people often have problems developing a firm understanding of self or in their relationships with other people. Studies have reported that abuse in childhood or losing a caregiver early in life has been linked to a high risk of developing a borderline personality disorder.

Some of the symptoms of BPD entail relationship challenges, an unstable sense of self. As a result, experts have recommended that such symptoms can be treated by developing better relationships which can be achieved through TFP. In the transference-focused therapy sessions, the emphasis is on the interaction between a patient and the therapist. It is rare for the therapist to provide any advice or instruct the patients on the next course of action. In its place, the therapist asks questions to assist patients to discover their responses in the course of the sessions. In TFP, the focus is primarily in the here and now instead of the past. Patients are encouraged to talk about their current relationship with the therapist rather than their past interaction with their caregivers. In most cases, during these sessions, the therapist remains neutral and avoids giving his view. Additionally, in transference-focused therapy, the therapist is rarely available when not in the therapy session unless when there is an emergency. Since the transference-focused treatment focuses on the present and tends to ignore the past, there is a likelihood that issues in the patient's history might not be addressed.

Some of the issues such as childhood abuse have been linked to the development of borderline personality disorder, and by ignoring such issues, the symptoms of the disorder might not be adequately addressed (Kaplan *et al.*, 2016). TFP might not be appropriate for all borderline personality disorder patients since some might not be comfortable with the interpersonal emotions raised during the therapy. Moreover, other patients might not tolerate being out of control. Transference-focused therapy involves many sessions, where some patients may not have the time or the finances to engage in. TFP therapists require extensive training, skills, and experience which lacks in most of them.

Conclusion

Currently, there are four psychosocial treatments for borderline personality disorder that have demonstrated some success in reducing

BPD psychopathology. The borderline personality disorder symptoms that have been reduced through the four psychosocial treatments include suicidal attempts and self-harming behaviours. Both patients and clinicians have four psychosocial therapies to choose from. This is necessary as one therapy may be more effective in a particular patient compared to others. Additionally, a clinician may have more experience in the use of one psychosocial treatment than others.

The dialectical behavioural therapy is more studied and widely used than the other treatments, especially in the United States. However, this does not signify that it is better than the other psychotherapies. Borderline personality disorder patients are responsive to various kinds of treatments. Regardless of the advances of these psychotherapies, more remains to be done (Zanarini, 2009). Several experts have concluded that all current therapies used in borderline personality disorders have considerable limitations. For instance, rarely do these therapies address both temperamental and acute symptoms. Moreover, most of these therapies take long periods and are intensive. The psychotherapies also require the therapists to have special training which in most situations is lacking. As a result, these therapies cannot be provided by a large number of mental health clinics, primary health centres, and private practitioners (Zanarini, 2009). Thus, there is a need to overhaul these treatments to address both kinds of symptom sin BPD patients. There is a need to develop more effective therapy in BPD treatment (Zanarini, 2009).

The psychological therapies run a risk of not helping all patients through issues in the relationship between the therapist and patient (Parry, 2016). A therapy's effectiveness is dependent on the therapist's skills in creating the likelihood of change in every patient. Therefore, a working relationship between the therapist and patient is a significant predictor of the results (Horvath *et al.*, 2011). Additionally, there is never a guarantee that the therapy will fulfil what the manual specifies (Parry, 2016). Studies have reported that over 50% of borderline personality disorder symptoms are acute, while the other 50% are temperamental (Zanarini *et al.*, 2009). Based on research, severe symptoms resolve quickly and are particular to BPD. These symptoms are frequently linked to costly therapies like psychiatric hospitalisations. On the contrary, temperamental symptoms resolve relatively slowly and are not specific to borderline personality disorder. Additionally, temperamental symptoms are linked to psychosocial impairments. Examples of temperamental symptoms include an intense fear of abandonment and extreme anger. On the other hand, self- harming and suicidal behaviours are examples of acute symptoms. An effective borderline personality disorder treatment should address both temperamental and acute symptoms. Currently, none of the psychosocial treatment used in BPD adequately address both symptoms; therefore, there is a need to overhaul these therapies. An example of a psychosocial treatment being used to address both acute and temperamental symptoms is the integrated modular treatment which integrates various treatment methods, strategies, and principles resulting from effective therapies and applies them in treating particular impairments. IMT enhances on models that focus on a few treatment methods. Therefore, the general treatment components in the integrated modular treatment entail a specific agreement on the treatment rules. The other module in IMT includes the therapy agreement between the therapist and patient. The regular observance by the therapist to the therapeutic framework and the motivation to change by the patient are also included in integrated modular treatment. Some treatment modules in IMT arise from treatment interventions that have been researched and tried. Others develop from the therapist's skills and experiences in the treatment of various personality disorders.

Integrated modular treatment guides on ways to match various symptoms of borderline personality disorder to a suitable treatment module. The integrated modular treatment is classified into general modules that exist in all therapies. Additionally, IMT is grouped into specific modules which are intended to treat particular impairments in all patients. Both categories are taken from the existing treatment models. Integrated modular treatment module phases include safety, modulation and regulation, containment, change and exploration, and synthesis and integration. Since the common modules targets are met, and their goals achieved, the therapist and patient move on to the specific therapy IMT modules. Specific modules are designed based on the patient's resilience level and symptoms. The integrated modular treatment practical approach provides the depth, scope, and flexibility of treatment which is absent in the current psychotherapies.

Effective Generalist Therapy BPD Approaches

Due to the limitations such as costs involved in the psychotherapies used in treating BPD patients, other general treatment approaches have been developed. These approaches include, among others, excellent clinical care, structured clinical management, general psychiatric management, and supportive psychotherapy.

Good Clinical Care

This is a cognitive behavioural therapy informed technique that integrates a problem-solving model as its primary treatment approach. Excellent clinical care emphasises the necessity of an efficient organisational structure. Trained psychologists provide cognitive behavioural therapy. A discussion is held on a weekly team meeting regarding the patients' progress. An excellent clinical care therapy is conducted once in every week. In cases where patients may require more sessions, the treatment is flexible. Case management is also provided flexibly. Furthermore, clinical trials range to around three in each therapy session (Bateman and Krawitz, 2013). A study conducted on the impact of good clinical therapy among adolescents with borderline personality disorder showed considerable improvement in various measures of clinical outcome (Chanen *et al.*, 2009).

Structured Clinical Management

Structured clinical management is founded on a counselling approach that is similar to supportive therapy. The therapy includes problem-solving, advocacy support, aggressive follow- up when a patient starts to miss appointments, crisis plan, case management, and review of medication. In the structured clinical management, medication is used as an addition, when indicated clinically. Non-professional clinicians, in most circumstances, are the ones who provide structured clinical management. This therapy is commonly conducted in either individual or group therapy sessions weekly (Batema and Krawitz, 2013).

General Psychiatric Management

This therapy is an approach that is psycho-dynamically informed, and that comprises adjunctive medication that target symptoms and case management. The psychodynamic approach emphasises that when a child's early attachments are disturbed, this can lead to the development of borderline personality disorder (Gunderson, 2009). The development of general psychiatric management was to give mental healthcare practitioners involved in the care of BPD patients' fundamental knowledge required in managing this group of patients. General psychiatric management does not need the professional to have intensive training.

General psychiatric management entails four crucial elements namely (Hopwood *et al.*, 2014). These elements are psychoeducation, constant focus on the life of the patient away from therapy.

The purpose of this focus is to connect the achievement of long-term goals with the requirement of learning self-harming and emotional control. The other element is the acknowledgement and use of the therapist's dual role both as a person and a professional. The personal part means the therapist discloses his feelings like apprehension or confusion, telling the patient of his desire to help. The professional role entails the provision of unemotional but concerned responses to the patient's emotions.

Additionally, the professional role involves endeavouring to understand the patients' persistent concerns regarding the trustworthiness, feelings, and motives of the therapist. The therapist, in his role as a professional, would also be required to share knowledge with the patient. The fourth element of the general psychiatric management entails a greatly interactive and an approach that directly engages the provider. General psychiatric management is delivered in four therapy phases (Hopwood *et al.*, 2014). The first phase is where a contractual agreement where the clinician and the patient agree on roles and goals.

The second phase in the general psychiatric management involves developing a relational agreement between the patient and the physician. In this phase which can last for a period between one to twelve months, the patient begins to trust and like the intentions of the therapist. The third phase entails a positive dependency; here, the patient attains some comfort linked to the therapist. The third phase can last between six months to five years. In the fourth phase patients begin to apply skills learned during therapy in all areas of their lives. This phase can last from two to ten years (Hopwood *et al.*, 2014). A study was conducted on comparing the outcome of borderline personality disorder patients receiving the supportive psychotherapy, transference-focused psychotherapy, or the dialectical behavioural therapy. The report demonstrated that all BPD patients in the three groups showed considerable improvement (Clarkin *et al.*, 2013). Borderline personality disorder patients on supportive psychotherapy were provided with one session each week. However, patients assigned to transference-focused psychotherapy or the dialectical behavioural therapy received two sessions per week. Therefore, the supportive psychotherapy compared to other therapies achieves the same result but at a lower cost (Batema and Krawitz, 2013).

Supportive Psychotherapy

This psychotherapy focuses on developing and upholding a therapeutic relationship that is relaxed, comfortable, and one that rarely uses interpretation. Supportive psychotherapy focuses on providing emotional support regarding current challenges the patient encounters. The therapist follows and manages transference while intentionally avoiding interpretation. The changes approach though supportive psychotherapy is believed to involve the patient identifying with constant attitudes. These attitudes include a non-judgemental acceptance by the therapist, kindness, interest, and benevolence. The supportive psychotherapy's sessions are offered every week, and at times additional sessions if required can be given (Bateman and Krawitz, 2013).

Pharmacotherapy for Borderline Personality Disorder

Generally, psychotherapy is the preferred treatment of borderline personality disorder compared to psychotropic medications and is often regarded as the first-line treatment of borderline personality disorder. Nevertheless, the impact of recognised psychotherapies are still few and exaggerated by publication bias (Stoffers-Winterling *et al.*, 2012). Over the years treating borderline personality disorder patients with medication has become common. However, there is no approved medicine in treating borderline personality disorder. Additionally, there is no specific medication that can be used to manage the disorder. However, there is an assumption that BPD can be treated with medication similar to other mental disorders. Pharmacotherapy is the treatment of borderline personality disorder founded on the view that some personality dimensions of BPD patients seem to be mediated by neurotransmitter physiology dysregulation and are responsive to drugs. Pharmacotherapy is utilised to treat borderline personality disorder symptoms during times of crisis (Stoffers *et al.*, 2010). During this period, drugs should not be changed; however, environmental measures should be taken until the time the patient has stabilised.

A borderline personality disorder is a chronic disorder, and although pharmacotherapy has shown considerable efficacy in reducing the severity of the symptoms, it can completely cure the disorder. Furthermore, the treatment of borderline personality disorder through pharmacotherapy is system based. Medicines focus on the behaviour of the **BPD** patient and not the disorder in its entirety (Stoffers *et al.*, 2010).

Evidence shows that since medicines are at the disposal of physicians, it is easy to prescribe them to **BPD** patients leading to over-prescription (Paris, 2008). It is easy to prescribe antidepressants; nevertheless, borderline personality disorder patients do not have classic depression. Furthermore, it is common for mood stabilisers to be prescribed to these patients without considering that the borderline personality disorder affective instability is different from bipolar disorder symptoms (Paris, 2008). Antipsychotics can also be prescribed to borderline personality disorder patients without considering that they do not have real psychosis.

The biological mechanisms associated with **BPD** symptoms can differ from those of other mental illnesses (Paris, 2008). That is the reason for using medications to treat borderline personality disorder is not always effective. It is necessary to state that drugs should not be entirely avoided in **BPD** treatment; however, care should be involved. The National Institute of Health and Clinical Excellence issued guidelines that drugs should not be used to treat borderline personality disorders and any related symptoms (Völlm *et al.*, 2012). Studies conducted in 2008 and 2010 estimated borderline personality disorder lifetime prevalence to be at 5.9% or 2.7% respectively (Trull *et al.*, 2010).

Epidemiological data report a high number of borderline personality disorder patients in the healthcare system. A study conducted reported that 50% of inpatients who had attempted suicide in the previous two years and between 15%–28% of patients in psychiatric hospitals or clinics were **BPD** patients (Ducasse *et al.*, 2019). Psychotropic drugs like mood stabilisers, antipsychotics, and antidepressants are considered an adjunctive treatment as there are no credible impacts of borderline personality disorder psychopathology (Stoffers *et al.*, 2010). In both the United States and Europe, there are no approved medications for the treatment of borderline personality disorder.

Nevertheless, patients diagnosed with various personality disorders are frequently prescribed medication compared to any other diagnostic group. A study was conducted in the United Kingdom in 2012 of 161 borderline personality disorder patients. The results showed that around 45% of these patients were prescribed second-generation antipsychotics (Völlm *et al.*, 2012). Furthermore, 20% of them were prescribed clozapine and 40% were given mood stabilisers.

Polypharmacy, according to the study, was also common among these BPD patients. Sixty-two per cent of the patients in this study were on more than one type of medication (Völlm *et al.*, 2012). Various factors frequently lead to polypharmacy in borderline personality disorder patients. Some of these factors include the notion that the right medications can correct the chemical imbalance in a person. Physicians may resort to agreeing with this idea, yet effective treatment of BPD is commonly psychosocial. Misdiagnosis of borderline personality disorder with other mental health disorders can also lead to polypharmacy.

Physicians at times may also feel they have to help their borderline personality disorder patients, thereby resorting to polypharmacy. There is minimal evidence supporting the efficacy of the heavy application of psychotropic agents in the treatment of borderline personality disorder. Although medication can help in some comorbid symptoms in borderline personality disorder patients, its efficacy regarding the disorder should be assumed. For instance, research has demonstrated that selective serotonin reuptake inhibitors can enhance anxiety or depression among BPD patients. Nevertheless, there are no accurate measures to show SSRIs impact on borderline personality disorder symptoms (May, Richardi, and Barth, 2016).

Although psychotherapy is necessary for determining long-term improvement in the personality and total functioning of BPD patient, pharmacotherapeutic agents are frequently prescribed in the management of the symptoms. Pharmacologic treatment can be started as an addition to psychotherapy among borderline personality disorder patients with symptoms of affective instability and impulsivity. Most individuals diagnosed with borderline personality disorder get medical treatment. Nevertheless, in most circumstances, there are no medicines which are specifically meant to treat BPD. There is no place in the world where psychotropic drugs have been approved for the treatment of borderline personality disorder (Völlm *et al.*, 2012). A particular drug is frequently used due to its known properties in the borderline personality disorder treatment. Additionally, a drug can also be used to treat other related disorders such as anxious, depressive, or psychotic disorders.

There are three significant factors of the BPD pharmacological treatment. They include the high frequency regarding the usage of these medications and the associated use of multiple drugs. The third feature is the inclination to administer multiple pharmacological agents. Studies have reported that between 90%–99% of individuals diagnosed with borderline personality disorder use medications (Bridler *et al.*, 2015).

Some of the most common drugs used to treat borderline personality disorder include mood stabilisers, antidepressants, and antipsychotics, among others. There is no definite research regarding these medications; in most cases, they are unlicensed and used off-label (Bellino *et al.*, 2008). The level in which these drugs are prescribed vary broadly; this can be due to factors like the kind of symptoms, BPD severity, frequency and type of co-occurring disorders. Other factors may entail diverse practices used in drug prescription in different countries and the prescribers' choice.

A study conducted showed that antidepressants were administered to 31%–79% of borderline personality disorder patients (Paton *et al.*, 2015). On the other hand, 35%–78% of borderline personality disorder patients, according to research, are on antipsychotics. The use of mood stabilisers among borderline personality disorder ranges between 20%–70% (Bridler *et al.*, 2015). Trends in using pharmacotherapy among BPD patients seem to be equivalent to pharmacotherapy trends of other mental disorders only to some degree. For instance, studies have reported a reduction in the use of antidepressants in treating borderline personality disorder (Zanarini *et al.*, 2015).

On the contrary, the use of mood stabilisers and second-generation antipsychotics in BPD treatment seems to be on the rise (Bridler *et al.*, 2015). Studies have also shown that 94% of borderline personality disorder patients received medication prescriptions from their psychiatrists. Ninety-nine per cent of these psychiatrists prescribed antidepressants, particularly the selective serotonin reuptake inhibitors (SSRI). Furthermore, 91 % of these psychiatrists prescribed second-generation antipsychotics (Knappich *et al.*, 2014).

It is a contradiction that extensive use of pharmacotherapy in the treatment of borderline personality disorder has happened with minimal evidence of the efficacy of the medication. Studies have demonstrated that there is mixed evidence regarding the effectiveness of drugs in the treatment of borderline personality disorder (Hancock-Johnson, Griffiths, and Picchioni, 2017). The UK National Institute for Health and Clinical Excellence has recommended that pharmacotherapy for borderline personality disorder should not be used unless there are co- occurring disorders (Starcevic and Janca, 2018). Clinicians often use pharmacotherapy to treat borderline personality disorder patients when there is inadequate psychotherapy. Clinicians also use pharmacotherapy when BPD patients get minimal or no psychological treatment. Borderline personality patients whose symptoms become worse through psychological therapy can also use pharmacotherapy. Therefore, in most cases, it is the self-harming behaviour, psychotic, agitation, or depressive symptoms that lead clinicians to administer drugs to people diagnosed with BPD.

It is necessary to note that medications in borderline personality disorder can lead to more problems than the ones they solve due to the risk of overdose, addiction, and side effects (Völlm *et al.*, 2012). As a result, the prescription of medication to borderline personality disorder patients should be done with caution. The use of drugs in treating borderline personality disorder patients at times can lead to more damage than good. For instance, individuals diagnosed with **BPD** might experience suicidal ideations similar to people with severe mental disorders. However, borderline personality disorder patients may be given more drugs, thereby experiencing additional side effects. Moreover, given how often **BPD** patients experience suicidal behaviours, much care should be taken to avoid medications that may be harmful when the patient overdoses.

Antidepressants

Studies in different countries have reported that antidepressants are a group of drugs commonly prescribed to borderline personality disorder patients (Paton *et al.*, 2015). Studies showed that 79.7% of **BPD** patients were on antidepressants drugs while 46.6% had been prescribed anxiolytics. According to the study, 35.9 % of **BPD** patients have been prescribed mood stabilisers and 38.6% were on neuroleptics (Zanarini, 2015). The study also reported that around 71% of **BPD** patients had used medications for six consecutive years. Additionally, the study revealed that other patients were likely to be on antipsychotics, mood stabilisers, and antidepressants (Zanarini, 2015).

These results show that most borderline personality disorder patients take psychotropic medications for long periods although the drugs are only to be used as an adjunctive to psychotherapy. Research has also shown that antidepressants assist individuals with borderline personality disorder who have also been diagnosed with depression (Zanarini, 2015).

Nevertheless, some depression symptoms connect to borderline personality disorder, and they may not be improved, for instance, extreme change of emotions which may be triggered by the situation or environment the patient is in.

Additionally, in circumstances where the patient does not take adhere to the prescription, the side effects and reactions are very harmful. Some of these side effects entail nausea, irritability, headaches, and agitation. Studies have demonstrated that depressive symptoms are common in people diagnosed with a borderline personality disorder. Researches have been done for many decades regarding the effectiveness of antidepressant in the treatment of borderline personality disorder. An example is the impact of selective serotonin reuptake inhibitors (SSRIs) have on the treatment of borderline personality disorder. Studies have reported that SSRIs have little effect on the impulsive aggression common among BPD patients (Paris, 2008).

The efficacy of serotonin reuptake inhibitors' widespread use among BPD patients has not been impressive (Paris, 2008). Studies have shown that most patients with different personality disorders have an inadequate response to antidepressants compared to those with no personality disorders. Antidepressants rarely work when an individual has depressive feelings even among people that do not have a comorbid diagnosis of personality disorders. One study reported that only 50% of patients with any kind of depression respond to antidepressants. Additionally, even a smaller percentage of the patients achieved complete remission (Rush, 2007).

Physicians and psychiatrists often switch from one antidepressant to another in search of the right one. This approach only works in a few borderline personalities disorder patients (Rush, 2007). Regrettably, many borderline personality disorder patients have been subjected to various antidepressants with no sign of improvement. When a patient remains in one kind of medicine, it becomes easier to assess its effectiveness. Due to the unstable mood linked to borderline personality disorder, there is a likelihood of placebo effects occurring. Additionally, research has shown that tricyclic antidepressants probably due to anticholinergic sequelae can worsen the effort to manage suicidality, aggression, and impulsivity (Ripoll, 2012).

The adverse cognitive sequelae often worsen the impulsivity experienced by borderline personality disorder patients (Mercer, 2009). Additionally, the use of tricyclic antidepressants in the treatment of BPD is often linked to the potential high risk of overdose. Treating borderline personality disorder through SSRIs can lead to other adverse effects such as weight gain and lack of motivation. Furthermore, the risk of suicide is also increased among adolescents who could be having both depression and borderline personality disorder. Tricyclic antidepressants, which include nortriptyline and amitryptiline, often worsen the symptoms of BPD in some patients.

For instance, amitryptiline has been linked to increased behavioural dysregulation, paranoia, assaultiveness, and suicidality in borderline personality disorder patients (Mercer *et al.*, 2009).

These side effects have been attributed to the lack of inhibition in affective and cognitive controls among BPD patients. Tricyclic antidepressants are rarely recommended for borderline personality disorder patients. These antidepressants slow down the metabolism and reuptake of norepinephrine and serotonin. Each of these drugs impact neurotransmitters in a different way (Carlstedt, 2009). Other side effects of tricyclic antidepressants include drops in blood pressure and heart arrhythmias.

An overdose of tricyclic antidepressants can lead to death. Studies have reported that tricyclic antidepressants worsen borderline personality disorder symptoms; therefore, they should be avoided (Carlstedt, 2009). Monoamine oxidase inhibitors (MAOIs) are another class of antidepressants frequently used in borderline personality disorder patients that are resistant to mood stabilisers and antipsychotics. Studies have shown that MAOI phenelzine can be useful in some BPD patients (Lieb, 2010). However, when administered orally, monoamine oxidase inhibitors can have severe and life-threatening side effects.

Some of the adverse effects associated with the use of MAOIs in the treatment of borderline personality disorder include an abrupt drop in blood pressure. Other side effects of monoamine oxidase inhibitors are changes in the patient's heart rhythm. MAOIs can also lead to fainting, twitching of muscles, weight gain, blurred vision, and changes in appetite among others. As a result, MAOIs are used by physicians to treat BPD patients only when other medications have been tried and failed. Currently, it is rare to meet BPD patients who are not on antidepressants.

Rarely do antidepressants treat borderline personality disorder; they only address the symptoms (Paris, 2008). Since antidepressants have not shown any considerable therapeutic benefit, they are not highly recommended in the treatment of borderline personality disorder. The antidepressants minimal therapeutic benefit in borderline personality disorder can be linked to the lack of specificity in the serotonin receptor. Furthermore, most antidepressants rarely target the mesocorticolimbic or receptors regions of the brain connected with clinically significant hyperactivity of the amygdala.

Antipsychotics

Antipsychotic drugs are commonly used in treating borderline personality disorders although they lack an adequately defined indication. The treatment of BPD with typical antipsychotic drugs makes it challenging to lessen self-harming behaviours and impulsivity. Atypical antipsychotics are commonly prescribed due to their broader therapeutic benefits and tolerability linked to noradrenergic and serotonergic activity. Atypical antipsychotics are believed to treat impulsive aggression in borderline personality disorder patients (Abraham and Calabrese, 2008). Nevertheless, high comorbidity of borderline personality disorder with obesity and eating disorders demonstrates that atypical antipsychotics treatment should be limited to steer clear of long-term health risks. An example of an antipsychotic that is used in the treatment of BPD is Haloperidol. This drug is most cases worsens the patient's overall status as it causes depression and sedation among other side effects (Ripoll, 2013). Another commonly atypical antipsychotic used in the treatment of borderline personality disorder is clozapine. Various studies have shown that medication reduces self-harming behaviour in borderline personality disorder patients (Carlstedt, 2009). However, the drug has been linked to a rare but grave drop in white blood cells. The treatment of this condition would necessitate a six-month weekly blood draws. Since most BPD patients have non-compliant behaviour, clozapine should only be used in a crisis.

Mood Stabilisers

Many studies have been conducted regarding the treatment of borderline personality disorders with mood stabilisers. There have been some positive results regarding this kind of treatment. However, when compared to antidepressants, the risk of toxicity from overdosing is higher. A borderline personality disorder is often characterised by instability and a high risk of self-harm. Additionally, borderline personality disorder patients are known for unstable moods which at times lead to misdiagnosis of the disorder as bipolar disorder (Paris, 2019). In most psychiatric practices, affective disorders like bipolar have been treated through mood stabilisers (Saunders and Hawton, 2009).

The use of mood stabilisers in the treatment of borderline personality disorder has been promoted by the idea that the disorder is similar to bipolar disorder. It is currently known that the two disorders are different and hardly ever evolve to become one (Gunderson *et al.*, 2014). Studies have shown that the brain of borderline personality disorder patients is distinctly different from that of people diagnosed with bipolar disorder (Das *et al.*, 2014). However, in clinical practice, borderline personality disorder patients are frequently misdiagnosed as having bipolar disorder. As a result, often these patients are provided with mood stabilisers for an extended period.

It is common for these patients due to the misdiagnosis and wrong prescriptions to experience side effects while the BPD symptoms become worse (Zanarini *et al.*, 2015). The side effects and risks of mood stabilisers differ depending on the kind of mood stabilisers the patient is using. For instance, every anticonvulsant mood stabiliser has its side effect profile. As a result, studies have been conducted on the impact of mood stabilisers in the treatment of borderline personality disorder symptom. An example of one of the mood stabilisers used in the treatment of BPD is lithium carbonate.

Lithium carbonate can lead to cognitive problems and gastrointestinal distress like weight gain, vomiting, tremors, and nausea. Lithium can also affect the patient's thyroid gland and kidneys. In high doses, lithium may be toxic; therefore, when prescribed to borderline personality disorder patients who are at a high risk of suicide, it can be detrimental. Carbamazepine another mood stabiliser when not monitored carefully can lead agranulocytosis, which is a rare condition that causes a considerable reduction in white blood cells. Carbamazepine can also worsen melancholic depression in borderline personality disorder patients. Lamotrigine another mood stabiliser can place BPD patients at risk of developing a life-threatening rush (Ripoll, 2013).

Mood stabilisers rarely reduce paranoia, dissociative episodes, and split-thinking commonly experienced by borderline personality disorder patients. Mood stabilisers are not effective in treating borderline personality disorder since the emotional deregulation witnessed in these patients differ entirely from the mood swings seen among bipolar disorder patients (Paris, 2019). Therefore, mood stabilisers are more effective among bipolar disorder patients than borderline personality disorder patients (Paris, 2019).

Anticonvulsants

Anticonvulsants also referred to as anti-seizure and antiepileptic drugs a group of pharmacological agents are commonly used to treat epileptic seizures. These drugs are gaining popularity in the treatment of bipolar and borderline personality disorders. The use of anticonvulsants in the treatment of BPD originates from a neurobehavioral aetiology theory (Paris, 2008). The theory tries to understand if the behavioural lack of control, perceptual and cognitive distortions, and affective dysregulation in borderline personality disorder patients are a reflection of the central nervous system. The similarity between symptoms in BPD patients and those with epileptic seizures suggests the likelihood of a common cause.

Anticonvulsants often act as mood stabilisers in treating neuropathic pain. The most commonly used antipsychotics include valproate, topiramate, lamotrigine, carbamazepine, gabapentin, and valproic acid. Some of these medications provide average to greater therapeutic benefits in the treatment of impulsivity, affective instability, and functioning in borderline personality disorder patients (Lieb *et al.*, 2010).

Topiramate has shown a broad range of therapeutic benefits, especially regarding interpersonal functioning and anger. Nevertheless, the cognitive sequelae in Topiramate can hamper with psychotherapies among some borderline personality disorder patients. Additionally, topiramate can lead to excessive weight loss which may harm some borderline personality disorder patients with comorbid eating disorders. Lamotrigine another type of anticonvulsant can enhance aggression, affective symptoms, and impulsivity. However, this medication has dangerous side effects, such as toxicity and life-threatening rash situations (Leiberich *et al.*, 2008).

Other Medications

Other medications commonly used to treat BPD include benzodiazepines and alprazolam. However, rather than enhancing the patient's mental health, these drugs worsen impulsivity and increase the risk of suicidality. Furthermore, borderline personality disorder patients are at a high risk of becoming dependent on benzodiazepine as they try to self-medicate refractory and chronic affective symptoms.

Conclusion

Currently, there is a broad agreement that no single medication can comprehensively treat borderline personality disorder (Biskin, 2012). Pharmacotherapy is often used to enhance particular symptoms a BPD patient could be experiencing. These symptoms could be specific to the definition provided by the *DSM-5* of borderline personality disorder. Other symptoms may not be specified and may include anxiety or depression, which is common in BPD. A particular kind of medication is often used depending on its identified efficacy in the treatment of similar symptoms in other mental health disorders. Consequently, various groups of drugs are used to treat borderline personality disorder (Zanarini, 2015).

When used as a component of integrated therapy, medication can be used to facilitate learning processes that are behaviorally mediated. In circumstances where BPD patients are misdiagnosed with bipolar disorder, they will probably be provided with psychopharmacological treatment (Parker, 2011). At times, patients associate the widespread use of drugs on borderline personality disorder treatment with clinicians' negative attitude towards the disorder. The lack of knowledge and understanding about BPD can lead clinicians to extensive use of medications in treating the disorder.

At times medications in the treatment of BPD can be as a result of lack of resources in the management of the disorder (Rogers and Acton, 2012). Therefore, there is a need to re-evaluate the common practice of giving medication automatically to borderline personality disorder patients when they experience a crisis. This might not be simple as it would need to consider changes in clinicians and patients' behaviour in a reformed healthcare system. Both clinicians and patients should be educated to enhance their knowledge regarding BPD.

Moreover, more focus should be on the significance of the therapeutic clinician-patient relationship. More emphasis should be made to promote combined treatment decision-making and develop easy practical ways of managing crisis among BPD patients. It would be wrong to fully lay blame on clinicians for the administration of medicines to borderline personality disorder patients. A singled-out pharmacotherapy approach supports clinicians to use drugs for borderline personality disorders symptoms that are responsive to medication.

Therefore, the use of medication in the treatment of BPD cannot be regarded as being against the acceptable clinical practice. However, there is a need for agreement and consistency in interpreting research regarding the efficacy of medication in borderline personality disorder treatment. There is a need for constant reviews concerning extended pharmacological borderline personality disorder treatment, particularly during times when the patient is experiencing symptomatic stability. These reviews, combined with the use of appropriate psychosocial approaches and specialised borderline disorder-focuses psychotherapy, can prevent the need for constant medication. Consequently, the adverse effects of the treatment, which may include negative effects of medicine, abuse, overdosing, or misuse can be avoided.

The use of polypharmacy should also be avoided or minimised. Since the use of medication on BPD is often a symptom-based method, it often leads to polypharmacy. Using multiple drugs in psychiatry often demonstrates the desperation of the clinician, suggesting that other therapeutic approaches are no longer effective. As a result, clinicians resort to the use of multiple medicines since there is nothing left to do. It is a principle in healthcare that clinicians should treat diseases but not symptoms. When multiple medicines are prescribed to borderline personality disorder patients, there is a tendency to forget what is being treated (Paris, 2008).

Furthermore, medicines from totally diverse groups create similar effects in borderline personality disorder patients (Paris, 2008). Therefore, one type of medicine is enough for symptomatic relief. There is no documented evidence of any benefit that accrues in treating borderline personality disorder through polypharmacy. Some of the adverse effects of this kind of treatment include higher severity or the risk of drug interactions. Additionally, if polypharmacy treatment is not effective in the short run, it is unlikely to become effective when used for a more extended period. Prescribing multiple drugs to borderline personality disorder patients increases the risk of them experiencing multiple side effects (Paris, 2019). There is a need for additional pharmacological trials regarding borderline personality disorder. The researches should focus on people diagnosed with BPD despite any co-occurring disorder. The impact of pharmacotherapy on the severity of borderline personality disorder symptoms should be measured in such trials.

The optimal period of the pharmacotherapy treatment should also be ascertained. These trials must determine if any particular drug combination is superior to the use of one drug. The trials can also be used to determine if combining pharmacotherapy and psychotherapy has any benefit. Flexibility is required to know when drugs should be used in the treatment of borderline personality disorder, for instance, for behavioural management and relief of symptoms. If not, drugs for the treatment of BPD should be avoided. Caution is necessary to make the best use of the benefits of pharmacotherapy and limit its harm. Currently, this means administering medication during crisis and aggravation (Paris, 2019). Psychiatrists should not stop administering medications to borderline personality disorder patients. However, both the clinicians and BPD patients should carefully evaluate the side effects versus the benefits of the drug. Borderline personality disorder patients should also develop a plan regarding how and when the medication should be discontinued after full benefits have been achieved. Furthermore, healthy scepticism is allowed regarding the administration of medications to borderline personality disorder patients. Research has shown that over 80% of BPD patients have remission with minimal rates of relapse even without any form of treatment (Gunderson *et al.*, 2011). Also, non-intensive treatments can be as quite effective as intensive therapies (Gunderson eta l., 2016). According to the National Institute for Health and Clinical Excellence (NICE) guidelines, medicines should not be used to specifically treat borderline personality disorder, individual symptoms, or behaviours linked to the disorder. Some of these behaviours include repeated self-harm, risk-taking behaviour, and emotional instability. However, drugs should be used to address comorbid conditions (NICE, 2009).

NICE further recommends that antipsychotics should not be used for the long or medium-term borderline personality disorder treatment. Nevertheless, regarding managing comorbidities, NICE states that treatment through medicine can be considered. In such cases, the NICE guidelines concerning each comorbid condition should be considered. Regarding treatment through medicine in times of crisis, NICE guidelines state that there should be an agreement between the prescriber and other professionals concerning the proposed treatment. Additionally, the main prescriber should be identified. The possible risks of prescribing, including illicit drug use and alcohol, should also be identified (NICE, 2009). The National Institute for Health and Clinical Excellence (NICE) emphasises that the prescriber's and patient's psychological role in prescribing should be considered. Additionally, NICE advocates that one kind of medicine should be used, and polypharmacy should be avoided entirely. In a crisis, the National Institute for Health and Clinical Excellence advocates that medicine with minimal side effects and has a low risk of overdose should be used. Moreover, after the crisis is over, a plan should be put in place to end the drug treatment. If this is difficult, a constant review of the side effects, dependency, misuse, and effectiveness of the medicine should be conducted (NICE, 2009).

The above guidelines are rarely adhered to; studies have shown that over 84.1% of borderline personality disorder patients are reported to be in constant use of psychotropic drugs (Zanarini, 2015). The study also reported that 92% of the patients reported using psychotropic medications for an undefined period (Paton *et al.*, 2015). It is common to find more borderline personality disorder patients using psychotropic medications than individuals with other mental disorders such as anxiety or major depressive disorders. A decision to use the medicine in treating borderline personality disorder should be done based on an honest discussion regarding the diagnosis and comorbid issues the patient has and which would require drugs. The patient, prescriber, and psychotherapist should make clear plans linked to self-harming behaviours and suicidal ideations. It is necessary for all the parties involved to realise that there are medications which are specifically meant to treat borderline personality disorder. Additionally, these parties should understand that there is a likelihood of error in treating BPD through medication. As a result, patients are often required to wait for a period of two to six weeks to evaluate the effectiveness of the medicines (NICE, 2009).

Changing the medication schedule due to minimal results entails careful consideration and thinking about reducing one medication and titrating to another. The prescription process is significant in setting up a trusting relationship founded on recognising the patient's pain alongside the restrictions of drugs. A vital clinical tool requires maintenance of a non-judgemental attitude. The clinicians must involve the BPD patient to assist in identifying therapeutic agents, enhance compliance, evaluate anticipated benefits against adverse side effects, and ensure safety. Clinicians or mental health professionals should prescribe pharmacotherapy only when the patient is under severe distress. In situations where the patient is distressed but refuses to take medications, the clinician should not force the patients but encourage them. When prescribing drugs such as selective serotonin reuptake inhibitors, the clinician should exercise caution. SSRIs, despite their benefits in enhancing some borderline personality disorder symptoms when overdosed, can pose health risks to the patient. When prescribing medication, clinicians should use their judgement to examine the benefits of the drugs. Borderline personality disorder patients can base their decisions regarding medications on the fear of being controlled, not feeling wanted, or their expectation of being restored to health.

REFERENCES

Abraham, P. F., and Calabrese, J. R. (2008) 'Evidenced-based pharmacologic treatment of borderline personality disorder: A shift from SSRIs to anticonvulsants and atypical antipsychotics?', *Journal of Affective Disorders*, *111*(1), pp. 21–30.

American Psychiatric Association (2013) 'Diagnostic and statistical manual of mental disorders', *BMC Med*, *17*, pp. 133–137.

Arntz, A., and Van Genderen, H. (2011) *Schema therapy for borderline personality disorder.* John Wiley and Sons.

Bateman, A. W., (2012) 'Treating borderline personality disorder in clinical practice'.

Bateman, A. W., and Fonagy, P. E., (2012). *Handbook of mentalizing in mental health practice.* American Psychiatric Publishing, Inc.

Bateman, A. W., and Krawitz, R. (2013) *Borderline personality disorder: an evidence-based guide for generalist mental health professionals*, Oxford University Press.

Bateman, A., and Fonagy, P. (2010) 'Mentalization based treatment for borderline personality Disorder', *World Psychiatry*, *9*(1), p. 11.

Bateman, A., and Fonagy, P. (2016) *Mentalization-Based Treatment for Personality Disorders: A Practical Guide*, Oxford University Press.

Bellino, S., Paradiso, E., and Bogetto, F. (2008) 'Efficacy and tolerability of pharmacotherapies for borderline personality disorder', *CNS Drugs*, *22*(8), pp. 671–692.

Bertsch, K., Schmidinger, I., Neumann, I. D., and Herpertz, S. C. (2013) 'Reduced plasma oxytocin levels in female patients with a borderline personality disorder', *Hormones and Behavior*, *63*(3), pp. 424–429.

Blum, N., St. John, D., Pfohl, B., Stuart, S., McCormick, B., Allen, J., . . . and Black, D. W. (2008) 'Systems Training for Emotional Predictability and Problem Solving (STEPPS) for outpatients with borderline personality disorder: a randomized controlled trial and 1-year follow-up', *American Journal of Psychiatry, 165*(4), pp. 468–478. *Borderline Personality Disorder,* Oxford University Press.

Bornovalova, M. A., Hicks, B. M., Iacono, W. G., and McGue, M. (2009) 'Stability, change, and heritability of borderline personality disorder traits from adolescence to adulthood: A longitudinal twin study', *Development and Psychopathology, 21*(4), pp. 1335–1353.

Bresin, K. (2014) 'Five indices of emotion regulation in participants with a history of nonsuicidal self-injury: A daily diary study', *Behavior Therapy, 45*(1), pp. 56–66.

Bridler, R., Häberle, A., Müller, S. T., Cattapan, K., Grohmann, R., Toto, S., . . . and Greil, W. (2015) Psychopharmacological treatment of 2195 in-patients with borderline personality disorder: a comparison with other psychiatric disorders', *European Neuropsychopharmacology, 25*(6), pp. 763–772.

Brown, J., Blum, N., and Black, D. W. (2013) 'Systems Training for Emotional Predictability and Problem Solving: An Advanced Understanding', *Journal of Law Enforcement, 3*(4).

Brüne, M., Dimaggio, G., and Edel, M. A. (2013) 'Mentalization-Based Group Therapy for Inpatients with Borderline Personality Disorder: Preliminary Findings', *Clinical Neuropsychiatry, 10*(5).

Brunner, R., Henze, R., Richter, J., and Kaess, M. (2015) 'Neurobiological findings in youth with a borderline personality disorder', *Scandinavian Journal of Child and Adolescent Psychiatry and Psychology, 3*(1), pp. 22–30.

Carlstedt, R. A. (2009) *Handbook of Integrative Clinical Psychology, Psychiatry, and Behavioral Medicine: Perspectives, Practices, and Research,* Springer Publishing Company.

Chalker, S. A., Carmel, A., Atkins, D. C., Landes, S. J., Kerbrat, A. H., and Comtois, K. A. (2015) 'Examining challenging behaviors of clients with a borderline personality Disorder', *Behavior Research and Therapy*, *75*, pp. 11–19.

Chanen, A. M., and McCutcheon, L. (2013) 'Prevention and early intervention for borderline personality disorder: current status and recent evidence', *The British Journal of Psychiatry*, *202*(s54), pp. s24–s29.

Chanen, A. M., Jackson, H. J., McCutcheon, L. K., Jovev, M., Dudgeon, P., Yuen, H. P., . . . and Clarkson, V. (2009) 'Early intervention for adolescents with borderline personality disorder: quasi-experimental comparison with treatment as usual', *Australian and New Zealand Journal of Psychiatry*, *43*(5), pp. 397–408.

Chanen, A. M., Jovev, M., Djaja, D., McDougall, E., Yuen, H. P., Rawlings, D., and Jackson, H. J. (2008) 'Screening for borderline personality disorder in outpatient youth', *Journal of Personality Disorders*, *22*(4), pp. 353–364.

Chanen, A. M., Jovev, M., McCutcheon, L. K., Jackson, H. J., and McGorry, P. D. (2008) 'Borderline personality disorder in young people and the prospects for prevention and early intervention', *Current Psychiatry Reviews*, *4*(1), pp. 48–57.

Chanen, A. M., Mccutcheon, L. K., Germano, D., Nistico, H., Jackson, H. J., and Mcgorry, P. D. (2009)'The HYPE Clinic: an early intervention service for borderline personality Disorder', *Journal of Psychiatric Practice*, *15*(3), pp. 163–172.

Chapman, A., and Gratz, K.(2007) *The Borderline Personality Disorder Survival Guide: Everything You Need to Know About Living With BPD*, New Harbinger Publications

Choi-Kain, L. W., and Gunderson, J. G. (eds.)(2019) *Applications of Good Psychiatric Management for Borderline Personality Disorder: A Practical Guide*, American Psychiatric Pub

Choi-Kain, L. W., Albert, E. B., and Gunderson, J. G.(2016) 'Evidence-based treatments for borderline personality disorder: implementation, integration, and stepped care', *Harvard Review of Psychiatry*, *24*(5), pp. 342–356.

Clarkin, J. F., Levy, K. N., Lenzenweger, M. F., and Kernberg, O. F.

(2013)'Evaluating three treatments for borderline personality disorder: A multiwave study', *Focus*, *11*(2), pp. 269–276.

Cloitre, M., Garvert, D. W., Weiss, B., Carlson, E. B., and Bryant, R. A. (2014)'Distinguishing PTSD, complex PTSD, and borderline personality disorder: A latent class Analysis', *European Journal of Psychotraumatology*, *5*(1), p. 25097.

Coyle, T. N., Shaver, J. A., and Linehan, M. M. (2018)'On the potential for iatrogenic effects of psychiatric crisis services: the example of dialectical behavioral therapy for adult women with a borderline personality disorder', *Journal of consulting and clinical psychology*, *86*(2), p. 116.

Crowell, S. E., and Kaufman, E. A. (2016)'Development of self-inflicted injury: Comorbidities and continuities with borderline and antisocial personality traits', *Development and Psychopathology*, *28*(4pt1), pp. 1071–1088.

Das, P., Calhoun, V., and Malhi, G. S. (2014)'Bipolar and borderline patients display differential patterns of functional connectivity among resting state networks', *Neuroimage*, *98*, pp. 73–81.

Dimeff, L. A., and Koerner, K. E. (2007)*Dialectical Behavior Therapy in Clinical Practice: Applications Across Disorders and Settings*, Guilford Press.

Douglas, B., and James, P.(2013) *Common Presenting Issues in Psychotherapeutic Practice*, Sage.

Ducasse, D., Lopez-Castroman, J., Dassa, D., Brand-Arpon, V., Dupuy-Maurin, K., Lacourt, L., . . . and Olié, E. (2019) 'Exploring the boundaries between borderline personality disorder and suicidal behavior disorder', *European Archives of Psychiatry and Clinical Neuroscience*, pp. 1–9.

Durand, V. M., and Barlow, D. H. (2012) *Essentials of Abnormal Psychology*. Cengage Learning. Edelstein, B. A., Hersen, M., and Thase, M. E. (eds.) (2013) *Handbook of Outpatient Treatment of Adults: Nonpsychotic Mental Disorders*, Springer Science+Business Media.

Gerull, F., Meares, R., Stevenson, J., Korner, A., and Newman,

L. (2008) 'The beneficial effect on family life in treating borderline personality', *Psychiatry*, *71*(1), pp. 59–70.

Guilé, J. M., Boissel, L., Alaux-Cantin, S., and de La Rivière, S. G. (2018) 'Borderline personality disorder in adolescents: prevalence, diagnosis, and treatment strategies', *Adolescent health, medicine, and therapeutics*, *9*, p. 199.

Gunderson, J. G. (2009) 'Borderline personality disorder: ontogeny of a diagnosis', *American Journal of Psychiatry*, *166*(5), pp. 530–539.

Gunderson, J. G. (2011) 'Borderline personality disorder', *New England Journal of Medicine*, *364*(21), pp. 2037–2042.

Gunderson, J. G. (2016) 'The emergence of a generalist model to meet public health needs for patients with borderline personality disorder', *American Journal of Psychiatry*, *173*(5), pp. 452–458.

Gunderson, J. G., Stout, R. L., McGlashan, T. H., Shea, M. T., Morey, L. C., Grilo, C. M., . . . and Ansell, E. (2011) 'The ten-year course of borderline personality disorder: psychopathology and function from the Collaborative Longitudinal Personality Disorders Study', *Archives of General Psychiatry*, *68*(8), pp. 827–837.

Gunderson, J. G., Stout, R. L., Shea, M. T., Grilo, C. M., Markowitz, J. C., Morey, L. C., . . . and McGlashan, T. H. (2014) 'Interactions of borderline personality disorder and mood disorders over ten years', *Journal of Clinical Psychiatry*, *75*(8), p. 829.

Gunderson, J. G., Weinberg, I., and Choi-Kain, L. (2013) 'Borderline personality disorder', *Focus*, *11*(2), pp. 129–145.

Gunderson, John G. (2009) 'Borderline personality disorder: ontogeny of a diagnosis.', *American Journal of Psychiatry* 166.5, pp. 530–539.

Hancock-Johnson, E., Griffiths, C., and Picchioni, M. (2017) 'A focused systematic review of pharmacological treatment for borderline personality disorder', *CNS Drugs*, *31*(5), pp. 345–356.

Harned, M. S., Rizvi, S. L., and Linehan, M. M. (2010) 'Impact of co-occurring posttraumatic stress disorder on suicidal women with a borderline personality disorder', *American Journal of Psychiatry*, *167*(10), pp. 1210–1217.

Herpertz, S. C., Zanarini, M., Schulz, C. S., Siever, L., Lieb, K., and Möller, H. J. (2007) 'Treatment of personality disorders: World Federation of Societies of Biological

Psychiatry (WFSBP) Guidelines for Biological Treatment of Personality Disorders', *The World Journal Biology of Psychiatry*, *8*(4), pp. 212–244.

Hirsh, J. B., Quilty, L. C., Bagby, R. M., and McMain, S. F. (2012) 'The relationship between agreeableness and the development of the working alliance in patients with a borderline personality disorder', *Journal of Personality Disorders*, *26*(4), pp. 616–627.

Hopwood, C. J., Swenson, C., Bateman, A., Yeomans, F. E., and Gunderson, J. G. (2014) 'Approaches to psychotherapy for borderline personality: Demonstrations by four master Clinicians', *Personality Disorders: Theory, Research, and Treatment*, *5*(1), p. 108.

Horvath, A. O., Del Re, A. C., Flückiger, C., and Symonds, D. (2011) 'Alliance in individual Psychotherapy', *Psychotherapy*, *48*(1), p. 9.

Kaess, M., von Ceumern-Lindenstjerna, I. A., Parzer, P., Chanen, A., Mundt, C., Resch, F., and Brunner, R. (2013) 'Axis I and II comorbidity and psychosocial functioning in female adolescents with a borderline personality disorder', *Psychopathology*, *46*(1), pp. 55–62.

Kaplan, C., Tarlow, N., Stewart, J. G., Aguirre, B., Galen, G., and Auerbach, R. P. (2016) 'Borderline personality disorder in youth: The prospective impact of child abuse on non- suicidal self-injury and suicidality', *Comprehensive Psychiatry*, *71*, pp. 86–94.

Kimmel, C. L., Alhassoon, O. M., Wollman, S. C., Stern, M. J., Perez-Figueroa, A., Hall, M. G., . . . and Radua, J. (2016) 'Age-related parieto-occipital and other gray matter changes in borderline personality disorder: a meta-analysis of cortical and subcortical structures', *Psychiatry Research: Neuroimaging,* *251*, pp. 15–25.

Kulacaoglu, F., and Kose, S. (2018) 'Borderline Personality Disorder (BPD): In the Midst of Vulnerability, Chaos, and Awe', *Brain Sciences, 8*(11), p. 201.

Laurenssen, E. M., Hutsebaut, J., Feenstra, D. J., Bales, D. L., Noom, M. J., Busschbach, J. J., . . . and Luyten, P. (2014) 'Feasibility of mentalization-based treatment for adolescents with borderline symptoms: A pilot study', *Psychotherapy, 51*(1), p. 159.

Leander, N. P., Moore, S. G., and Chartrand, T. L. (2009) *Mystery Moods: Their Origins and Consequences.* Na.

Leiberich, P., Nickel, M. K., Tritt, K., and Gil, F. P. (2008) 'Lamotrigine treatment of aggression in female borderline patients, Part II: an 18-month follow-up', *Journal of Psychopharmacology, 22*(7), pp. 805–808.

Lieb, K., Völlm, B., Rücker, G., Timmer, A., and Stoffers, J. M. (2010) 'Pharmacotherapy for borderline personality disorder: Cochrane systematic review of randomised trials', *The British Journal of Psychiatry, 196*(1), pp. 4–12.

Linehan, M. M. (2018) *Cognitive-Behavioral Treatment of Borderline Personality Disorder,* Guilford Publications.

Linehan, M. M., Korslund, K. E., Harned, M. S., Gallop, R. J., Lungu, A., Neacsiu, A. D., . . . and Murray-Gregory, A. M., 'Dialectical behavior therapy for high suicide risk in individuals with borderline personality disorder: a randomized clinical trial and component analysis', *JAMA Psychiatry, 72*(5), pp. 475–482.

Livesley, J. (2008) 'Toward a genetically-informed model of borderline personality disorder', *Journal of Personality Disorders, 22*(1), pp. 42–71.

Lopez-Castroman, J., Galfalvy, H., Currier, D., Stanley, B., Blasco-Fontecilla, H., Baca-Garcia, E., . . . and Oquendo, M. A. (2012) 'Personality disorder assessments in acute depressive episodes: stability at follow-up', *The Journal of Nervous and Mental Disease, 200*(6), p. 526.

May, J. M., Richardi, T. M., and Barth, K. S. (2016) 'Dialectical behavior therapy as treatment for borderline personality disorder', *Mental Health Clinician, 6*(2), pp. 62–67, 'Borderline personality disorder in adolescents', *Clinical Psychology Review, 28*(6), pp. 969–981.

McMain, S. F., Links, P. S., Gnam, W. H., Guimond, T., Cardish, R. J., Korman, L., and Streiner, D. L. (2009) 'A randomized trial of dialectical behavior therapy versus general psychiatric management for borderline personality disorder', *American Journal of Psychiatry, 166*(12), pp. 1365–1374.

Mercer, D., Douglass, A. B., and Links, P. S. (2009) 'Meta-analyses of mood stabilizers, antidepressants and antipsychotics in the treatment of borderline personality disorder: effectiveness for depression and anger symptoms', *Journal of Personality Disorders, 23*(2), pp. 156–174.

Miller, A. L., Muehlenkamp, J. J., and Jacobson, C. M. (2008) 'Fact or fiction: Diagnosing'.

Moffitt, T. E., in alphabetical order, Arseneault, L., Jaffee, S. R., Kim-Cohen, J., Koenen, K. C., . . . and Viding, E. (2008) 'Research review: DSM-V conduct disorder: Research needs for an evidence base', *Journal of Child Psychology and Psychiatry, 49*(1), pp. 3–33.

Neacsiu, A. D., Rizvi, S. L., and Linehan, M. M. (2010) 'Dialectical behavior therapy skills use as a mediator and outcome of treatment for borderline personality in order', *Behavior Research and Therapy, 48*(9), pp. 832–839.

Oumaya, M., Friedman, S., Pham, A., Abou, T. A., Guelfi, J. D., and Rouillon, F. (2008) 'Borderline personality disorder, self-mutilation, and suicide: a literature review', *L'Encephale, 34*(5), pp. 452–458.

Paris, J. (2008) 'Clinical trials of treatment for personality disorders', *Psychiatric Clinics of North America, 31*(3), pp. 517–526.

Paris, J. (2009) 'The treatment of borderline personality disorder:

implications of research on diagnosis, etiology, and outcome', *Annual Review of Clinical Psychology*, *5*, pp. 277–290.

Paris, J. (2010) 'Estimating the prevalence of personality disorders in the community', *Journal of personality disorders*, *24*(4), pp. 405–411.

Paris, J. (2019) *Treatment Of Borderline Personality Disorder: A Guide to Evidence-Based Practice*, Guilford Publications.

Parker, G. (2011) 'Clinical differentiation of bipolar II disorder from personality-based "emotional dysregulation" conditions', *Journal of Affective Disorders*, *133*(1–2), pp. 16–21.

Parry, G. D., Crawford, M. J., and Duggan, C. (2016) 'Iatrogenic harm from psychological therapies–time to move on', *The British Journal of Psychiatry*, *208*(3), pp. 210–212.

Paton, C., Crawford, M. J., Bhatti, S. F., Patel, M. X., and Barnes, T. R. (2015) 'The use of psychotropic medication in patients with emotionally unstable personality disorder under the care of UK mental health services', *The Journal of Clinical Psychiatry*, *76*(4), pp. 512–518.

Porr, V. (2010) *Overcoming Borderline Personality Disorder: A Family Guide for Healing and Change*, Oxford University Press.

Rausch, J., Gäbel, A., Nagy, K., Kleindienst, N., Herpertz, S. C., and Bertsch, K. (2015) 'Increased testosterone levels and cortisol awakening responses in patients with borderline personality disorder: gender and trait aggressiveness matter', *Psychoneuroendocrinology*, *55*, pp. 116–127.

Reddy, M. S., and Vijay, M. S. (2017) 'Empirical reality of dialectical behavioral therapy in borderline personality', *Indian Journal of Psychological Medicine*, *39*(2), p. 105.

Ripoll, L. H. (2012) 'Clinical psychopharmacology of borderline personality disorder: an update on the available evidence in light of the Diagnostic and Statistical Manual of Mental Disorders–5', *Current Opinion in Psychiatry*, *25*(1), pp. 52–58.

Ripoll, L. H. (2013) 'Psychopharmacologic treatment of borderline personality disorder', *Dialogues in Clinical Neuroscience*, *15*(2), p. 213.

Rogers, B., and Acton, T. (2012) '"I think we're all guinea pigs really": a qualitative study of medication and borderline personality disorder', *Journal of Psychiatric and Mental Health Nursing*, 19(4), pp. 341–347.

Ruocco, A. C., Amirthavasagam, S., Choi-Kain, L. W., and McMain, S. F. (2013) 'Neural correlates of negative emotionality in borderline personality disorder: an activation-likelihood-estimation meta-analysis', *Biological Psychiatry*, 73(2), pp. 153–160.

Sadock, B. J., Sadock, V. A., and Levin, Z. E. (eds.) (2007) *Kaplan and Sadock's Study Guide and Self-Examination Review in Psychiatry*, Lippincott Williams and Wilkins.

Schulze, L., Schmahl, C., and Niedtfeld, I. (2016) 'Neural correlates of disturbed emotion processing in borderline personality disorder: a multimodal meta-analysis', *Biological Psychiatry*, 79(2), pp. 97–106.

Shaffer, D., and Jacobson, C. (2009) 'Proposal to the DSM-V childhood disorder and mood disorder work groups to include non-suicidal self-injury (NSSI) as a DSM-V disorder', *American Psychiatric Association*, pp. 1–21.

Siever, L. J. (2008) 'Neurobiology of aggression and violence', *American Journal of Psychiatry*, 165(4), pp. 429–442.

Silk, K. R. (2008) 'Personality disorder in adolescence: The diagnosis that dare not speak its Name.

Silvers, J. A., Hubbard, A. D., Biggs, E., Shu, J., Fertuck, E., Chaudhury, S., . . . and Brodsky, B. S. (2016) 'Affective lability and difficulties with regulation are differentially associated with the amygdala and prefrontal response in women with Borderline Personality Disorder', *Psychiatry Research: Neuroimaging*, 254, pp. 74–82.

Skodol, A. E., Gunderson, J. G., Shea, M. T., McGlashan, T. H., Morey, L. C., Sanislow, C. A., . . . and Pagano, M. E. (2005) 'The collaborative longitudinal personality disorders study (CLPDS): Overview and implications', *Journal of Personality Disorders*, 19(5), pp. 487–504.

Soloff, P., Nutche, J., Goradia, D., and Diwadkar, V. (2008) 'Structural brain abnormalities in borderline personality disorder: a voxel-based morphometry study', *Psychiatry Research: Neuroimaging*, *164*(3), pp. 223–236.

Stanley, B., and New, A. (eds.) (2017) *Borderline Personality Disorder*, Oxford University Press.

Stanley, B., and Siever, L. J. (2009) 'The interpersonal dimension of borderline personality disorder: toward a neuropeptide model', *American Journal of Psychiatry*, *167*(1), pp. 24–39.

Starcevic, V., and Janca, A. (2018) 'Pharmacotherapy of borderline personality disorder: replacing confusion with prudent pragmatism', *Current opinion in psychiatry*, *31*(1), pp. 69–73.

Steele, H., and Siever, L. (2010) 'An attachment perspective on borderline personality disorder: Advances in gene–environment considerations', *Current Psychiatry Reports*, *12*(1), pp. 61–67.

Stoffers-Winterling, J. M., Völlm, B. A., Rücker, G., Timmer, A., Huband, N., and Lieb, K. (2012) 'Psychological therapies for people with borderline personality disorder', *Cochrane Database of Systematic Reviews*, (8).

Torgersen, S., Myers, J., Reichborn-Kjennerud, T., Røysamb, E., Kubarych, T. S., and Kendler, K. S. (2012) 'The heritability of Cluster B personality disorders assessed both by personal interview and questionnaire', *Journal of Personality Disorders*, *26*(6), pp. 848–866.

Tottenham, N., Hare, T. A., Quinn, B. T., McCarry, T. W., Nurse, M., Gilhooly, T., . . . and

Thomas, K. M. (2010) 'Prolonged institutional rearing is associated with atypically large amygdala volume and difficulties in emotion regulation', *Developmental Science*, *13*(1), pp. 46–61.

Trull, T. J., Jahng, S., Tomko, R. L., Wood, P. K., and Sher, K. J. (2010) 'Revised NESARC personality disorder diagnoses: gender, prevalence, and comorbidity with substance dependence disorders', *Journal of Personality Disorders*, *24*(4), pp. 412–426.

Völlm, B. A., Chadwick, K., Abdelrazek, T., and Smith, J. (2012)

'Prescribing of psychotropic medication for personality disordered patients in secure forensic settings', *The Journal of Forensic Psychiatry and Psychology*, *23*(2), pp. 200–216.

Walsh, C., Ryan, P., and Flynn, D. (2018) 'Exploring dialectical behaviour therapy clinicians' experiences of team consultation meetings', *Borderline Personality Disorder and Emotion Dysregulation*, *5*(1), p. 3.

Wang, L., Ross, C. A., Zhang, T., Dai, Y., Zhang, H., Tao, M., . . . and Xiao, Z. (2012) 'Frequency of borderline personality disorder among psychiatric outpatients in Shanghai', *Journal of Personality Disorders*, *26*(3), pp. 393–401.

Wedig, M. M., Frankenburg, F. R., Reich, D. B., Fitzmaurice, G., and Zanarini, M. C. (2013) 'Predictors of suicide threats in patients with borderline personality disorder over 16 years of prospective follow-up', *Psychiatry Research*, *208*(3), pp. 252–256.

Weniger, G., Lange, C., Sachsse, U., and Irle, E. (2009) 'Reduced amygdala and hippocampus size in trauma-exposed women with borderline personality disorder and without posttraumatic stress disorder', *Journal of Psychiatry and Neuroscience*, 34, pp. 383–388.

Widiger, T. A. (ed.) (2012) *The Oxford Handbook of Personality Disorders*, Oxford University Press.

Wingenfeld, K., Spitzer, C., Rullkötter, N., and Löwe, B. (2010) 'Borderline personality disorder: hypothalamus pituitary adrenal axis and findings from neuroimaging studies', *Psychoneuroendocrinology*, *35*(1), pp. 154–170.

Winograd, G., Cohen, P., and Chen, H. (2008) 'Adolescent borderline symptoms in the community: prognosis for functioning over 20 years', *Journal of Child Psychology and Psychiatry*, *49*(9), pp. 933–941.

Zanarini, M. C., Frankenburg, F. R., Reich, D. B., and Fitzmaurice, G. (2010) 'Time to the attainment of recovery from borderline personality disorder and stability of recovery: A 10-year prospective follow-up study', *American Journal of Psychiatry*, *167*(6), pp. 663–667.

Zanarini, M. C., Frankenburg, F. R., Reich, D. B., Harned, A. L., and Fitzmaurice, G. M. (2015) 'Rates of psychotropic medication use reported by borderline patients and axis II comparison subjects over 16 years of prospective follow-up', *Journal of Clinical Psychopharmacology*, *35*(1), 63. 'English 11-year-olds and 34,653 American adults', *Journal of Personality Disorders*, *25*(5), pp. 607–619.

Zanarini, M. C., Frankenburg, F. R., Reich, D. B., Harned, A. L., and Fitzmaurice, G. M. (2015) 'Rates of psychotropic medication use reported by borderline patients and axis II comparison subjects over 16 years of prospective follow-up', *Journal of Clinical Psychopharmacology*, *35*(1), p. 63.

Zanarini, M. C., Horwood, J., Wolke, D., Waylen, A., Fitzmaurice, G., and Grant, B. F. (2011) 'Prevalence of DSM-IV borderline personality disorder in two community samples: 6,330'.

Zimmerman, M., Chelminski, I., and Young, D. (2008) 'The frequency of personality disorders in psychiatric patients', *Psychiatric Clinics of North America*, *31*(3), pp. 405–420.

CHAPTER 9

Promising Treatments for BPD

The current treatment of borderline personality disorder comprises pharmacological and disorder has remained a challenge both in its treatment and management. Pharmacology has demonstrated a promising impact in treating BPD; however, it has not helped in completely eradicating the symptoms of the disorder. The effectiveness of psychotherapies, such as dialectical behavioural therapy on BPD, has been minimal. As a result, the need to develop alternative therapies for the treatment of borderline personality disorder is critical and necessary. The increased understanding of the neurobiology and neuropsychiatry of major mental disorders has led investigators to develop new treatments that can directly stimulate the brain. The goal of these treatments is to improve the symptoms of various psychiatric disorders. Neurostimulation techniques such as repetitive transcranial magnetic stimulation, deep brain stimulation, and vagus nerve stimulation have therefore been developed in trying to treat psychiatric disorders.

These interventions have helped improve some of the borderline personality disorder symptoms, such as impulsivity and suicidal ideations (Cristea *et al.*, 2017).

Neurostimulation Techniques

Neurostimulation refers to the therapeutic modulation or stimulation of some regions of the nervous system. Neurostimulation, just like surgery, targets particular anatomical areas. Nevertheless, distinct from medicine, neurostimulation is reversible and adjustable. The stimulation devices, when required, can also be turned off. Neurostimulation is recommended since it does not have the adverse effects of pharmacotherapy. Brain stimulation treatment entails transmitting electric pulses to the brain to activate neural activity to treat a psychiatric condition such as obsessive compulsive disorder, anxiety, borderline personality disorder, and depression among others.

Neurostimulation involves modulating the activity of the nervous system using either non- invasive or invasive procedures. Neurostimulation treatments are used as a substitute for patients who are not responsive to either psychotherapy or pharmacotherapy. Most of these therapies entail the placement of electrodes on the exterior part of the scalp. At times brain stimulation therapy can involve surgical procedures where a device is inserted under the skin; this kind of procedure is more invasive. Brain stimulation techniques are frequently used in the treatment of psychiatric disorders where medicine and psychotherapies, such as cognitive behavioural therapy, have not been effective.

Brain stimulation therapies can be traced as far as the 1700s when machines for transcranial electrical stimulation were used to treat various mental health conditions. These devices used static, friction, or battery to produce a minimal electrical current. Therapists, physicians, and patients administered brain stimulation therapy in the 1800s and 1900s. These groups claimed that the treatment produced euphoric feelings and enhanced the mental performance of the patient. Nevertheless, no regulations were guiding the therapy; this caused adverse effects such as nausea, dizziness, and headaches.

In 1801, Giovanni Aldini, an Italian physicist, used an earlier form of transcranial direct stimulation (tDCS). This procedure is usually non-invasive and is commonly regarded as being safe. Additionally, tDCS, in comparison to other brain stimulation methods, is less painful. Giovanni Aldini used transcranial direct stimulation to enhance a farmer's mood, who earlier on had been diagnosed with melancholia, which is a type of depression. Nevertheless, the lack of scientific knowledge and technology caused transcranial direct stimulation to be left behind by other discoveries.

Another neurostimulation therapy earlier used in the treatment of psychiatric disorders is electroconvulsive therapy (ECT). This therapy was initially used to treat mental disorders in the 1930s. ECT has remained the first line of treatment for patients with depressive symptoms and acute suicidal thoughts and behaviours. ECT can also be used in the treatment of a major depressive disorder that has no psychotic symptoms. Electroconvulsive therapy is often used when antidepressants have failed. Despite its favourable outcome, the use of ECT has been limited by the availability of anaesthetists and equipment, patients' perception, and side effects such as short-term amnesia (Kennedy and Giacobbe, 2007). Over the years, other brain stimulation therapies have emerged in the treatment of psychiatric disorders. Some of them include transcranial direct current stimulation, transcranial magnetic stimulation, deep brain stimulation, and the vagus nerve stimulation.

Transcranial Magnetic Stimulation Therapy

Transcranial magnetic stimulation (TMS) is a procedure that does not use medication and is non-invasive. This therapy is based on the electromagnetic induction principle, where an electric current is passed through a coil. When the generated magnetic field comes into contact with the brain, it generates a secondary electric field. The magnetic field produced by TMS varies within milliseconds. As a result, an electric field is induced in the area under the coil. The magnetic field goes through the fat, bone, and skin with minimal resistance and little deviation. This ensures the current that is induced is relatively central.

Nevertheless, there is a reduction in intensity when the distance from the coil's centre is increased (Hallet, 2007). The magnetic fields are generated with flux lines perpendicular to the coil's plane. Circular coils have a higher concentration of magnetic fields on the coil's inner margin; additionally, no current is generated at the centre. The secondary electric current produced in neurons is generated parallel to the magnetic field (Hallet, 2007). Electromyography (EMG) is used to measure the impact of a single transcranial magnetic stimulation pulse on the motor cortex.

Each transcranial magnetic stimulation pulse randomly activates all neurons in areas where the stimulus is generated. However, depending on the depolarisation proximity, orientation, and threshold of the coil, they might or might not fire. When firing, the stimulation of the cortical-spinal pyramidal neurons can generate direct waves generated first. Stimulating interneurons, on the other hand, produces indirect waves that appear at regular intervals with amplitude smaller following the direct waves. Different pulse coil positions and pulse intensities can trigger diverse indirect and direct waves.

Transcranial magnetic stimulation directs repeated magnetic energy pulses at particular areas of the brain that are involved in the regulation of mood. The magnetic pulses are then passed through the skull to activate brain cells. This procedure is painless and is known to enhance communication in various regions of the brain. This procedure does not involve surgery, and its impact is rarely experienced in the whole body. Anaesthesia is also not used in transcranial magnetic stimulation since it is not a surgical procedure.

The transcranial magnetic stimulation principle is founded on Faraday's principle regarding electromagnetic induction. Transcranial magnetic stimulation activates hemodynamic, metabolic, neurons, and behavioural modification (Ustohal, 2018). The procedure is well tolerated by borderline personality disorder patients in comparison to the adverse effects of medications. Some of the rare negative effects of transcranial magnetic stimulation on borderline personality disorder are seizures.

In the treatment of borderline personality disorder, transcranial magnetic stimulation can be applied alone or together with other therapies such as behavioural therapies and drugs. TMS, which was first developed in 1985, can be beneficial in the treatment of mood disorders. Transcranial magnetic stimulation uses magnetic energy to stimulate regions of the brain adversely impacted by psychiatric disorders.

In borderline personality disorder, transcranial magnetic stimulation is used in conjunction with other therapies. Studies have shown that when TMS is used, there is a significant reduction of borderline personality disorder symptoms. The impact is mostly felt when TMS is used as an addition to current treatment approaches. Studies have also reported a decrease in suicidal and self-injurious tendencies among borderline personality disorder patients when transcranial magnetic stimulation is used. TMS is a treatment approach that can be used to reduce impulsivity among borderline personality disorder patients. Transcranial magnetic stimulation commonly comprises thirty-six therapy sessions, which last for three months. Each session usually takes between twenty to thirty minutes. Most borderline personality disorder patients begin with five sessions per week. As the BPD symptoms start to improve, the sessions are reduced to two per week. During TMS sessions, BPD patients recline in a chair used for treatment where they are required to remain alert and awake throughout the session. A transcranial magnetic stimulation magnet is then placed over the head of the patient to transmit pulses to particular regions of the brain. After each therapy session, borderline personality disorder patients may immediately go back to their regular routines. The administration of transcranial magnetic stimulation can either be done individually (single-pulse TMS) or through repetitive transcranial magnetic stimulation (rTMS) (Ustohal, 2018). Single-pulse TMS is used mainly in different neuroscience research models jointly with electroencephalography,

PET, and functional MRI. Single-pulse TMS is used in examining basic neural and cognitive functions.

The repetitive transcranial magnetic stimulation has more impact although its likelihood to cause seizures is high. Transcranial magnetic stimulation can be used in psychiatric treatment as an approach to evaluate the central motor conduction. TMS can also be used as a tool for researching various human brain physiology features, which may include language, vision, and function. Studies have reported that transcranial magnetic stimulation effectively influences the cognitive and affective states, both in the long and short term. Therefore, TMS can be viewed as a potential therapy in reducing suicidality (Wasserman *et al.*, 2008).

Repetitive Transcranial Magnetic Stimulation Therapy for Depression

Many borderline personality disorder patients also have problems with depressive symptoms. It is common for BPD to co-occur with depression. The comorbidity rate between depression and borderline personality disorder is high (Beatson and Rao, 2013). It is necessary to note that depression is not just normal sadness. Several psychophysiological changes are associated with depression, such as the inability to experience pleasure, sleep disturbance, and suicidal thoughts and behaviours. The depressive mood is a common and potentially risky mental complication in psychiatric disorders. Depression often worsens the clinical condition of mental disorder.

Depression in borderline personality disorder presents itself differently than people without the disorder (Yoshimatsu and Palmer, 2014). For instance, although depression is usually associated with emotions of guilt and sadness, in BPD, it is described as being connected to feelings of shame, emptiness, loneliness, and anger. Borderline personality disorder patients when depressed portray feelings of intense restlessness, loneliness, and boredom. Additionally, depressive episodes in **BPD** patients are frequently caused by interpersonal losses, such as relationship break-ups.

Depression has a significant impact on a patient's life and can restrict the social activities of the affected individual. Depression frequently leads to withdrawal from family, community, and friends. There are several mental health disorders which can include symptoms of depression. They include schizoaffective disorder, mood disorders, and personality disorders like a borderline personality disorder. People who have several depressed mood episodes can be diagnosed as having a major depressive disorder.

Over the years, the clinical approach of patients with depression has evolved and commonly entails psychotherapy, pharmacotherapy, and supportive care. Therapy for depression includes short-term approaches to activate remission and long-term techniques to inhibit recurrence. Available medication for depression involves tricyclic antidepressants (**TCA**), selective serotonin reuptake inhibitors (**SSRI**), monoamine oxidase inhibitors (**MAOI**), and selective norepinephrine reuptake inhibitors (**NRI**). Nonetheless, only a few patients respond positively to antidepressant treatment. Furthermore, studies have shown that 50% of patients who often remit relapse within six to twelve months (Meguins, 2012). As a result, although antidepressants are widely used as a treatment for depression, they have minimal impact on reducing depressive symptoms.

The number of patients diagnosed with treatment-resistant depression is increasing (Yoshimatsu and Palmer, 2014). Most of these patients are at a high risk of suicide; effective therapy is necessary for this disorder. Patients that are not responsive to antidepressants are often referred to the electroconvulsive therapy. Although ECT has some positive effects in treating depressive symptoms, its side effects, such as cognitive impairment, restrict its clinical application. Additionally, electroconvulsive therapy has been linked to a high rate of relapse (Minichino et al., 2012).

Studies have reported that patients with depression and personality disorder often have inadequate responses to conventional treatment such as psychotherapy and medications than people without such disorders (Yoshimatsu and Palmer, 2014). As a result, neurostimulation techniques such as repetitive transcranial magnetic stimulation have proven effective. The FDA in 2008 conducted intensive research before approving repetitive transcranial magnetic stimulation as a therapy for depression, especially one that is treatment-resistant. In many countries, rTMS is an approved therapy for major depressive disorder and is regarded as a first- line treatment (Perera *et al.*, 2016).

Anthony Barker, a physicist from Sheffield, was the one who invented the first repetitive transcranial magnetic stimulation machine in 1985 for the treatment of depression. Repetitive transcranial magnetic stimulation is a technique that stimulates the brain and depends on the production of brief magnetic fields through a coil that is placed on the scalp. The rTMS entails the transmission of constant electric current bursts to activate neural activity in the brain region, linked to mood regulation. The magnetic pulses produce an electric current that temporarily stimulates neurons at the stimulation site.

Additionally, this therapy, compared to electroconvulsive therapy, is more effective. Repetitive transcranial magnetic stimulation also has lesser risks than those experienced through electroconvulsive therapy (Minichino *et al.*, 2012). In major depressive disorder, repeated transcranial magnetic stimulation therapy targets the dorsolateral prefrontal cortex, an area involved in regulating various processes like attention, decision-making, and working memory.

When a person is clinically depressed, their dorsolateral prefrontal cortex tends to become hypoactive (Kaiser *et al.*, 2015). The hypoconnectivity of the frontoparietal network has been linked to the default mode network's hyperconnectivity. As a result, an increase in adverse emotional bias, rumination, and dysfunctional self-referential processing may occur (Williams, 2016).

Repetitive transcranial magnetic stimulation stimulates the left dorsolateral prefrontal cortex, and this is viewed as being necessary for normalising the functional balance among the neural networks. For instance, rTMS down-regulates connections in the default mode network.

Additionally, through rTMS, the connectivity within the insula and left dorsolateral prefrontal cortex is regulated. Repetitive transcranial magnetic stimulation therapy also helps control the connectivity between the hippocampus and the salience network, which has been linked to the reduction of depressive symptoms (Philip et al., 2018). Patients that experience improvement of their depressive symptoms for a short period can benefit from regular treatment. Dosing in repetitive transcranial magnetic stimulation refers to the number of pulses and stimulation intensity used in a particular session. The intensity is linked to the strength of the generated magnetic field, which can be controlled by the operator. A study was conducted on borderline personality disorders that were exposed to repetitive transcranial magnetic stimulation (Calihol et al., 2014). The results showed that BPD patients tolerated the stimulation and did not experience any adverse effects.

Repetitive transcranial magnetic stimulation therapy uses several sessions per day with a minimum of six hundred pulses for every session, which leads to the reduction of the total therapy period. The rTMS was introduced as a treatment for depression to challenge the remission and response rate often witnessed in electroconvulsive therapy. When the number of rTMS sessions on the left dorsolateral prefrontal cortex are increased from one session to two per day, studies have shown enhanced clinical results, reducing the therapy period (Modirrousta et al., 2018).

Minimal changes in the coil positioning can lead to considerable differences in the brain regions being stimulated. It is, therefore, necessary throughout the therapy period to stimulate the identified regions only. Diverse approaches on the coil positions are often utilised, and they have varying levels of clinical effectiveness versus cost. These entail the five-centimetre rule, neuronavigation stimulation, stimulation over F3. The five-centimetre principle is usually the most straightforward technique. Nonetheless, this method has been criticised since it does not account for the size of the head and individual variances in brain anatomy.

However, this limitation is addressed by the stimulation over F3. The transcranial magnetic stimulation is placed at electroencephalography (EEG) electrodeposition F3 that is believed to connect to the dorsolateral prefrontal cortex (DLPFC). The ideal personalised approach in positioning the coil is founded on frameless stereotactic systems that allow accurate neuronavigation of the brain region predefined. Transcranial magnetic stimulation neuronavigation is considered superior regarding precision. Nonetheless, whether TMS neuronavigation enhances clinical efficacy in treating depression is still debatable (Sack *et al.*, 2009). In most cases, patients with depression undergoing repetitive transcranial magnetic stimulation therapy continue using antidepressants. However, studies have reported that repetitive transcranial magnetic stimulation therapy is more effective than medication. It is also noted that rTMS might cost less than most medicines used in treating depression (Voigt *et al.*, 2017).

Repetitive Transcranial Magnetic Stimulation Therapy in Treating Impulsivity in Borderline Personality Disorder

Based on *DSM*-5, some of the symptoms of borderline personality disorder include instability in interpersonal relationships and impulsivity. Borderline personality disorder impairs the psychosocial functioning of those affected (Schulze, Schmahl, and Niedtfeld, 2016). Borderline personality disorder patients are characterised by their inability to regulate their emotions and often experience emotional vulnerability. Studies have demonstrated that BPD patients have frontal parts and front-limbic connections that are impaired.

These brain regions are necessary for emotional regulation, decision-making, and behavioural inhibition. BPD patients also have greater amygdala reactivity while their PFC responses are altered. Studies have shown that the volume of the grey matter, orbitofrontal cortex, and insula in borderline personality disorder patients is smaller than that of their healthy counterparts (Schulze, Schmahl, and Niedtfeld, 2016).

Impulsive aggression among borderline personality disorder patients has been linked to serotonin neurotransmission that is also affected by the prefrontal cortex. Neuroimaging studies show that an overactive amygdala can be as a result of damaged inhibitory control of the reactivity of limbic emotion by PFC regions. Research has shown positive results when repetitive transcranial magnetic stimulation is used in treating borderline personality disorder symptoms. For instance, rTMS leads to a greater desire to change self-esteem, planning ability, happiness, and sociability in borderline personality disorder patients.

Studies have demonstrated that repetitive transcranial magnetic stimulation can regulate mood.

Improved moods as a result of rTMS often lead to better memory, executive functions, and attention. Consequently, rTMS enhances a more rational and balanced thought pattern. TMS can also assist in normalising the mood of a borderline personality disorder patient. The procedure can also lead to a healthier brain by preventing mind states that are mostly linked to aggression, impulsivity, and despair.

Studies have reported that rTMS is a well-tolerated and safe procedure that does not require surgery and can be successful in treating psychiatric disorders. Repetitive transcranial magnetic stimulation utilises an electromagnetic coil that is placed beneath the patient's scalp. The coil is used to transmit electromagnetic pulses that are painless. The treatment duration varies from one patient to another. Some patients may experience improvement for a short period only. Other patients may experience long-term improvement while others may not experience any change.

The study also showed that the activity of the prefrontal cortex could be enhanced by rTMS neuromodulation. Consequently, the repetitive transcranial magnetic stimulation downregulated the subcortical structures (Calihol et al., 2014). This hypothesis thereby could explain the impact of rTMS on impulsivity, affect instability, and anger. Repetitive transcranial magnetic stimulation has also been effective in reducing borderline personality disorder symptoms, including anger, emotional instability, fear of abandonment, and impulsivity. Repetitive transcranial magnetic stimulation by targeting the PFC region can enhance borderline personality disorder symptoms. Stimulating the cerebellum under low frequency can also decrease BPD symptoms.

Repetitive Transcranial Magnetic Stimulation Therapy in Treating Suicidality in Borderline Personality Disorder

According to the World Health Organization, the clinical problems of self-harm, suicidal thoughts, and suicide have led to the deaths of millions of people annually (Caine, 2012). Despite the efficacy of current psychological and pharmacological treatments, the problem of suicidality has persisted. Suicidality can be both a disabling and chronic disorder for many individuals, especially those diagnosed with mental health disorders. There is an urgent need to change focus from managing suicidality through comprehensive psychiatric treatments. Furthermore, there is a need to have an enhanced understanding of the neurophysiology and neuropsychology of suicidal behaviour to assist in targeted interventions.

Suicidal behaviour and thoughts are a common symptom of people diagnosed with various psychiatric disorders such as schizophrenia, borderline personality disorder, and bipolar disorder. Over ninety per cent of individuals who die due to suicide are often diagnosed with mental disorders (Caine, 2012). Suicidal behaviour is multi-factorial, complex behaviours that involve various cultural, psychosocial, and medical-biologic components. Studies have shown that there is a high prevalence of suicidal ideations in patients with psychiatric disorders. Among these disorders, mood disorders such as borderline personality disorder represent a high-risk factor for suicide attempts and suicide ideations. Self-harm and suicidal behaviour occur with diverse psychiatric disorders and entail endangering one's life, passive neglect, and putting oneself in risky situations. The reduction of suicidality lies in effectively treating the underlying psychiatric disorder through medications and other psychosocial interventions such as psychotherapy. Nevertheless, several challenges exist relating to the effective treatment of suicidality (Maltsberger *et al.*, 2015). One of the challenges is that neither psychotherapy nor pharmacotherapies are fast enough to reduce suicidal ideation. Moreover, studies have reported that even well-established medications and therapies for suicidality, such as dialectical behavioural therapy, clozapine, and lithium, are limited in their effectiveness (Sher, Mindes, and Novakovic, 2010).

Another factor includes the fact that antidepressants prescribed to depressed patients can become a potential method of suicide, for instance, through intoxication. The lack of success of various treatments in the treatment of suicidal behaviour and ideation shows the need for more effective interventions. The current therapies for suicidality are ineffective and inadequate. Therefore, there is an urgent need to develop new treatment approaches to prevent suicide risk among psychiatric patients (Desmyter *et al.*, 2016). As a result, transcranial magnetic stimulation is gradually being adopted as a new approach in the treatment of suicidality.

Repetitive transcranial magnetic stimulation is highly tolerable and is free from the adverse effects that are common in antidepressant mediations. Consequently, repetitive transcranial magnetic stimulation is attractive to psychiatric patients who are unwilling to take medications (Rasmussen, 2011). Transcranial magnetic stimulation has been reported to influence the cognitive and affective states in both short and long time frames. Therefore, rTMS can be considered a possible treatment for decreasing suicidality (Sher, Mindes, and Novakovic, 2010). Furthermore, unlike other brain stimulation techniques such as ECT, repetitive transcranial magnetic stimulation does not use anaesthesia. The magnetic stimulation is delivered in a focal way at a selected cortical target instead of affecting the whole brain as is common in electroconvulsive therapy. As a result, side effects through rTMS are significantly reduced (Dougherty and Widge, 2017). Transcranial magnetic stimulation has also not been linked to cognitive impairment, and its side effects range from mild to modest. Some studies have reported reduced suicidal behaviour and ideations after psychiatric patients were treated with repetitive transcranial magnetic stimulation (Levkovitz *et al.*, 2015). Evidence has shown that most severe psychiatric disorders linked to suicidal behaviour and ideations, such as major depressive disorder and schizophrenia, can be managed through rTMS.

Repetitive transcranial magnetic stimulation affects the cortico-limbic imbalances linked to depression. Suicidality entails disturbed executive function and emotional regulation in the cortico-limbic networks. Transcranial magnetic stimulation restores the cortical network balance; therefore, it is a logical brain stimulation method for suicidality and depression (Levkovitz *et al.*, 2015). Studies have reported that repetitive transcranial magnetic stimulation delivered in high doses on the left prefrontal cortex can be used to reduce suicidal ideation rapidly.

Furthermore, TMS can also offer secondary benefits like constant interaction between the patient and psychiatrist. This interaction can assist the mental health practitioner in recognising the signs of potential suicidal behaviour and attempts. Repetitive transcranial magnetic stimulation is regarded as safer than other invasive neurostimulation therapies. Although transcranial magnetic stimulation is not a direct treatment for suicidality, it is a significant treatment of depression which can exhibit suicidal ideations. However, the technique is linked to some side effects, which include light-headedness and headaches after the procedure.

Combining Pharmacotherapy with Repetitive Transcranial Magnetic Stimulation

In most circumstances, patients undergoing repetitive transcranial magnetic stimulation continue with the use of antidepressants. Nonetheless, much remains unknown regarding the effect of pharmacotherapy on the efficacy of rTMS. Some studies propose that benzodiazepines, anticonvulsants, and antidepressants impact cortical excitability. Antidepressants in humans seem to expedite the neuroplastic impact of brain stimulation. On the other hand, benzodiazepines and anticonvulsants appear to have an inhibitory effect (Hunter *et al.*, 2019).

The studies on repetitive transcranial magnetic stimulation on major depressive disorder are very varied regarding concomitant medication. As a result, it becomes challenging to determine a superior combined impact of these approaches. The likely interaction of particular pharmacological treatment and repetitive transcranial magnetic stimulation cannot be exploited or excluded in attaining better clinical results. More future research is required in evaluating the effect of pharmacotherapy on the efficacy of rTMS.

Combining Psychotherapy with Repetitive Transcranial Magnetic Stimulation

The combination of repetitive transcranial magnetic stimulation with psychotherapy can enhance the remission and response rate. A study that was conducted showed that simultaneously applying psychotherapy and rTMS in the treatment-resistant depression led to a 56% remission rate and a 66% response rate after the treatment had ended. Additionally, combining these two treatments led to a 60% constant remission after a six-month follow-up (Donse *et al.*, 2018). Although combining the two treatments seems promising, there is a need for systematic research and clinical trials on both approaches.

Combining Cognitive Training with Repetitive Transcranial Magnetic Stimulation

Over fifty per cent of patients with depression have cognitive impairments. A recent study examining the cognitive-enhancing impact of repetitive transcranial magnetic stimulation alone reported an average improvement in the trail making test performance. This test is used to examine cognitive flexibility, visual scanning, and psychomotor speed (Martin *et al.*, 2017).

When cognitive training is performed alone, the results appear promising (Motter *et al.*, 2016). However, combining both approaches might lead to a more cognitive-enhancing impact. There has been a view that devoid of cognitively relevant brain activity; repetitive transcranial magnetic stimulation can lead to cognitive enhancement. During repetitive transcranial magnetic stimulation treatment, patients remain unengaged. Therefore, it would be reasonable to complement cognitive training with rTMS. Studies in the future should consequently evaluate if such an approach can lead to a decrease in depressive symptoms while also enhancing cognition. Unveiling cognitive effects, a wide variety of cognitive functions should be evaluated with sensitive, reliable, and valid techniques.

Maintenance of Repetitive Transcranial Magnetic Stimulation

Even though there are no clearly laid down rules, maintenance of repetitive transcranial magnetic stimulation applied after a positive response to an acute rTMS course has been proposed to extend its positive clinical impact. However, studies are greatly varied regarding the design due to sample sizes that are small and lack placebo control. The regularity of repetitive transcranial magnetic stimulation maintenance varies from distributed distinct sessions that can be conducted weekly, monthly, biweekly, or bimonthly. These sessions can be spread over two to three months.

Maintenance of rTMS can also be based on short treatment phases conducted daily, for instance, one week every month. The maintenance can also be clustered, for example, in every fifth week. Nevertheless, most patients exhibit average success with repetitive transcranial magnetic stimulation maintenance compared to when there is no treatment. Studies have reported that these patients attain remission ranging from three months to five years (Haesebaert *et al.*, 2018). More studies are required in the future to explore the ability of rTMS maintenance in preventing relapses. Additionally, these studies should assess the long-term efficacy and safety of this kind of maintenance.

Deep Brain Stimulation

There is a long history of neurosurgical approaches for psychiatric disorders. Nevertheless, previous attempts were significantly limited due to the primitiveness of neuroanatomical models and the available strategies employed. Deep brain stimulation has developed as an intervention that can enhance symptoms of patients with severe psychiatric disorders (Holtzheimer and Mayberg, 2011). Developing neurosurgical approaches for stimulation and focal ablation historically have been motivated by endeavours to treat complex mental disorders (HarIz, Blomstedt, and Zrinzo, 2010). Before the 1950s, there was no medication for severe mental disorders. The aggressive and disabling nature of these disorders led to the adoption of invasive treatments such as hypoglycaemic coma, electroconvulsive therapy, neurosurgery, and malarial pyrotherapy. The first surgery to treat patients that were severely psychotic had limited success.

Over time, neurosurgical therapies shifted to interrupting the white matter linking brain regions related to behaviour and mood regulation. This process was later referred to as the prefrontal lobotomy. The surgical techniques used to severe these areas were limited and were often conducted blindly and led to large lesions. Medications that had antidepressant, antipsychotic, and anti-manic effects in the mid-twentieth century, eventually terminated the lobotomy era. As early as the 1950s, investigators began to look at the impact of intracranial stimulation in patients with psychiatric disorders (Hariz *et al.*, 2010).

Deep brain stimulation is a neuromodulation technique that entails surgically implanting a neuro- stimulating device (Gold and Frierson, 2017). DBS is a technique whose purpose is to treat psychiatric or neurological disorders by implanting electrodes into a specific area of the brain. The electrodes are inserted through a neurosurgical process and later linked to a pulse generator that is placed on the wall of the chest. The pulse generator is used to allow constant stimulation of the relevant regions of the brain. Deep brain stimulation has been extensively used in the last few decades to treat several neurological disorders such as Parkinson's disease.

Before 1999, deep brain stimulation was not viewed as a viable therapy in the treatment of psychiatric disorders (Holtzheimer and Mayberg, 2011). Presently deep brain stimulation is seen as a potential therapy in the treatment of essential tremor, Parkinson's disease, chronic dystonia, and obsessive compulsive disorder. It is necessary to note that researchers are looking at the efficacy of DBS in treating various psychiatric disorders. Multiple studies have reported that deep brain stimulation can be an effective and safe approach to treating depression.

The DBS device, which is commonly referred to as a neurostimulator, comprises three elements, namely the impulse generator, electrode, and extension. The impulse generator is a device that is operated through a battery. The device is usually placed below the patient's clavicle. However, some impulse generators can be placed in a cavity in the patient's skull since they are small. A clinician can outwardly regulate the device to ensure maximum benefits and minimal side effects (Higgins and George, 2019). The extension, on the other hand, transfers the electrical signal from the generator's impulses to the electrodes.

The application of deep brain stimulation in treating psychiatric disorders is based on two widely recognised research traditions. They include brain imaging and ablation/lesion surgeries; both try to identify the circuits behind psychiatric disorders (Marks, 2015). Ablation/lesion surgeries are criticised because of clinical privilege abuses associated with the procedure in the early and mid-twentieth century. Some of the factors that led to the abuse of these clinical privileges comprised the absence of proper infrastructure in guarding human research subjects. Classification of psychiatric disorders used by mental health practitioners was another factor that led to the abuse. Psychiatric neurosurgery in the current era started with a British neurosurgeon named Geoffrey Knight. In his surgery, Geoffrey destroyed large parts of the orbitofrontal white matter (Marks, 2015). The surgery was a success, and it led to the development and adoption of deep brain stimulation as a treatment method for several psychiatric disorders. Psychotherapy, medications, and other therapies are useful to some extent in treating psychiatric disorders like a borderline personality disorder. However, in most situations, the rate of relapse is high, and there is a low resolution of symptoms.

Consequently, advanced techniques that alter neural activity, such as deep brain stimulation (DBS), have been developed. Deep brain stimulation is a neurosurgical approach that is invasive; it is currently being evaluated for the treatment of various mental disorders, including BPD and depression among others.

Deep brain stimulation uses probes that are commonly placed jointly in the subcortical parts of the brain. By placing them there, the probes release electrical stimulation (Higgins and George, 2019). After this procedure, the probes can be positioned in any part of the brain even on the extradural (the surface under the skull). Sometimes the neurosurgery for implanting the device is done under a general and local anaesthesia combination. The preference for using local anaesthesia over general anaesthesia is to help the patient become involved in enhancing the electrode's correct placement.

The use of deep brain stimulation in the treatment of mental disorders is founded on its success.

DBS involves the implantation of one electrode or more into particular parts of the brain by burring holes in the skull (Holtzheimerand Mayberg, 2011). Implanting the electrodes is done during a neurosurgical procedure. Subsequently, it is linked to a pulse generator that is placed on a chest to enable electric stimulation of the specific areas of the brain. Various factors have led to an interest in the likelihood of using deep brain stimulation in the treatment of mental disorders. One of the factors entailed the use of surgical methods in the past in the treatment of mental disorders. Historically, severe mental disorders like depression and obsessive compulsive disorders were treated through lesioning procedures. Some of the procedures historically used to treat such psychiatric disorders included limbic leucotomy, subcaudal tractotomy, and anterior capsulotomy among others. The purpose of such procedures was to interrupt links between cortical and subcortical parts of the brain that were involved in most symptoms of psychiatric disorders.

Another factor that has increased the interest of DBS as a technique in the treatment of psychiatric disorders is the mood material impact experienced by borderline personality disorder patients when this approach is used. Furthermore, studies have recognised continuously that most mental disorders entail interruption of the brain system that is involved in several dysfunctional brain parts. A treatment approach such as deep brain stimulation, therefore, target particular nodes in the brain system is therefore required.

Deep Brain Stimulation for Treatment-Resistant Depression

Depression is common among people diagnosed with a borderline personality disorder.

Treatments for depression entail antidepressant medication, psychotherapy, and other somatic therapies such as light therapy and electroconvulsive therapy. Despite these therapies, studies have shown that two-thirds of patients diagnosed with depression do not become symptom-free. Additionally, one-third of the patients do not remit even with several treatments while a minimum of 20% despite aggressive treatments remain symptomatic (Holtzheimerand Mayberg, 2011). For patients who are responsive to treatment, it is common for them to experience a depressive relapse.

At times patients can have treatment-resistant depression, which has a higher risk of relapse.

Often, such patients are treated using electroconvulsive therapy (ECT). Although ECT is effective in patients with treatment-resistant depression, it has several drawbacks. The first is that ECT can only be conducted in a facility that can give anaesthesia, thereby limiting its access. Additionally, ECT is linked to cognitive side effects and can also lead to memory loss.

These and other limitations have made **DBS** a potential approach in patients with treatment resistant depression (Delaloye and Holtzheimer, 2014). Studies evaluating whether deep brain stimulation is an effective therapy for depression that is treatment-resistant has demonstrated positive results (Gold and Frierson, 2017). The function of **DBS** can be compared to that of a pacemaker; however, it is used in the brain and not the heart.

In treating depression, deep brain stimulation targets several brain regions for electrode placement. The areas of the brain targeted by deep brain stimulation are the habenula, posterior gyrus rectus, inferior thalamic peduncle, nucleus accumbens, and the ventral capsule. Electrodes are bilaterally placed in the subcallosal cingulate gyrus during **DBS** treatment of depression (Accolla *et al.*, 2016). The subcallosal cingulate gyrus is often linked in mood regulation. The subcallosal cingulate gyrus is a brain region that has been studied extensively regarding its relation to depression. Patients with depression demonstrate increased activity in the subcallosal cingulate gyrus as a reaction to adverse stimuli. Normalising the subcallosal cingulate activity can be linked to enhancing the depressive symptoms.

Studies show that the hyperactivity of the subcallosal cingulate gyrus diminishes through successful psychotherapy, pharmacotherapy, transcranial magnetic stimulation (Konarski *et al.*, 2009). Another study was conducted that showed that using tractography and high-resolution magnetic resonance imagery can guide on the best region for placing the electrode. Additionally, this can give a personalised surgical approach to deep brain stimulation placement in patients with treatment-resistant depression. The study further reported that individualised placement enhanced the treatment's efficacy to 73% response in six months and 82% at one year (Riva- Posse *et al.*, 2018).

The treatment of depression through deep brain stimulation helps regulate irregular impulses (Pattern *et al.*, 2016). During this procedure, electrodes are implanted in the brain parts that control moods. These brain regions, which are hyperactive due to the depletion of tryptophan, include the anterior cingulate, thalamus, orbitofrontal cortex, and ventral striatum. Research has shown that deep brain stimulation of the subcallosal cingulate white matter can enhance the functional neuroanatomical modifications previously linked with antidepressant response (Mayberg, 2009). Additionally, the researchers reported that DBS of the subcallosal cingulate in patients with treatment-resistant depression could lead to symptomatic improvement.

Long-term follow-up reported a response rate of 45% and a 15% rate of remission after two years. A three-year continuing stimulation reported a response rate of 60% while there was a remission rate of 50% (Kennedy *et al.*, 2011). However, there were side effects of the treatment, such as infection and worsening irritability, not related to the manageable situation. Studies have also shown that individuals prone to depression often have an overactive emotion-regulating brain circuit. The purpose of deep brain stimulation is necessary among depressed patients is because they have low chemical messenger.

In the treatment of depression, DBS targets the nucleus accumbens septi as this helps in eliminating the primary symptom of depression, which is a loss of interest in activities previously enjoyed. The nucleus accumbens are neurons that are situated in the vagus nerve. The connection between nucleus accumbens and depression is a functional and structural correlation between nucleus accumbens and the level of anhedonia, which is a symptom of depression. The severity of the anhedonia depends on the size of the nucleus. Severe anhedonia is linked to a smaller nucleus and little activation of the nucleus accumbens.

Increased activity in the nucleus accumbens has been associated with reward-seeking behaviours, drug abuse, and monetary reward, viewing faces that are attractive and pleasurable music. The pleasure response of humans to stimuli like faces or music is linked to the nucleus accumbens' activity (Wacker, Dillon, and Pizzagalli, 2009). Therefore, a change in the nucleus accumbens activity can reduce depressive symptoms. Studies have been conducted to stimulate the nucleus accumbens (Bewenirck *et al.*, 2010). These studies have shown patients with anhedonia who had their nucleus accumbens stimulated experienced an increase in their reward-seeking thoughts.

Furthermore, stimulating the NACC demonstrated a bilateral rise in the dorsolateral prefrontal Cortex's metabolic function, a structure that is commonly hypoactive in depression. Additionally, reduced activity was witnessed in the study of the ventromedial prefrontal activity that was shown to be overactive during the depression (Koenigs and Grafman, 2009). Therefore, a pathological function reversal due to the stimulation of the nucleus accumbens was witnessed parallel to the reduction of depressive symptoms (Schlaepfer *et al.*, 2009).

Evidence has shown that patients with major depressive disorder have reduced responsiveness to pleasurable stimuli, especially the capacity to incorporate the history of reward reinforcement over time (Pizzagalli *et al.*, 2008). This has been linked to reduced activity in the nucleus accumbens region among these patients. Looking at the nucleus accumbens function in hedonic reactions, researchers believed that DBS of this region could reduce anhedonia in patients with treatment-resistant depression (Schlaepfer *et al.*, 2008). Deep brain stimulation of the nucleus accumbens can affect anhedonia, a primary symptom of depression. As a result, the stimulation can lead to an antidepressant effect in patients with treatment-resistant depression.

A study was done on patients with treatment-resistant depression receiving deep brain stimulation if the nucleus accumbens. The study reported that these patients experienced improved hedonic response during the stimulation, and the response was turned off when the stimulation was reversed (Schlaepfer *et al.*, 2008). In managing treatment-resistant depression among psychiatric patients, DBS also targets the lateral habenula, a midbrain structure comprising of various small nuclei that lie caudal and dorsal to dorsal thalamus main structure. The lateral habenula coordinates monoaminergic neurotransmission and gets input from subcortical and cortical structures through the stria medullaris thalami.

Studies have reported overactivity of the lateral habenula in depressed patients (Rant *et al.*, 2010). The lateral habenula has a role in controlling reward through the ventral tegmentum (Li *et al.*, 2011). The activity of the lateral habenula correlates adversely to the expectation of reward and response of reward. Firing in the lateral habenula neurons is enhanced in the opposite circumstances. The lateral habenula inhibits the dopamine neurons of the ventral striatum, active in the expectation and response of rewards. An increase in the activity of the lateral habenula can hence explain some depressive symptoms such as an increase in pain sensation and reduced reward-seeking behaviour (Loonen and Ivanova, 2016).

Based on this theory, a quick reduction of plasma tryptophan, a drug used to alleviate the worsening of depressive symptoms, demonstrated an increase of the blood flowing into the habenular region. Deep brain stimulation can reduce depressive symptoms by inhibiting the function of the lateral habenula. Deep brain stimulation of the lateral habenula led to remission after a patient with the major depressive disorder was stimulated for four months. Furthermore, based on its anatomy, the habenula is a likely target for deep brain transmission for treatment- resistant depression (Sartorious *et al.*, 2010).

The ventral capsule is also targeted in the treatment of depression as it is often linked in regulating the reward system neural network (Greenberg *et al.*, 2010). The high functional connectedness of the ventral striatum with several brain regions has been associated with depressive symptoms (Quevedo *et al.*, 2017). For instance, increased networks from the left ventral striatum to the left caudate have been linked with anhedonia. Moreover, increased links from the left ventral striatum to the right superior and mid anterior cingulate cortex and prefrontal cortex were associated with more suicidality.

The severity of depression also correlates to the connection of the left ventral striatum with the right precuneus and the mid and left cingulate. Studies have reported that intensity in the functional connectivity between the default mode network and the ventral striatum is positively correlated with the Center for Epidemiologic Studies Depression Scale (Hwang *et al.*, 2016). The study of the anterior limb of the internal capsule has shown brain areas linked to depressive symptoms (Hwang *et al.*, 2016). Reduced interest in pleasurable activities among patients diagnosed with depression has been connected to decreased bilateral ventral striatum activation in responding to positive stimuli (Epstein *et al.*, 2006).

A study was conducted that showed the efficacy of deep brain stimulation in the ventral striatum in treating patients with the treatment-resistant disorder (Dougherty *et al.*, 2015). Another study conducted on patients with depression treated with deep brain stimulation on the ventral capsule showed that 40% of them had curative effects six months after surgery. The ventral striatum and ventral capsule was originally a target in the treatment of the obsessive compulsive disorder.

The idea that deep brain stimulation could be used in the treatment of depression by targeting the ventral striatum and ventral capsule arose from the reports of stimulating patients with obsessive compulsive disorder. These reports indicated that patients with obsessive compulsive disorder who also had depression improved after DBS targeted the ventral striatum and ventral capsule in their treatment. Most of these patients improved in their social functioning and resumed school, work, and independent living.

Search for the Ideal Target Brain Region for Deep Brain Stimulation

The clinical trial for deep brain stimulation for treatment-resistant depression has provided safety and efficacy for different brain targets. Studies have shown that after stimulation of the subgenual anterior cingulate cortex, one-third of patients achieved complete remission through deep brain stimulation. Another third of the patients demonstrated improvement while a third did not experience any benefit from the stimulation (Lozano *et al.*, 2012). Going forward, the effectiveness of deep brain stimulation therapy on treatment-resistant depression can be ascertained through active-sham designed studies. Designing these trails, adequate duration such as six months should be provided with the prospect of examining the setting of the deep brain stimulation parameter.

It is necessary to have at least one week before the crossover stage (Bergfeld *et al.*, 2016). By doing this, the efficacy of the clinical trials can be ensured. The primary condition for deep brain stimulation therapy of depression involves identifying the right target accurately. Finding an ideal node which can decrease or eliminate the functional treatment-resistant depression abnormality is vital. Finding an ideal deep brain stimulation target is crucial; nonetheless, consideration should be put in place that there is no one ideal DBS target in the treatment of depression.

The stimulation effect of antidepressants can be attained through different targets; this supports the idea that depression is a neurocircuitry disorder that involves disrupting numerous extensive neural networks instead of damage to a single brain region. Neurocircuitry of depression is viewed as involving the dorsal, ventral, and modulatory components. Each deep brain stimulation-treatment resistant depression target structure has a unique functional and anatomical position within the networks. These networks regulate the DBS capacity to enhance depressive symptoms during stimulation. For example, it was assumed that deep brain stimulation was applied in a region where fibres from the dorsal and ventral compartments meet. For example, the nucleus accumbens could enhance simulation inhibition and excitation in the ventral and dorsal compartments.

Another example of a specific role of the stimulated region in extensive communication is the anterior cingulate cortex. The integrative activity of the anterior cingulate cortex in cognitive processing can explain the efficacy of deep brain stimulation of the subgenual anterior cingulate cortex in the treatment of depression (Kibleur *et al.*, 2017). Different brain regions ought to be used in various stages due to the presence of diverse underlying abnormalities in the brain.

Personalising Deep Brain Stimulation in the Treatment of Depression

Dependable biomarkers of the brain abnormalities are required to identify the efficacy and suitability of deep brain stimulation. Custom-made DBS therapy that can include the precise needs of the patient can enhance the total efficacy of deep brain stimulation techniques. Individualised deep brain stimulation therapy requires a specific assessment of the patient's brain impairment and personalised DBS protocol. A registry for future clinical studies has been proposed as one way of developing individualised treatment (Morishita *et al.*, 2014).

Morishita and colleagues recommend that future DBS clinical studies for treatment-resistant depression should be gathered in an organised way. The data will then be used to create a shared register of factors linked to the patient's clinical status before commencing treatment. This data can also be used to determine stimulation parameters, the exact placing of the electrode in the brain structure, and postoperative results, including adverse effects. Extensive meta-analyses can be performed based on the gathered information, and the deep brain stimulation is personalised to match the pre-surgical traits of each patient (Zhou *et al.*, 2018).

It is necessary to receive a precise assessment of the impairment of each patient. Additionally, it is essential to objectively measure the brain's abnormality as this would help differentiate the various categories of depression as this would enhance efficacy. The diagnostic tools currently used, such as psychometric techniques and structured diagnostic interviews, cannot adequately measure the functional or structural abnormalities in the brain. These tools focus on the symptoms outcome of the disease. Additionally, using direct neuroimaging tools like electroencephalography and the standard clinical magnetic resonance imaging is primarily constrained to a different diagnosis of depression. These tools only identify or eliminate epilepsy and brain lesions. Electroencephalogram analysis is a possible solution as an objective biomarker of brain abnormalities in depression. This technique is a piece of promising neurophysiological equipment for comprehending and evaluating the dynamics of the brain network on a sub-second timescale (Michel and Koenig, 2018).

Potential Risks of Deep Brain Stimulation

There are critical kinds of safety issues linked with the administration of deep brain stimulation.

The first safety concern is directly connected to the implanted device, and the second is associated with the side effects that arise from the neurosurgical procedure.

Device and Procedure-Related Risks

Complications associated with the neurosurgical procedure include seizures and bleeding in the brain after the surgery. Other adverse effects can entail the wound becoming infected after the surgery. It is necessary to note that diverse target areas in the brain need different deep brain stimulation implantation routes. There is a likelihood of higher levels of haemorrhage arising from implanting electrodes in less accessible regions of the brain. For instance, implanting these devices in brain regions with high numbers of blood vessels can lead to haemorrhage.

Nonetheless, there are no studies on the safety of deep brain stimulation in the major regions targeted in the treatment of psychiatric disorders. Side effects related to the neurosurgical procedure depend on the experience and competency of the surgical team. Side effects associated with the device being can occur if the neurostimulator becomes faulty (Bewernick et al., 2010).

Stimulation-Related Risks

Side effects arising from stimulation are common and are linked to the neuroanatomical stimulation site. These effects frequently arise at stimulation and contact parameters, which are not ideal for therapeutic benefits. The trial causes these adverse effects-and-error approach search for ideal stimulation location. The two commonly witnessed stimulation side effects are anxiety/agitation and transient hypomania induction (Goodman *et al.*, 2010). Additionally, insomnia has been reported after an increase in voltage and may require an increase in sedative drugs. Patients should be closely monitored for temporal worsening of psychiatric symptoms like increased aggression, reduced mood, and obsession. Stimulation can also lead to other adverse effects such as hot and cold flushes and tingling sensation. Many implantation regions have also been reported to lead to changes in blood pressure, dizziness, nausea, and sweating. Motor effects that can occur include temporal motor slowing, orofacial muscle contractions, and oculomotor disturbance (Schlaepfer *et al.*, 2013).

Some deep brain stimulation parameters have also been associated with memory disturbance and transient confusion. However, the occurrence of these side effects is minimal. Therefore, deep brain stimulation is a better treatment for depression in borderline personality disorder than other therapies.

Recommendations

Deep brain stimulation, as a treatment for psychiatric disorders, should occur for patients who have enrolled in a clinical trial. Implantation of the deep brain stimulation device should be performed by a neurosurgeon that has fundamental expertise in DBS processes. Additionally, it is necessary that the neurosurgeon involved in DBS procedures be involved in such processes regularly. Programming of the deep brain stimulation device should be closely supervised by a psychiatrist with adequate experience in clinically managing patients with the psychiatric disorder being treated.

Before deep brain stimulation is fully adopted as a treatment approach for psychiatric disorders such as borderline personality disorder and depression, patients must provide their consent first before the procedure is undertaken. An autonomous body must review the personal suitability and consent of these patients before commencing the procedure. The review process should incorporate the psychiatric suitability of the treatment and the neurosurgical experience of the surgeon conducting the deep brain stimulation.

The review should consider the quality of the team involved in long-term care for the patient.

Additionally, the patient's capacity to give informed consent and participate in the treatment procedure should also be reviewed. Deep brain stimulation is an emerging and promising treatment for a wide range of psychiatric and neurological disorders. Nonetheless, more research is required to justify the clinical practice of deep brain stimulation in psychiatric conditions.

Vagus Nerve Stimulation

In the last twenty years, there has been an emergence of new effective neurostimulation treatments for depression. It is necessary to note that patients with borderline personality disorder are prone to depressive symptoms. One of the neurostimulation approaches that have emerged in the treatment of depressive symptoms is the vagus nerve stimulation. This therapy targets the vagus nerve, one of the most significant nerves in the body of a human. The nerve is a part of the nervous system that regulates unconscious and involuntary body functions such as control of digestion and maintaining the heart rate.

The vagus nerve goes through the neck to the chest, abdomen, and lower brain regions. This nerve is related to motor functions in the stomach, diaphragm, and sensory functions in the tongue and ear, heart, and voice box. The nerve is also linked to the sensory and motor functions in the oesophagus and sinuses. The vagus nerve is involved in emotional response and regulation. Vagus nerve stimulation is a new technique used to treat neuropsychiatric and neurological diseases (George and Aston-Jones, 2010).

VNS is a procedure done surgically as therapy for treatment-resistant depression, which is common in personality disorders such as borderline personality disorders. Vagus nerve stimulation was initially introduced as a treatment for epilepsy that was drug-resistant. The first vagus nerve stimulation surgeries for the treatment of epilepsy were done in the 1980s. The surgery involved enfolding an electrode around the left vagus nerve, which was linked to an implant pulse generator that was transmitting low-frequency electrical signals to the nerve (Andrew, 2010). Studies later showed that these patients after VNS were experiencing improved social functioning and mood.

These reports led to more studies regarding whether vagus nerve stimulation could be beneficial in treatment-resistant depression. The results from these studies led the United States, in 2005, to approve vagus nerve stimulation to treat recurring and chronic depression and other personality disorders. After several years, healthcare agencies in several countries, including Canada, South and Central America, Australia, and the European Union, approved vagus nerve stimulation for the treatment-resistant depression (de Leon et al., 2019). As part of the FDA approval in the United States, the VNS device manufacturer agreed to develop a treatment-resistant depression registry that would gather data on patients followed over several years (Aaronson et al., 2017).

To qualify for vagus nerve stimulation, a patient should have tried a minimum of four anti-depressants in two diverse categories (Aaronson et al., 2017). This means that the drugs should have a minimum of two different techniques of action in the chemistry of the body. The therapies ought also to entail two kinds of augmentation therapy, which is a combination of two drugs that act differently hen put together. Before beginning the vagus nerve stimulation, it is also necessary for patients to have been subjected to psychotherapies such as interpersonal therapy and cognitive behavioural therapy.

Some mental health conditions eliminate psychiatric patients from vagus nerve stimulation.

Some of these conditions include suicidal behaviours and thoughts, schizophrenia, alcohol and substance abuse, and schizoaffective disorder. Since the vagus nerve is linked to various major organs, some health conditions exclude psychiatric patients from vagus nerve stimulation. Some of these medical conditions include severe lung disorders, ulcers, previous brain injury, and heart arrhythmias among others. Additionally, patients whose vagus nerve is removed cannot be considered for vagus nerve stimulation.

During the VNS surgical procedure, a device that is similar to a pacemaker is implanted in the patient's body and connected to a stimulating wire that is wound along the vagus nerve. This nerve goes up the neck and into the brain, where it links to regions believed to regulate mood.

After the device is implanted, it continuously transmits impulses to the vagus nerve. During the surgical procedure of the vagus nerve stimulation, the surgeon inserts a small device that is battery powered and works like a pacemaker into the patient's chest (Andrew, 2010).

Two small incisions are performed; one is on the left side of the neck, a thin wire that is placed under the patient's skin and runs from the equipment to a large vagus nerve in the neck. The other incision is in the upper area of the chest; the pulse generator is placed there (O'Reardon, Cristancho, and Peshek, 2006). The incisions are small; therefore, they heal with minimal noticeable scarring. The device then begins to and electrical pulses into the nerve then transmitted into the brain.

A week or two after the procedure, the doctor turns on the stimulator and progressively adjusts the stimulation strength over several weeks (O'Reardon, Cristancho, and Peshek, 2006). The vagus nerve stimulation procedure often takes one to two hours to be completed (Andrew, 2010). The procedure can be performed on an outpatient basis, or the patient may stay at the hospital overnight. VNS can use local or general anaesthesia. In most cases, the vagus nerve stimulation device is set to go off at systematic interludes. The stimulator is programmed to transmit to the electrical nerve impulses consistently throughout the day.

The stimulations carry on for thirty seconds and occur at an interlude of five minutes (Andrew, 2010). After the device has been implanted, it becomes permanent, not automatic. Patients are provided with a magnet which they can use to turn off the device temporarily. Patients can turn off the device if the timed stimulation becomes disruptive during some of their activities such as singing, giving a speech, or exercising. The batteries can be replaced after several years through a surgical procedure that takes a short period. It is possible to remove the pulse generator; however, the wires are permanently connected to the vagus nerve. For reasons that have not yet been proven or identified scientifically, the electrical pulses sent to the brain through the vagus nerve relieve the depressive symptoms. The impulses can impact how the nerve cell circuits send signals in brain regions that regulate mood.

Nevertheless, it might take some time before the patient experiences these effects. Studies have reported a positive impact of vagus nerve stimulation on patients with treatment- resistant depression. VNS therapy is approved for patients with depressive symptoms who have failed to respond to a minimum of at least four antidepressants in the course of the illness (Aaronson *et al.*, 2017). This is a degree of treatment that is above the scope of most current clinical trials. Furthermore, patients with treatment-resistant depression comorbid with bipolar depression and have not benefited from electroconvulsive therapy are candidates for VNS. Patients who have experienced depression for more than three years can also qualify for vagus nerve stimulation.

Patients who have not received relief from chronic, recurrent, or severe depression symptoms can benefit from VNS. To qualify for vagus nerve stimulation, a patient must have tried several therapies, including medications, cognitive behavioural therapy with no success (O'Reardon, Cristancho, and Peshek, 2006). VNS therapy is linked to various significant organs; therefore, some health conditions such as lung disorders, previous brain injury, and ulcers exclude some patients from this therapy.

It is necessary to note that vagus nerve stimulation is a long-term treatment. Although most patients might need fewer medications after VNS, drug therapy would still be required to manage some of the depressive symptoms. Vagus nerve stimulation targets brain regions that influence the production of serotonin and norepinephrine. It is believed these chemicals are involved in depression. Most antidepressants enhance the availability of the two chemicals. The vagus nerve transmits sensory information to the locus coeruleus from the body. The locus coeruleus is a primary source of norepinephrine while the raphe nucleus produces serotonin (Andrews, 2010).

VNS applies its beneficial impact by stimulating the solitary tract nucleus that has secondary projections to cortical and limbic structures responsible for mood regulation. When these brain structures are activated, they trigger several neurochemical changes. These changes include processes linked to neurotransmission and generation of growth factors. Studies have shown that vagus nerve stimulation triggers acute changes in the amygdala, medial prefrontal cortex, hippocampus, hypothalamus, and insula. VNS, similar to other treatments for depression, deactivates the ventromedial prefrontal cortex (Ressler and Mayberg, 2007).

Researchers also suggest that the positive impact of vagus nerve stimulation in depressed patients is partially an outcome of stimulating the vagal efferent pathway (Das, 2007). Studies have reported that the vagus nerve afferent pathways impact the transmission of monoaminergic into the brain. The non-systemic nature of VNS allows it to be combined with almost all other treatments for affective disorders. Combining vagus nerve stimulation with other treatments helps if the patient's response is slow.

Vagus nerve stimulation can generate long-term benefits and may decrease the number of depressive episodes. VNS can also reduce the severity and duration of affective episodes. Therefore, through VNS, the quality of life of patients with treatment-resistant depression is enhanced. In selecting Vagus nerve stimulation as an intervention for patients with treatment- resistant severe depression, clinicians should be careful. VNS takes a long period before the patient can see its full benefit. Therefore, patients requiring critical intervention such as acute suicidality cannot be regarded as potential candidates for vagus nerve stimulation (Aaronson et al., 2017).

Neuroimaging and clinical studies have demonstrated that the impact of vagus nerve stimulation on treatment-resistant depression occurs gradually (Mertens *et al.*, 2018). Therefore, the clinician needs to inform patients of the extended period involved before they can experience any long- lasting benefits from VNS. Although vagus nerve stimulation is considered safe, there are some side effects connected to initial surgery and brain stimulation. Potential complications that may arise from the surgery include infection, pain, nausea, damage to the vagus nerve, scarring, lung, or heart problems (Andrew, 2010).

Vagus nerve stimulation can also lead to breathing problems, skin tingling, difficulties swallowing, chest or neck pain, tickling in the throat, and changes in the patient's voice. In rare cases, vagus nerve stimulation can worsen depression and trigger suicidal behaviours and thoughts. Additionally, the pulse generator is at risk of malfunctioning or moving out of place, leading to more surgery. Most of these side effects are mild and can be reduced by having the physician adjust the strength or timing of the electrical pulses. However, if the side effects persist, the device may be temporarily or permanently shut off (Andrew, 2010).

Vagus nerve stimulation seems to be a valued addition to current psychiatric treatment. Evidence shows that this therapy is a well-tolerated and promising intervention that is effective in patients diagnosed with treatment-resistant depression. Clinical trials regarding vagus nerve stimulation in treating depression keep growing. Vagus nerve stimulation is a research tool that provides hope of enhanced knowledge in treating various psychiatric disorders. Currently, the technology underlying the efficacy of VNS in treatment-resistant depression is not yet wholly understood.

One explanation concerning the efficacy of vagus nerve stimulation in the treatment of psychiatric disorders states that this therapy is mediated by the recognised direct and secondary vagus nerve projections to the brain parts involved in mood regulation. Since it is non-systemic, vagus nerve stimulation can be combined with all current psychiatric disorder treatments. Studies have demonstrated the safety and efficacy of VNS when combined with other therapies. More research in the future is required to increase the understanding of the mechanism of vagus nerve stimulation in treatment-resistant depression.

REFERENCES

Aaronson, S. T., Sears, P., Ruvuna, F., Bunker, M., Conway, C. R., Dougherty, D. D., . . . and Zajecka, J. M. (2017) 'A 5-year observational study of patients with treatment-resistant depression treated with vagus nerve stimulation or treatment as usual: comparison of response, remission, and suicidality', *American Journal of Psychiatry*, *174*(7), pp. 640–648.

Abraham, P. F., and Calabrese, J. R. (2008) 'Evidenced-based pharmacologic treatment of borderline personality disorder: A shift from SSRIs to anticonvulsants and atypical antipsychotics?', *Journal of Affective Disorders*, *111*(1), pp. 21–30.

American Psychiatric Association (2013) 'Diagnostic and statistical manual of mental Disorders', *BMC Med*, *17*, pp. 133–137.

Andrews, L. W. (2010) *Encyclopedia of Depression* (2 volumes), ABC-CLIO.

Arntz, A., and Van Genderen, H. (2011) *Schema Therapy for Borderline Personality Disorder*, John Wiley & Sons.

Bateman, A. W. (2012) 'Treating borderline personality disorder in clinical practice'.

Bateman, A. W., and Fonagy, P. E. (2012) *Handbook of Mentalizing in Mental Health Practice*, American Psychiatric Publishing, Inc.

Bateman, A. W., and Krawitz, R. (2013) *Borderline Personality Disorder: An Evidence-Based Guide for Generalist Mental Health Professionals*, Oxford University Press.

Bateman, A., and Fonagy, P. (2010) 'Mentalization based treatment for borderline personality Disorder', *World Psychiatry*, *9*(1), p. 11.

Bateman, A., and Fonagy, P. (2016) *Mentalization-Based Treatment for Personality Disorders: A Practical Guide*, Oxford University Press.

Beatson, J. A., and Rao, S. (2013) 'Depression and borderline personality disorder', *Medical Journal of Australia*, *199*, pp. s24–s27.

Bellino, S., Paradiso, E., and Bogetto, F. (2008) 'Efficacy and tolerability of pharmacotherapies for borderline personality disorder', *CNS Drugs*, *22*(8), pp. 671–692.

Bergfeld, I. O., Mantione, M., Figee, M., Schuurman, P. R., Lok, A., and Denys, D. (2018) 'Treatment-resistant depression and suicidality', *Journal of Affective Disorders*, *235*, pp. 362–367.

Bertsch, K., Schmidinger, I., Neumann, I. D., and Herpertz, S. C. (2013) 'Reduced plasma oxytocin levels in female patients with a borderline personality disorder', *Hormones and Behavior*, *63*(3), pp. 424–429.

Bewernick, B. H., Hurlemann, R., Matusch, A., Kayser, S., Grubert, C., Hadrysiewicz, B., . . . and Brockmann, H. (2010) 'Nucleus accumbens deep brain stimulation decreases ratings of depression and anxiety in treatment-resistant depression', *Biological Psychiatry*, *67*(2), pp. 110–116.

Blum, N., St. John, D., Pfohl, B., Stuart, S., McCormick, B., Allen, J., . . . and Black, D. W. (2008) 'Systems Training for Emotional Predictability and Problem Solving (STEPPS) for outpatients with borderline personality disorder: a randomized controlled trial and 1-year follow-up', *American Journal of Psychiatry*, *165*(4), pp. 468–478.

Boisseau, C. L., Yen, S., Markowitz, J. C., Grilo, C. M., Sanislow, C. A., Shea, M. T., . . . and

McGlashan, T. H. (2013) 'Individuals with single versus multiple suicide attempts over 10 years of prospective follow-up', *Comprehensive Psychiatry*, *54*(3), pp. 238–242. *Borderline Personality Disorder*, Oxford University Press.

Bornovalova, M. A., Hicks, B. M., Iacono, W. G., and McGue, M. (2009) 'Stability, change, and heritability of borderline personality disorder traits from adolescence to adulthood: A longitudinal twin study', *Development and Psychopathology*, *21*(4), pp. 1335–1353.

Bresin, K. (2014) 'Five indices of emotion regulation in participants with a history of nonsuicidal self-injury: A daily diary study', *Behavior Therapy*, *45*(1), pp. 56–66.

Bridler, R., Häberle, A., Müller, S. T., Cattapan, K., Grohmann, R., Toto, S., . . . and Greil, W. (2015) 'Psychopharmacological treatment of 2195 in-patients with borderline personality disorder: a comparison with other psychiatric disorders', *European Neuropsychopharmacology*, *25*(6), pp. 763–772.

Brown, J., Blum, N., and Black, D. W. (2013) 'Systems Training for Emotional Predictability and Problem Solving: An Advanced Understanding', *Journal of Law Enforcement*, *3*(4).

Brüne, M., Dimaggio, G., and Edel, M. A. (2013) 'Mentalization-Based Group Therapy for Inpatients with Borderline Personality Disorder: Preliminary Findings', *Clinical Neuropsychiatry*, *10*(5).

Brunner, R., Henze, R., Richter, J., and Kaess, M. (2015) 'Neurobiological findings in youth with a borderline personality disorder', *Scandinavian Journal of Child and Adolescent Psychiatry and Psychology*, *3*(1), pp. 22–30. Cailhol, L., Roussignol, B., Klein, R., Bousquet, B., Simonetta-Moreau, M., Schmitt, L., . . . and

Birmes, P. (2014) 'Borderline personality disorder and rTMS: a pilot trial', *Psychiatry Research*, *216*(1), pp. 155–157.

Caine, E. D. (2012) 'Suicide prevention is a winnable battle', *American Journal of Public Health*, *102*(S1), pp. S1–S6.

Carlstedt, R. A. (2009) *Handbook of Integrative Clinical Psychology, Psychiatry, And Behavioral Medicine: Perspectives, Practices, and Research*, Springer Publishing Company.

Carrion, V. G., Weems, C. F., Watson, C., Eliez, S., Menon, V., and Reiss, A. L. (2009) 'Converging evidence for abnormalities of the prefrontal cortex and evaluation of midsagittal structures in pediatric posttraumatic stress disorder: an MRI study', *Psychiatry Research: Neuroimaging*, *172*(3), pp. 226–234.

Chalker, S. A., Carmel, A., Atkins, D. C., Landes, S. J., Kerbrat,

A. H., and Comtois, K. A. (2015) 'Examining challenging behaviors of clients with a borderline personality disorder', *Behavior Research and Therapy*, *75*, pp. 11–19.

Chanen, A. M., and McCutcheon, L. (2013) 'Prevention and early intervention for borderline personality disorder: current status and recent evidence', *The British Journal of Psychiatry*, *202*(s54), pp. s24–s29.

Chanen, A. M., Jackson, H. J., McCutcheon, L. K., Jovev, M., Dudgeon, P., Yuen, H. P., . . . and Clarkson, V. (2009) 'Early intervention for adolescents with borderline personality disorder: quasi-experimental comparison with treatment as usual', *Australian and New Zealand Journal of Psychiatry*, *43*(5), pp. 397–408.

Chanen, A. M., Jovev, M., Djaja, D., McDougall, E., Yuen, H. P., Rawlings, D., and Jackson, H. J. (2008) 'Screening for borderline personality disorder in outpatient youth', *Journal of Personality Disorders*, *22*(4), pp. 353–364.

Chanen, A. M., Jovev, M., McCutcheon, L. K., Jackson, H. J., and McGorry, P. D. (2008) 'Borderline personality disorder in young people and the prospects for prevention and early intervention', *Current Psychiatry Reviews*, *4*(1), pp. 48–57.

Chanen, A. M., Mccutcheon, L. K., Germano, D., Nistico, H., Jackson, H. J., and Mcgorry, P. D. (2009) 'The HYPE Clinic: an early intervention service for borderline personality Disorder', *Journal of Psychiatric Practice*, *15*(3), pp. 163–172.

Chapman, A., and Gratz, K. (2007) *The Borderline Personality Disorder Survival Guide: Everything You Need to Know About Living with BPD*, New Harbinger Publications.

Choi-Kain, L. W., and Gunderson, J. G. (eds.) (2019) *Applications of Good Psychiatric Management for Borderline Personality Disorder: A Practical Guide*, American Psychiatric Pub.

Choi-Kain, L. W., Albert, E. B., and Gunderson, J. G. (2016) 'Evidence-based treatments for borderline personality disorder: implementation, integration, and stepped care', *Harvard Review of Psychiatry*, *24*(5), pp. 342–356.

Clarkin, J. F., Levy, K. N., Lenzenweger, M. F., and Kernberg, O. F. (2013) 'Evaluating three treatments for borderline personality disorder: A multiwave study', *Focus*, *11*(2), pp. 269–276.

Cloitre, M., Garvert, D. W., Weiss, B., Carlson, E. B., and Bryant, R. A. (2014) 'Distinguishing PTSD, complex PTSD, and borderline personality disorder: A latent class analysis', *European Journal of Psychotraumatology*, *5*(1), p. 25097.

Coyle, T. N., Shaver, J. A., and Linehan, M. M. (2018) 'On the potential for iatrogenic effects of psychiatric crisis services: the example of dialectical behavioral therapy for adult women with a borderline personality disorder', *Journal of Consulting and Clinical Psychology*, *86*(2), p. 116.

Cristea, I. A., Gentili, C., Cotet, C. D., Palomba, D., Barbui, C., and Cuijpers, P. (2017) 'Efficacy of psychotherapies for borderline personality disorder: a systematic review and meta-analysis', *JAMA Psychiatry*, *74*(4), pp. 319–328.

Crowell, S. E., and Kaufman, E. A. (2016) 'Development of self-inflicted injury: Comorbidities and continuities with borderline and antisocial personality traits', *Development and Psychopathology*, *28*(4pt1), pp. 1071–1088.

Cyprien, F., Courtet, P., Malafosse, A., Maller, J., Meslin, C., Bonafé, A., . . . and Artero, S. (2011) 'Suicidal behavior is associated with reduced corpus callosum area', *Biological Psychiatry*, *70*(4), pp. 320–326.

Das, P., Calhoun, V., and Malhi, G. S. (2014) 'Bipolar and borderline patients display differential patterns of functional connectivity among resting state networks', *Neuroimage*, *98*, pp. 73–81. de Leon, V. C., Drysdale, A. T., Conway, C. R., and Aaronson, S. T. (2019) 'Predictors of response for vagus nerve stimulation in treatment-resistant depression', *Personalized Medicine in Psychiatry*.

Delaloye, S., and Holtzheimer, P. E. (2014) 'Deep brain stimulation in the treatment of

Depression', *Dialogues in Clinical Neuroscience*, *16*(1), p. 83.

Desmyter, S., Duprat, R., Baeken, C., Van Autreve, S., Audenaert,

K., and van Heeringen, K. (2016) 'Accelerated intermittent theta burst stimulation for suicide risk in therapy- resistant depressed patients: a randomized, sham-controlled trial', *Frontiers in Human Neuroscience*, *10*, p. 480.

Dimeff, L. A., and Koerner, K. E. (2007) *Dialectical Behavior Therapy in Clinical Practice: Applications Across Disorders and Settings*, Guilford Press.

Donse, L., Padberg, F., Sack, A. T., Rush, A. J., and Arns, M. (2018) 'Simultaneous rTMS and psychotherapy in major depressive disorder: clinical outcomes and predictors from a large naturalistic study', *Brain Stimulation*, *11*(2), pp. 337–345.

Dougherty, D. D., and Widge, A. S. (2017) 'Neurotherapeutic interventions for psychiatric Illness', *Harvard Review of Psychiatry*, *25*(6), p. 253.

Dougherty, D. D., Rezai, A. R., Carpenter, L. L., Howland, R. H., Bhati, M. T., O'Reardon, J. P., . . . and Cusin, C. (2015) 'A randomized sham-controlled trial of deep brain stimulation of the ventral capsule/ventral striatum for chronic treatment-resistant depression', *Biological Psychiatry*, *78*(4), pp. 240–248.

Douglas, B., and James, P. (2013) *Common Presenting Issues in Psychotherapeutic Practice*, Sage.

Ducasse, D., Lopez-Castroman, J., Dassa, D., Brand-Arpon, V., Dupuy-Maurin, K., Lacourt, L., . . . and Olié, E. (2019) 'Exploring the boundaries between borderline personality disorder and suicidal behavior disorder', *European Archives of Psychiatry and Clinical Neuroscience*, pp. 1–9.

Durand, V. M., and Barlow, D. H. (2012) *Essentials of Abnormal Psychology*, Cengage Learning.

Edelstein, B. A., Hersen, M., and Thase, M. E. (eds.) (2013) *Handbook of Outpatient Treatment of Adults: Nonpsychotic Mental Disorders*, Springer Science+Business Media.

Emsell, L., Leemans, A., Langan, C., Van Hecke, W., Barker, G. J., McCarthy, P., . . . and McDonald, C. (2013) 'Limbic and callosal white matter changes in euthymic bipolar I disorder: an advanced diffusion magnetic resonance imaging tractography study', *Biological Psychiatry*, *73*(2), pp. 194–201.

Epstein, J., Pan, H., Kocsis, J. H., Yang, Y., Butler, T., Chusid, J., . . . and Silbersweig, D. A. (2006) 'Lack of ventral striatal response to positive stimuli in depressed versus normal Subjects', *American Journal of Psychiatry*, *163*(10), pp. 1784–1790.

Gan, J., Yi, J., Zhong, M., Cao, X., Jin, X., Liu, W., and Zhu, X. (2016) 'Abnormal white matter structural connectivity in treatment-naïve young adults with borderline personality disorder', *Acta Psychiatrica Scandinavica*, *134*(6), pp. 494–503.

Gerull, F., Meares, R., Stevenson, J., Korner, A., and Newman, L. (2008) 'The beneficial effect on family life in treating borderline personality', *Psychiatry*, *71*(1), pp. 59–70.

Gerull, F., Meares, R., Stevenson, J., Korner, A., and Newman, L. (2008). The beneficial effect on family life in treating borderline personality. *Psychiatry*, *71*(1), 59-70.

Gold, L. H., and Frierson, R. L. (eds.) (2017) *The American Psychiatric Publishing Textbook of Forensic Psychiatry*, American Psychiatric Pub.

Goodman, W. K., Foote, K. D., Greenberg, B. D., Ricciuti, N., Bauer, R., Ward, H., . . . and Okun, M. S. (2010) 'Deep brain stimulation for intractable obsessive compulsive disorder: pilot study using a blinded, staggered-onset design', *Biological Psychiatry*, *67*(6), pp. 535–542.

Greenberg, B. D., Gabriels, L. A., Malone, D. A., Rezai, A. R., Friehs, G. M., Okun, M. S., . . . and Malloy, P. F. (2010) 'Deep brain stimulation of the ventral internal capsule/ventral striatum for obsessive-compulsive disorder: worldwide experience', *Molecular Psychiatry*, *15*(1), pp. 64–79.

Guilé, J. M., Boissel, L., Alaux-Cantin, S., and de La Rivière, S. G. (2018) 'Borderline personality disorder in adolescents: prevalence, diagnosis, and treatment strategies', *Adolescent Health, Medicine, and Therapeutics*, *9*, p. 199.

Gunderson, J. G. (2009) 'Borderline personality disorder: ontogeny of a diagnosis', *American Journal of Psychiatry*, *166*(5), pp. 530–539.

Gunderson, J. G. (2011) 'Borderline personality disorder', *New England Journal of Medicine, 364*(21), pp. 2037–2042.

Gunderson, J. G. (2016) 'The emergence of a generalist model to meet public health needs for patients with borderline personality disorder', *American Journal of Psychiatry, 173*(5), pp. 452–458.

Gunderson, J. G., Stout, R. L., McGlashan, T. H., Shea, M. T., Morey, L. C., Grilo, C. M., . . . and Ansell, E. (2011) 'The ten-year course of borderline personality disorder: psychopathology and function from the Collaborative Longitudinal Personality Disorders Study', *Archives of General Psychiatry, 68*(8), pp. 827–837.

Gunderson, J. G., Stout, R. L., Shea, M. T., Grilo, C. M., Markowitz, J. C., Morey, L. C., . . . and McGlashan, T. H. (2014) 'Interactions of borderline personality disorder and mood disorders over ten years', *Journal of Clinical Psychiatry, 75*(8), p. 829.

Gunderson, J. G., Weinberg, I., and Choi-Kain, L. (2013) 'Borderline personality disorder', *Focus, 11*(2), pp. 129–145.

Gunderson, John G. (2009) 'Borderline personality disorder: ontogeny of a diagnosis', *American Journal of Psychiatry* 166.5, pp. 530–539.

Haesebaert, F., Moirand, R., Schott-Pethelaz, A. M., Brunelin, J., and Poulet, E. (2018) 'Usefulness of repetitive transcranial magnetic stimulation as a maintenance treatment in patients with major depression', *The World Journal of Biological Psychiatry, 19*(1), pp. 74–78.

Hallett, M. (2007) 'Transcranial magnetic stimulation: a primer', *Neuron, 55*(2), pp. 187–199.

Hancock-Johnson, E., Griffiths, C., and Picchioni, M. (2017) 'A focused systematic review of pharmacological treatment for borderline personality disorder', *CNS Drugs, 31*(5), pp. 345–356.

HarIz, M. I., Blomstedt, P., and Zrinzo, L. (2010) 'Deep brain stimulation between 1947 and 1987: the untold story', *Neurosurgical Focus, 29*(2), E1.

Harned, M. S., Rizvi, S. L., and Linehan, M. M. (2010) 'Impact of co-occurring posttraumatic stress disorder on suicidal women with a borderline personality disorder', *American Journal of Psychiatry, 167*(10), pp. 1210–1217.

Herpertz, S. C., Zanarini, M., Schulz, C. S., Siever, L., Lieb, K., and Möller, H. J. (2007) 'Treatment of personality disorders: World Federation of Societies of Biological Psychiatry (WFSBP) Guidelines for Biological Treatment of Personality Disorders', *World J Biol Psychiatry, 8*(4), pp. 212–244.

Higgins, E. S., and George, M. S. (2019) *Brain Stimulation Therapies for Clinicians*, American Psychiatric Pub.

Hirsh, J. B., Quilty, L. C., Bagby, R. M., and McMain, S. F. (2012) 'The relationship between agreeableness and the development of the working alliance in patients with a borderline personality disorder', *Journal of Personality Disorders, 26*(4), pp. 616–627.

Holtzheimer, P. E., and Mayberg, H. S. (2011) 'Deep brain stimulation for psychiatric Disorders', *Annual review of Neuroscience, 34*, pp. 289–307.

Hopwood, C. J., Swenson, C., Bateman, A., Yeomans, F. E., and Gunderson, J. G. (2014) 'Approaches to psychotherapy for borderline personality: Demonstrations by four master Clinicians', *Personality Disorders: Theory, Research, and Treatment, 5*(1), p. 108.

Horvath, A. O., Del Re, A. C., Flückiger, C., and Symonds, D. (2011) 'Alliance in individual Psychotherapy', *Psychotherapy, 48*(1), p. 9.

Hwang, J. W., Xin, S. C., Ou, Y. M., Zhang, W. Y., Liang, Y. L., Chen, J., . . . and Ma, W. H. (2016) 'Enhanced default mode network connectivity with ventral striatum in subthreshold depression in Kaess, M., von Ceumern-Lindenstjerna, I. A., Parzer, P., Chanen, A., Mundt, C., Resch, F., and Brunner, R. (2013) 'Axis I and II comorbidity and psychosocial functioning in female adolescents with a borderline personality disorder', *Psychopathology, 46*(1), pp. 55–62.

Kaiser, R. H., Andrews-Hanna, J. R., Wager, T. D., and Pizzagalli,

D. A. (2015) 'Large-scale network dysfunction in major depressive disorder: a meta-analysis of resting-state functional connectivity'; *JAMA Psychiatry, 72*(6), pp. 603–611.

Kaplan, C., Tarlow, N., Stewart, J. G., Aguirre, B., Galen, G., and Auerbach, R. P. (2016) 'Borderline personality disorder in youth: The prospective impact of child abuse on non- suicidal self-injury and suicidality', *Comprehensive Psychiatry, 71*, pp. 86–94.

Kennedy, S. H., and Giacobbe, P. (2007) 'Treatment resistant depression—advances in somatic Therapies', *Annals of Clinical Psychiatry, 19*(4), pp. 279–287.

Kibleur, A., Polosan, M., Favre, P., Rudrauf, D., Bougerol, T., Chabardès, S., and David, O. (2017) 'Stimulation of subgenual cingulate area decreases limbic top-down effect on ventral visual stream: A DBS-EEG pilot study', *NeuroImage, 146*, pp. 544–553.

Kimmel, C. L., Alhassoon, O. M., Wollman, S. C., Stern, M. J., Perez-Figueroa, A., Hall, M. G., . . . and Radua, J. (2016) 'Age-related parieto-occipital and other gray matter changes in borderline personality disorder: a meta-analysis of cortical and subcortical structures', *Psychiatry Research: Neuroimaging, 251*, pp. 15–25.

Koenigs, M., and Grafman, J. (2009) 'The functional neuroanatomy of depression: distinct roles for ventromedial and dorsolateral prefrontal cortex', *Behavioural Brain Research, 201*(2), pp. 239–243.

Kulacaoglu, F., and Kose, S. (2018) 'Borderline Personality Disorder (BPD): In the Midst of Vulnerability, Chaos, and Awe', *Brain Sciences, 8*(11), p. 201.

Laurenssen, E. M., Hutsebaut, J., Feenstra, D. J., Bales, D. L., Noom, M. J., Busschbach, J. J., . . . and Luyten, P. (2014) 'Feasibility of mentalization-based treatment for adolescents with borderline symptoms: A pilot study', *Psychotherapy, 51*(1), p. 159.

Leander, N. P., Moore, S. G., and Chartrand, T. L. (2009) *Mystery Moods: Their Origins and Consequences*, Na.

Leiberich, P., Nickel, M. K., Tritt, K., and Gil, F. P. (2008) 'Lamotrigine treatment of aggression in female borderline patients, Part II: an 18-month follow-up', *Journal of Psychopharmacology*, 22(7), pp. 805–808.

Levkovitz, Y., Isserles, M., Padberg, F., Lisanby, S. H., Bystritsky, A., Xia, G., . . . and Hafez, H. M. (2015) 'Efficacy and safety of deep transcranial magnetic stimulation for major depression: a prospective multicenter randomized controlled trial', *World Psychiatry*, 14(1), pp. 64–73.

Li, B., Piriz, J., Mirrione, M., Chung, C., Proulx, C. D., Schulz, D., . . . and Malinow, R. (2011) 'Synaptic potentiation onto habenula neurons in the learned helplessness model of Depression', *Nature*, 470(7335), pp. 535–539.

Lieb, K., Völlm, B., Rücker, G., Timmer, A., and Stoffers, J. M. (2010) 'Pharmacotherapy for borderline personality disorder: Cochrane systematic review of randomised trials', *The British Journal of Psychiatry*, 196(1), pp. 4–12.

Linehan, M. M. (2018) *Cognitive-Behavioral Treatment of Borderline Personality Disorder*, Guilford Publications.

Linehan, M. M., Korslund, K. E., Harned, M. S., Gallop, R. J., Lungu, A., Neacsiu, A. D., . . . and Murray-Gregory, A. M. (2015) 'Dialectical behavior therapy for high suicide risk in individuals with borderline personality disorder: a randomized clinical trial and component analysis', *JAMA Psychiatry*, 72(5), pp. 475–482.

Livesley, J. (2008) 'Toward a genetically-informed model of borderline personality Disorder', *Journal of Personality Disorders*, 22(1), pp. 42–71.

Loonen, A. J., and Ivanova, S. A. (2016) 'Circuits regulating pleasure and happiness—Mechanisms of depression', *Frontiers in Human Neuroscience*, 10, p. 571.

Lopez-Castroman, J., Galfalvy, H., Currier, D., Stanley, B., Blasco-Fontecilla, H., Baca-Garcia, E., . . . and Oquendo, M. A.

(2012) 'Personality disorder assessments in acute depressive episodes: stability at follow-up', *The Journal of Nervous and Mental Disease, 200*(6), p. 526.

Lozano, A. M., Giacobbe, P., Hamani, C., Rizvi, S. J., Kennedy, S. H., Kolivakis, T. T., . . . and Ilcewicz-Klimek, M. (2012) 'A multicenter pilot study of subcallosal cingulate area deep brain stimulation for treatment-resistant depression', *Journal of Neurosurgery, 116*(2), pp. 315–322.

Maltsberger, J. T., Schechter, M., Herbstman, B., Ronningstam, E., and Goldblatt, M. J. (2015) 'Suicide studies today'.

Marks Jr, W. J. (ed.) (2015) *Deep Brain Stimulation Management*, Cambridge University Press.

Martin, Donel M., Shawn M. McClintock, Jane J. Forster, Tin Yan Lo, and Colleen K. Loo. (2017) 'Cognitive enhancing effects of rTMS administered to the prefrontal cortex in patients with depression: A systematic review and meta-analysis of individual task effects', *Depression and Anxiety* 34, no. 11, pp. 1029–1039.

May, J. M., Richardi, T. M., and Barth, K. S. (2016) 'Dialectical behavior therapy as treatment for borderline personality disorder', *Mental Health Clinician, 6*(2), pp. 62–67. 'Borderline personality disorder in adolescents', *Clinical Psychology Review, 28*(6), pp. 969–981.

McMain, S. F., Links, P. S., Gnam, W. H., Guimond, T., Cardish, R. J., Korman, L., and Streiner, D. L. (2009) 'A randomized trial of dialectical behavior therapy versus general psychiatric management for borderline personality disorder', *American Journal of Psychiatry, 166*(12), pp. 1365–1374.

Meguins, L. C. (2012) 'Deep brain stimulation for treatment-resistant depression: a state-of-the- art review', *Juruena MF. Clinical, Research and Treatment Approaches to Affective Disorders*, pp. 357–64.

Mercer, D., Douglass, A. B., and Links, P. S. (2009) 'Meta-analyses of mood stabilizers, antidepressants and antipsychotics in the treatment of borderline personality disorder: effectiveness for depression and anger symptoms', *Journal of Personality Disorders, 23*(2), pp. 156–174.

Mertens, A., Raedt, R., Gadeyne, S., Carrette, E., Boon, P., and Vonck, K. (2018) 'Recent advances in devices for vagus nerve stimulation', *Expert review of medical devices, 15*(8), pp. 527–539.

Miller, A. L., Muehlenkamp, J. J., and Jacobson, C. M. (2008), 'Fact or fiction: Diagnosing'.

Minichino, A., Bersani, F. S., Capra, E., Pannese, R., Bonanno, C., Salviati, M., . . . and Biondi, M. (2012) 'ECT, rTMS, and deepTMS in pharmacoresistant drug-free patients with unipolar depression: a comparative review', *Neuropsychiatric disease and treatment, 8*, pp. 55.

Modirrousta, M., Meek, B. P., and Wikstrom, S. L. (2018) 'Efficacy of twice-daily vs once-daily sessions of repetitive transcranial magnetic stimulation in the treatment of major depressive disorder: a retrospective study', *Neuropsychiatric Disease and Treatment, 14*, p. 309.

Moffitt, T. E., in alphabetical order, Arseneault, L., Jaffee, S. R., Kim-Cohen, J., Koenen, K. C., . . . and Viding, E. (2008) 'Research review: DSM-V conduct disorder: Research needs for an evidence base', *Journal of Child Psychology and Psychiatry, 49*(1), pp. 3–33.

Morishita, T., Fayad, S. M., Higuchi, M. A., Nestor, K. A., and Foote, K. D. (2014) 'Deep brain stimulation for treatment-resistant depression: systematic review of clinical outcomes', *Neurotherapeutics, 11*(3), pp. 475–484.

Motter, J. N., Pimontel, M. A., Rindskopf, D., Devanand, D. P., Doraiswamy, P. M., and Sneed, J. R. (2016) 'Computerized cognitive training and functional recovery in major depressive disorder: a meta-analysis', *Journal of Affective Disorders, 189*, pp. 184–191.

Naidich, T. P., Castillo, M., Cha, S., and Smirniotopoulos, J. G. (2012) *Imaging of the Brain: Expert Radiology Series*, Elsevier Health Sciences.

Neacsiu, A. D., Rizvi, S. L., and Linehan, M. M. (2010) 'Dialectical behavior therapy skills use as a mediator and outcome of treatment for borderline personality disorder', *Behavior research and therapy*, *48*(9), pp. 832–839.

Niedtfeld, I., Schulze, L., Krause-Utz, A., Demirakca, T., Bohus, M., and Schmahl, C. (2013) 'Voxel-based morphometry in women with borderline personality disorder with and without comorbid posttraumatic stress disorder', *PloS One*, *8*(6).

O'Reardon, J. P., Cristancho, P., and Peshek, A. D. (2006) 'Vagus nerve stimulation (VNS) and treatment of depression: to the brainstem and beyond', *Psychiatry (Edgmont)*, *3*(5), p. 54.

Oumaya, M., Friedman, S., Pham, A., Abou, T. A., Guelfi, J. D., and Rouillon, F. (2008) 'Borderline personality disorder, self-mutilation, and suicide: a literature review', *L'Encephale*, *34*(5), pp. 452–458.

Paris, J. (2008) 'Clinical trials of treatment for personality disorders', *Psychiatric Clinics of North America*, *31*(3), pp. 517–526.

Paris, J. (2009) 'The treatment of borderline personality disorder: implications of research on diagnosis, etiology, and outcome', *Annual Review of Clinical Psychology*, *5*, pp. 277–290.

Paris, J. (2010) 'Estimating the prevalence of personality disorders in the community', *Journal of Personality Disorders*, *24*(4), pp. 405–411.

Paris, J. (2019) *Treatment of Borderline Personality Disorder: A Guide to Evidence-Based Practice*, Guilford Publications.

Parker, G. (2011) 'Clinical differentiation of bipolar II disorder from personality-based "emotional dysregulation" conditions', *Journal of Affective Disorders*, *133*(1–2), pp. 16–21.

Parry, G. D., Crawford, M. J., and Duggan, C. (2016) 'Iatrogenic harm from psychological therapies–time to move on', *The British Journal of Psychiatry*, *208*(3), pp. 210–212.

Paton, C., Crawford, M. J., Bhatti, S. F., Patel, M. X., and Barnes, T. R. (2015) 'The use of psychotropic medication in patients with emotionally unstable personality disorder under the care of UK mental health services', *The Journal of Clinical Psychiatry*, *76*(4), pp. 512–518.

Patten, C. A., Goggin, K., Harris, K. J., Richter, K. P., Williams, K., Decker, P. A., . . . and Catley, D. (2016) 'Relationship of autonomy social support to quitting motivation in diverse smokers', *Addiction Research and Theory*, *24*(6), pp. 477–482.

Perera, T., George, M. S., Grammer, G., Janicak, P. G., Pascual-Leone, A., and Wirecki, T. S. (2016) 'The clinical TMS society consensus review and treatment recommendations for TMS therapy for major depressive disorder', *Brain Stimulation*, *9*(3), pp. 336–34.

Philip, N. S., Barredo, J., van't Wout-Frank, M., Tyrka, A. R., Price, L. H., and Carpenter, L. L. (2018) 'Network mechanisms of clinical response to transcranial magnetic stimulation in posttraumatic stress disorder and major depressive disorder', *Biological Psychiatry*, *83*(3), pp. 263–272.

Porr, V. (2010) *Overcoming Borderline Personality Disorder: A Family Guide for Healing and Change*, Oxford University Press. Quevedo, K., Ng, R., Scott, H., Kodavaganti, S., Smyda, G., Diwadkar, V., and Phillips, M. (2017) 'Ventral striatum functional connectivity during rewards and losses and symptomatology in depressed patients', *Biological Psychology*, *123*, 62–73.

Ranft, K., Dobrowolny, H., Krell, D., Bielau, H., Bogerts, B., and Bernstein, H. G. (2010) 'Evidence for structural abnormalities of the human habenular complex in affective disorders but not in schizophrenia', *Psychological Medicine*, *40*(4), pp. 557–567.

Rasmussen, K. G. (2011) 'Some considerations in choosing electroconvulsive therapy versus transcranial magnetic stimulation for depression', *The Journal of ECT*, *27*(1), pp. 51–54.

Rausch, J., Gäbel, A., Nagy, K., Kleindienst, N., Herpertz, S. C., and Bertsch, K. (2015) 'Increased testosterone levels and cortisol awakening responses in patients with borderline personality disorder: gender and trait aggressiveness matter', *Psychoneuroendocrinology*, *55*, pp. 116–127.

Reddy, M. S., and Vijay, M. S. (2017) 'Empirical reality of dialectical behavioral therapy in borderline personality', *Indian Journal of Psychological Medicine*, *39*(2), p. 105.

Ripoll, L. H. (2012) 'Clinical psychopharmacology of borderline personality disorder: an update on the available evidence in light of the Diagnostic and Statistical Manual of Mental Disorders–5', *Current Opinion in Psychiatry*, *25*(1), pp. 52–58.

Ripoll, L. H. (2013) 'Psychopharmacologic treatment of borderline personality disorder', *Dialogues in Clinical Neuroscience*, *15*(2), p. 213.

Rogers, B., and Acton, T. (2012) '"I think we're all guinea pigs really": a qualitative study of medication and borderline personality disorder', *Journal of Psychiatric and Mental Health Nursing*, *19*(4), pp. 341–347.

Ruocco, A. C., Amirthavasagam, S., Choi-Kain, L. W., and McMain, S. F. (2013) 'Neural correlates of negative emotionality in borderline personality disorder: an activation-likelihood-estimation meta-analysis;, *Biological Psychiatry*, *73*(2), pp. 153–160.

Sack, A. T., Cohen Kadosh, R., Schuhmann, T., Moerel, M., Walsh, V., and Goebel, R. (2009) 'Optimizing functional accuracy of TMS in cognitive studies: a comparison of Methods', *Journal of Cognitive Neuroscience*, *21*(2), pp. 207–221.

Sadock, B. J., Sadock, V. A., and Levin, Z. E. (eds.) (2007) *Kaplan and Sadock's Study Guide and Self-Examination Review in Psychiatry*, Lippincott Williams and Wilkins.

Sartorius, A., Kiening, K. L., Kirsch, P., von Gall, C. C., Haberkorn, U., Unterberg, A. W., . . . and Meyer-Lindenberg, A. (2010) 'Remission of major depression under deep brain stimulation of the lateral habenula in a therapy-refractory patient', *Biological Psychiatry*, *67*(2), pp. e9–e11.

Schlaepfer, T. E., Bewernick, B. H., Kayser, S., Mädler, B., and Coenen, V. A. (2013) 'Rapid effects of deep brain stimulation for treatment-resistant major depression', *Biological Psychiatry*, *73*(12), pp. 1204–1212.

Schlaepfer, T. E., Cohen, M. X., Frick, C., Kosel, M., Brodesser,

D., Axmacher, N., . . . and Sturm, V. (2008) 'Deep brain stimulation to reward circuitry alleviates anhedonia in refractory major depression', *Neuropsychopharmacology*, *33*(2), pp. 368–377.

Schulze, L., Schmahl, C., and Niedtfeld, I. (2016) 'Neural correlates of disturbed emotion processing in borderline personality disorder: a multimodal meta-analysis', *Biological Psychiatry*, *79*(2), pp. 97–106.

Shaffer, D., and Jacobson, C. (2009) 'Proposal to the DSM-V childhood disorder and mood disorder work groups to include non-suicidal self-injury (NSSI) as a DSM-V disorder', *American Psychiatric Association*, pp. 1–21.

Sher, L., Mindes, J., and Novakovic, V. (2010) 'Transcranial magnetic stimulation and the treatment of suicidality', *Expert Review of Neurotherapeutics*, *10*(12), pp. 1781–1784.

Siever, L. J. (2008) 'Neurobiology of aggression and violence', *American Journal of Psychiatry*, *165*(4), pp. 429–442.

Silk, K. R. (2008) 'Personality disorder in adolescence: The diagnosis that dare not speak its Name'.

Silvers, J. A., Hubbard, A. D., Biggs, E., Shu, J., Fertuck, E., Chaudhury, S., . . . and Brodsky, B. S. (2016) 'Affective lability and difficulties with regulation are differentially associated with the amygdala and prefrontal response in women with Borderline Personality Disorder', *Psychiatry Research: Neuroimaging*, *254*, pp. 74–82.

Skodol, A. E., Gunderson, J. G., Shea, M. T., McGlashan, T. H., Morey, L. C., Sanislow, C. A., . . . and Pagano, M. E. (2005) 'The collaborative longitudinal personality disorders study (CLPS): Overview and implications', *Journal of Personality Disorders*, *19*(5), pp. 487–504.

Smoski, M. J., Salsman, N., Wang, L., Smith, V., Lynch, T. R., Dager, S. R., . . . and Linehan, M. M. (2011) 'Functional imaging of emotion reactivity in opiate-dependent borderline personality disorder', *Personality Disorders: Theory, Research, and Treatment*, *2*(3), p. 230.

Soloff, P., Nutche, J., Goradia, D., and Diwadkar, V. (2008) 'Structural brain abnormalities in borderline personality disorder: a voxel-based morphometry study', *Psychiatry Research: Neuroimaging, 164*(3), pp. 223–236.

Stanley, B., and New, A. (eds.) (2017) *Borderline Personality Disorder*, Oxford University Press.

Stanley, B., and Siever, L. J. (2009) 'The interpersonal dimension of borderline personality disorder: toward a neuropeptide model', *American Journal of Psychiatry, 167*(1), pp. 24–39.

Starcevic, V., and Janca, A. (2018) 'Pharmacotherapy of borderline personality disorder: replacing confusion with prudent pragmatism', *Current Opinion in Psychiatry, 31*(1), pp. 69–73.

Steele, H., and Siever, L. (2010) 'An attachment perspective on borderline personality disorder: Advances in gene–environment considerations', *Current Psychiatry Reports, 12*(1), pp. 61–67.

Stoffers-Winterling, J. M., Völlm, B. A., Rücker, G., Timmer, A., Huband, N., and Lieb, K. (2012) 'Psychological therapies for people with borderline personality disorder', *Cochrane Database of Systematic Reviews*, (8).

Torgersen, S., Myers, J., Reichborn-Kjennerud, T., Røysamb, E., Kubarych, T. S., and Kendler, K. S. (2012) 'The heritability of Cluster B personality disorders assessed both by personal interview and questionnaire', *Journal of Personality Disorders, 26*(6), pp. 848–866.

Tottenham, N., Hare, T. A., Quinn, B. T., McCarry, T. W., Nurse, M., Gilhooly, T., . . . and

Thomas, K. M. (2010) 'Prolonged institutional rearing is associated with atypically large amygdala volume and difficulties in emotion regulation', *Developmental Science, 13*(1), pp. 46–61.

Trull, T. J., Jahng, S., Tomko, R. L., Wood, P. K., and Sher, K. J. (2010) 'Revised NESARC personality disorder diagnoses: gender, prevalence, and comorbidity with substance dependence disorders', *Journal of Personality Disorders, 24*(4), pp. 412–426.

Ustohal, L. (Ed.). (2018) *Transcranial Magnetic Stimulation in Neuropsychiatry*. BoD–Books on Demand.

Voigt, J., Carpenter, L., and Leuchter, A. (2017) 'Cost effectiveness analysis comparing repetitive transcranial magnetic stimulation to antidepressant medications after a first treatment failure for major depressive disorder in newly diagnosed patients–A lifetime analysis', *PLoS One, 12*(10).

Völlm, B. A., Chadwick, K., Abdelrazek, T., and Smith, J. (2012) 'Prescribing of psychotropic medication for personality disordered patients in secure forensic settings', *The Journal of Forensic Psychiatry and Psychology, 23*(2), pp. 200–216.

Wacker, J., Dillon, D. G., and Pizzagalli, D. A. (2009) 'The role of the nucleus accumbens and rostral anterior cingulate cortex in anhedonia: integration of resting EEG, fMRI, and volumetric techniques', *Neuroimage, 46*(1), pp. 327–337.

Walsh, C., Ryan, P., and Flynn, D. (2018) 'Exploring dialectical behaviour therapy clinicians' experiences of team consultation meetings', *Borderline Personality Disorder and Emotion Dysregulation, 5*(1), p. 3.

Wang, L., Ross, C. A., Zhang, T., Dai, Y., Zhang, H., Tao, M., . . . and Xiao, Z. (2012) 'Frequency of borderline personality disorder among psychiatric outpatients in Shanghai', *Journal of Personality Disorders, 26*(3), pp. 393–401.

Wedig, M. M., Frankenburg, F. R., Reich, D. B., Fitzmaurice, G., and Zanarini, M. C. (2013) 'Predictors of suicide threats in patients with borderline personality disorder over 16 years of prospective follow-up', *Psychiatry Research, 208*(3), pp. 252–256.

Weniger, G., Lange, C., Sachsse, U., and Irle, E. (2009) 'Reduced amygdala and hippocampus size in trauma-exposed women with borderline personality disorder and without posttraumatic stress disorder', *Journal of Psychiatry and Neuroscience*, 34, pp. 383–388

Widiger, T. A. (ed.) (2012) *The Oxford Handbook of Personality Disorders*, Oxford University Press.

Williams, L. M. (2016) 'Precision psychiatry: a neural circuit taxonomy for depression and Anxiety', *The Lancet Psychiatry*, *3*(5), pp. 472–480.

Wingenfeld, K., Spitzer, C., Rullkötter, N., and Löwe, B. (2010) 'Borderline personality disorder: hypothalamus pituitary adrenal axis and findings from neuroimaging studies', *Psychoneuroendocrinology*, *35*(1), pp. 154–170.

Winograd, G., Cohen, P., and Chen, H. (2008) 'Adolescent borderline symptoms in the community: prognosis for functioning over 20 years', *Journal of Child Psychology and Psychiatry*, *49*(9), pp. 933–941.

Yoshimatsu, K., and Palmer, B. (2014) 'Depression in patients with borderline personality Disorder', *Harvard Review of Psychiatry*, *22*(5), pp. 266–273.

Zanarini, M. C., Frankenburg, F. R., Reich, D. B., and Fitzmaurice, G. (2010) 'Time to the attainment of recovery from borderline personality disorder and stability of recovery: A 10-year prospective follow-up study', *American Journal of Psychiatry*, *167*(6), pp. 663–667.

Zanarini, M. C., Frankenburg, F. R., Reich, D. B., Harned, A. L., and Fitzmaurice, G. M. (2015) 'Rates of psychotropic medication use reported by borderline patients and axis II comparison subjects over 16 years of prospective follow-up', *Journal of Clinical Psychopharmacology*, *35*(1), pp. 63. 'English 11-year-olds and 34,653 American adults', *Journal of Personality Disorders*, *25*(5), pp. 607–619.

Zanarini, M. C., Frankenburg, F. R., Reich, D. B., Harned, A. L., and Fitzmaurice, G. M. (2015) 'Rates of psychotropic medication use reported by borderline patients and axis II comparison subjects over 16 years of prospective follow-up', *Journal of Clinical Psychopharmacology*, *35*(1), p. 63.

Zanarini, M. C., Horwood, J., Wolke, D., Waylen, A., Fitzmaurice, G., and Grant, B. F. (2011) 'Prevalence of DSM-IV borderline personality disorder in two community samples: 6,330'.

Zhou, C., Zhang, H., Qin, Y., Tian, T., Xu, B., Chen, J., . . . and

Lian, B. (2018) 'A systematic review and meta-analysis of deep brain stimulation in treatment-resistant depression', *Progress in Neuro-Psychopharmacology and Biological Psychiatry, 82*, pp. 224–232.

Zimmerman, M., Chelminski, I., and Young, D. (2008) 'The frequency of personality disorders in psychiatric patients', *Psychiatric Clinics of North America, 31*(3), pp. 405–420.

CHAPTER 10

Post-Traumatic Stress Disorder

PTSD is not about what is wrong with people, it is about what happened to people and how to move on!

According to *DSM*-5, the most important aspect of post-traumatic stress disorder is the onset of the disorder after the exposure to one or more traumatic events. In contrast to intrusive depressive memories, the traumatic events are usually re-experienced by involuntary and intrusive recollection of the event, most commonly during distressing dreams and flashbacks episodes.

Physical sensations such as sweating, dizziness, and rapid heartbeat are the most common somatic presentations. Amnesia (inability to remember an important aspect of the traumatic event) is commonly reported by people suffering from PTSD. In most of the cases, patients try to avoid any trigger that could remind them of the event, and they unwillingly talk about the event (internal reminders).

Individuals diagnosed with PTSD are usually short-fused and very aggressive with any valid reasons, often involved in self-harming behaviours such as excessive alcohol and illegal drugs use, negligent driving, physical fights and injuries, and suicidal behaviour. Depersonalisation is a common feeling among people suffering from PTSD. They describe this phenomenon by having feelings that the world around them is not real and their life is a movie.

Current treatment for PTSD is CBT (exposure in vivo) and

medications called selective serotonin reuptake inhibitors (SSRIs) and selective norepinephrine reuptake inhibitors (SNRIs).

Unfortunately, not every individual is responding to these treatments; therefore, a new, promising therapeutic substance called ketamine has been tested, and so far it shows promising results in treating anxiety disorders, suicide, and PTSD (Feder 2014, and Murrough 2015). In the next study, I have pinpointed the importance of a hidden relationship between a silent stroke and PTSD symptoms, which is often ignored due to its complex nature.

REFERENCES

AMERICAN PSYCHIATRIC ASSOCIATION (2013) *DIAGNOSTIC AND STATISTICAL MANUAL OF MENTAL Disorders* (5th ed.), Washington, DC.

Feder, A., Parides, M., Murrough, J. W., *et al.* (2014) 'Efficacy of intravenous ketamine for treatment of chronic posttraumatic stress disorder: a randomized clinical trial', *JAMA Psychiatry*, 71(6), pp. 661–688.

Murrough, J. W., Soleimani, L., DeWilde, K. E., *et al.* (2015) 'Ketamine for rapid reduction of suicidal Ideation: a randomized controlled trial', *Psychological Medicine*, 45(16), pp. 3571–3580.

PTSD, Associated Symptoms and Silent Stroke: A Hidden Relationship

Abstract

Auditory hallucinations and language impairments such as aphasia have historically been largely attributed to psychosis and traumatic brain injury respectively. Research suggests, however, that these may, in fact, be discrete symptoms in some cases of post-traumatic stress disorder (PTSD). More recent research has also revealed a relationship between PTSD, auditory hallucinations and language impairments in that up to one-third of sufferers have also experienced a silent (ie, asymptomatic) stroke. Although the sequence of these conditions and symptoms may vary widely among sufferers, findings suggest that future research could assist with early identification of possible comorbidities to improve health outcomes. The present study reviews existing research regarding the antecedents to the development of PTSD, auditory hallucinations, and aphasia and the complex symptoms experienced by suffers. Furthermore, in examining specific regions of the brain affected by these conditions, the present study explores the possibility that silent stoke may be involved in a significant proportion of cases and may represent a currently under-researched factor related to the presentation of PTSD and its associated symptoms.

Future research may be able to provide further guidance and assist in pinpointing a common pattern of symptom development. This may contribute to reducing the onset and severity of these potentially comorbid conditions through monitoring and early intervention.

PTSD, Its Associated Symptoms and Silent
Stroke: A Hidden Relationship

Research suggests that on average, 7.8% of adults will suffer from post-traumatic stress disorder (PTSD) at some point in their lives (Hart *et al.*, 2008). The prevalence of PTSD among several sub-populations, such as veterans from the United States, United Kingdom, and Australia returning from wars in Iraq and Afghanistan is believed to be significantly higher than the general population (Brewin and Patel, 2010). PTSD's main symptoms include problematic and vivid recollections of a traumatic event, intrusive thoughts of the event, an exaggerated reaction to stimuli reminiscent of the trauma, and an overactive fight-or-flight response to stressful situations (van der Kolk, 2012). Two lesser-known symptoms of the condition are language impairment-based: pseudo-auditory hallucinations, or *hearing things* and transcortical motor aphasia (TMA), a type of non- fluent aphasia where speech production is characterised as halting and effortful (McCarthy-Jones, 2012). Historically, auditory hallucinations have been associated with psychosis and schizophrenia (Moskowitz and Corstens, 2008). Recent research, has identified, however, that auditory hallucinations are a discrete symptom that is only connected to psychosis in some cases (Choong, Hunter, and Woodruff, 2007).

Hallucinations that a person realises are hallucinations even as they occur are referred to as *pseudo-hallucinations* (Taylor, 1981). Although research in this area is limited, pseudo-auditory hallucinations may also be set apart from more common auditory hallucinations in other ways (de Leede-Smith and Barkus, 2013). It has been posited that both pseudo-auditory hallucinations (Kindler *et al.*, 2013) and TMA (Freedman, Alexander and Naeser, 1984) may be neurologically connected to the superior temporal gyrus, the part of the brain that houses the primary auditory cortex and is connected to Broca's area, an important language centre (Kendel, Schwartz, and Jessell, 2014). Given this similarity in origin, these two conditions that have been found to be associated with PTSD may be interrelated (Lezak, Howieson, Loring, Hannay, and Fischer, 2004). Furthermore, both of the conditions have been observed in patients who have suffered a *silent stroke* (ie, asymptomatic) believed to be caused by structural changes in the temporal lobe as the result of reduced blood supply through the middle cerebral artery (Vermeel *et al.*, 2002; Leff *et al.*,

2009). Bruggimann *et al.* (2016) found that one in every five patents who suffers from PTSD has also suffered from a silent stroke. The present paper seeks to review the available literature to determine the relationship, if any, between PTSD, pseudo-auditory hallucinations, transcortical motor aphasia, and the occurrence of silent stroke.

PTSD

PTSD can be caused by a variety of psychologically traumatic stressors, as well as physical trauma such as a serious injury or illness, including stroke (Edmondson *et al.*, 2013). The development of PTSD among specific sub-populations such as war veterans may be attributed to experiences that simultaneously combine multiple types of trauma such as deployment to an area of active conflict (Steenkamp, Litz, Hoge, and Marmar, 2015). The specific causes of PTSD are related to the outcomes experienced because the primary symptoms of PTSD are directly connected to the re-invocation of the initial trauma (Hart, 2015). Therefore, thoughts of the trauma may become pervasive and intrude upon a person's life to a significant degree (Hart, 2015). The most common manifestation of this is an exaggerated reaction to any stimulus which mimics the original, for example, explosion's loud sound could trigger traumatic war memories for a former soldier (Hoffer *et al.*, 2009). In this sense, PTSD is problematic in that it makes returning to normal life more difficult, often leaving sufferers socially isolated (Haller, Angkaw, Hendricks, and Norman, 2016). In addition to the re-invocation symptoms of PTSD other symptoms have been linked, however inconsistently, to conditions including deficits in memory (Dekel, Solomon, and Ein-Dor, 2016), attention (Badura-Brack *et al.*, 2015), and dysexecutive syndromes (Clark *et al.*, 2016). The nature of the relationship between these symptoms and PTSD is presently unclear—they may represent pre-trauma risk factors for PTSD, symptoms of PTSD, or post-traumatic comorbidities (Hart *et al.*, 2008).

Pseudo-Auditory Hallucinations

Under certain circumstances, the symptoms of PTSD may include hallucinations (Wade, Brewin, Howell, White, Mythen, and Weinman, 2015), some of which may be auditory (Brewin and Patel, 2010). Hallucinations refer to the phenomenon of illusory sensation (Taylor, 1981). Although the word hallucination most commonly associated with visual hallucinations, hallucinations can also be auditory (McCarthy-Jones, 2012). The most well-known forms of auditory hallucinations are the illusory voices associated with schizophrenia and other forms of psychosis (Moskowitz and Corstens, 2008). Historically, hearing voices was considered a psychotic symptom (Choong *et al.*, 2007). More recent research, however, has established auditory hallucinations as being a distinct symptom (Choong *et al.*, 2007; Moskowitz and Corstens, 2008). Auditory hallucinations may be linked to Psychosis; however, they are not necessarily indicative of psychosis (Lezak, Howieson, Loring, Hannay, and Fischer, 2004). Thus, their association with PTSD under certain circumstances does not imply a connection between PTSD and psychosis (Steel, 2015). Auditory hallucinations may manifest in a number of forms. The well-known *hearing-voices* form of hallucinating is referred to as audio-verbal hallucination (de Leede-Smith, and Barkus, 2013). Others suffering from auditory hallucinations may instead perceive music or other sounds, for example, hallucinations known as *musical ear syndrome* (Mahendran, 2007). Differences between types of hallucination include the perception of sound and whether it originates from within a person's head or appears to be from an external source (Copolov, Trauer, and Mackinnon, 2004). Internal hallucinations have often been considered more benign, being more akin to normal thought, but empirical results do not support the hypothesis that they significantly differ in effect (Copolov *et al.*, 2004).

When the person experiencing the illusory sound is aware that it is a hallucination even while experiencing it, the term *pseudo-hallucination* is used (Taylor, 1981). Pseudo- hallucinations can sometimes be associated with hearing impairment, especially under significant stress, such as military combat (Balan *et al.*, 1996). Other researchers have connected auditory hallucination to stress in general, hypothesising that they represent *false positives* in terms of hearing detection, evolved from a mechanism that serves to reduce the chance of *false negatives* (ie, dismissing a real sound as imagined) under stressful or dangerous circumstances (Dodgson and Gordon, 2009). In this light, the connection of auditory hallucinations to PTSD seems logical but not emphatically supported by current research. Although auditory hallucinations as a symptom of PTSD have been observed in both military personnel and civilians (Brewin and Patel, 2010), the specific nature of the relationship between stress, trauma, and hallucination is not entirely clear. At present, research has not yet been able to explicitly link the content of auditory hallucinations to sources of trauma associated with the development of PTSD (Steel, 2015).

The phenomenon of auditory hallucination has not yet been conclusively explained from a neurological perspective (Steel, 2015). Research has, however, traced the genesis of auditory verbal pseudo-hallucinations back to Heschl's gyrus, within the general area of the temporal gyri (Hubl *et al.*, 2010). Results indicated, based on brain scans, that patients with auditory pseudo-hallucinations had a significantly higher chance of exhibiting duplication in Heschl's gyrus, along with higher than average levels of white matter within the gyrus (Hubl *et al.*, 2010). Although Hubl *et al.*'s (2010) sample included participants who had been diagnosed with schizophrenia, researchers hypothesised that the underlying effects on the Heschl's gyrus were not the result of a symptom of schizophrenia. In another study by Kindler *et al.* (2013), the researchers sought to compare pre- and post-therapeutic brain scans relative to an electromagnetic treatment for auditory pseudo-hallucinations. Their results indicated that in patients for whom the therapy was effective the post-treatment scans showed reduced cerebral blood flow in the primary auditory cortex, the left Broca's area, and cingulate gyrus (Kindler *et al.*, 2013).

These regions of the brain are associated with language function and provide support for the hypothesis of Homan, Kindler, Hauf,

Hubl, and Dierks (2012) that blood flow within the language centres of the brain are associated with auditory pseudo-hallucinations. These results link pseudo-auditory hallucinations to various locations within or connected to the superior temporal gyrus (see appendix A), specifically the Heschl's gyrus and auditory cortex. This correlates with the hypothesis in Balan *et al.* (1996) that hearing impairments could contribute to experiencing auditory hallucinations. Research suggests, however, that the left posterior superior temporal gyrus is associated with the functions of both language production and language comprehension (Buchsbaum, Hickok, and Humphries, 2001). In other studies, the left posterior superior temporal gyrus was also found to play a role in multiple types of aphasia (Hickok *et al.*, 2000).

Transcortical Motor Aphasia

Aphasia is, in general, an inability to formulate and comprehend language (ASHA, 2018). Aphasias are classified in terms of fluency or non-fluency (ie, a patient can or cannot produce fluent-sounding speech), comprehension, and repetition (ASHA, n.d.). Within this broad categorisation, transcortical motor aphasia (TMA) represents a relatively rare form, constituting a small percentage of all aphasias (Pedersen, Vinter, and Olsen, 2004). TMA is characterised as a type of non-fluent aphasia, so called because speech production is halting and effortful. Neurological injury, resulting in TMA is typically located in the anterior portion of the left hemisphere (Kendel, Schwartz, and Jessell, 2014). The dominant feature of TMA is agrammatism (impaired syntax), and although the use of content words (nouns and verbs) may be preserved, sentences are difficult to produce due to the problems with grammar and result in *telegraphic speech*, as well as difficulty initiating speech or carrying on a conversation (ASHA, 2018, n.p.; Lezak, Howieson, Loring, Hannay, and Fischer, 2004). TMA, however, only affects outgoing speech, not hearing or language comprehension (Swanberg, Nasreddine,

Mendez, and Cummings, 2007). This results in a situation wherein a person can comprehend language normally but cannot speak fluently although their (grammatically broken) words will likely still retain meaningful content (Swanberg *et al.*, 2007).

Like most aphasias, TMA is generally caused by a traumatic event such as a stroke (Stewart and Riedel, 2016) or head trauma (Yourganov, Smith, Fridriksson, and Rorden, 2015). The specific pathology of this linkage lies in either a loss of connectivity between the brain's language centres or damage to the anterior frontal lobe (Freedman *et al.*, 1984). Since the superior temporal gyrus represents a significant portion of the contents of the frontal lobe (Friederici, Rueschemeyer, Hahne, and Fiebach, 2003) and is significantly linked to both language comprehension and speech (Buchsbaum *et al.*, 2001), it can naturally be linked to aphasias (Hickok *et al.*, 2000). Emphasising this connection, TMA is sometimes also referred to as *white-matter dysphasia* (Manasco, 2017). Additionally, TMA is often encountered as a stage during the recovery from Broca's aphasia (Swanberg *et al.*, 2007). Broca's aphasia is characterised by symptoms similar to those of TMA, except that the patient is also unable to repeat speech (ASHA, 2018). Broca's aphasia is generally caused by a stroke affecting Broca's area of the brain, which is associated with language processing and creation (Stewart and Riedel, 2016). Broca's area is adjacent to the superior temporal gyrus and connected thereto (Kindler et al., 2013).

Silent Stroke

According to Furst *et al.* (2001), silent stroke is present in more than 30% of people who suffer from carotic diseases such as carotid artery stenosis caused by narrowing of the blood vessels in the neck. More often the symptoms are not distinguishable and patients are not aware of the condition (Kendel, Schwartz, and Jessell, 2014). As many as one in four stroke survivors experience PTSD (Edmondson *et al.*, 2013). Bruggimann *et al.*, (2016) found that one in every five patents who suffers from PTSD has also suffered from a silent stroke. Further, approximately 32% of silent stroke survivors experience aphasia (Pedersen et al, 2004). A study undertaken by Leff *et al.*, (2009) found a strong correlation between TMA and pseudo-auditory hallucinations in 210 patients who were found to have suffered a silent stroke. The study also identified that short-term memory, auditory and speech comprehension impairments were caused by damage to the structural integrity of a posterior region of the superior temporal gyrus and sulcus.

If there is an association between PTSD, TMA, pseudo-auditory hallucinations, and silent stroke, given that a silent stroke is by virtue asymptomatic, it would be difficult to determine if there is an identifiable sequence in these conditions occurring. Furthermore, silent strokes may be identified as having occurred in many patients who seek treatment for a number of disorders or conditions unrelated to PTSD, aphasias, or hallucinations. The incidence of silent stroke in the general population in comparison to those suffering from PTSD or pseudo-auditory hallucinations may inevitably be found to be unremarkable.

Stroke and brain injury, the two main causes of aphasia, are however, both psychically and psychologically traumatic events which may lead to the development of PTSD. These findings suggest that although the sequence is unknown, there could be a genuine relationship between PTSD, TMA, pseudo-auditory hallucinations and stroke (whether asymptomatic or not). It may well be that these are comorbid conditions although research in this area would need to progress before the strength of any possible association could be determined.

Conclusion

PTSD has been characterised as having a significant (if inconsistently reported) association with certain dysexecutive syndromes (Hart *et al.*, 2008), and notably, TMA may also be characterised as a dysexecutive syndrome in the sense that it represents a partial loss of executive function regarding language (ASHA, 2018). Research further suggests that pseudo-auditory hallucinations are associated with PTSD and TMA, both having strong connections to the superior temporal gyrus. It is, therefore, reasonable to consider that these conditions, both influenced by the same part of the brain and both linked to pseudo-auditory hallucinations, might have a deeper relationship with one another. Furthermore, it could also be posited that there might be a connection between TMA and pseudo-auditory hallucinations in the context of PTSD and unremarked silent stroke. Future studies may be able to provide further guidance and assist in pinpointing sequence to determine causality of language deficits and potentially even a wider range of language disorders associated with stroke and PTSD.

REFERENCES

ASHA (2018) ASHA glossary, *Asha.org*, https://www.asha.org.

ASHA (n.d). Common classifications of aphasia, *Asha.org*, https://www.asha.org/uploadedFiles/ASHA/Practice_Portal/Clinical_Topics/A phasia/Common-Classifications-of-Aphasia.pdf.

Badura-Brack, A. S., Naim, R., Ryan, T. J., Levy, O., Abend, R., Khanna, M. M., . . . and

Bar-Haim, Y. (2015) 'Effect of attention training on attention bias variability and

PTSD symptoms: randomized controlled trials in Israeli and US combat veterans', *American Journal of Psychiatry*, *172*(12), pp. 1233–1241, http://doi:10.1176/appi.ajp.2015.14121578.

Balan, S., Spivak, B., Nachshoni, T., Kron, S., Mester, R., and Weizman, A. (1996)

'Auditory pseudohallucinations induced by a combination of hearing impairment and environmental stress', *Psychopathology*, *29*(3), pp. 198–200, http://doi: 10.1159/000284992.

Bruggimann, J., Annoni, A. J, Staub, F. J, Von Steinbüchel, N., Van der Linden M, *et al.* (2016) 'Chronic posttraumatic stress symptoms after non severe stroke', *Neurology 301*, pp. 9–18.

Buchsbaum, B. R., Hickok, G., and Humphries, C. (2001) 'Role of left posterior superior temporal gyrus in phonological processing for speech perception and production', *Cognitive Science*, *25*(5), pp. 663–678, http://doi: 10.1016/S0364- 0213(01)00048-9.

Brewin, C. R., and Patel, T. (2010) 'Auditory pseudo hallucinations in United Kingdom

was veterans and civilians with posttraumatic stress disorder', *The*

Journal of Clinical Psychiatry, *71(4)*, pp. 419–425, http://doi: 10.4088/JCP.09m05469blu.

Choong, C., Hunter, M. D., and Woodruff, P. W. R. (2007) 'Auditory hallucinations in those populations that do not suffer from schizophrenia;, *Current Psychiatry Reports*, *9*(3), pp. 206–212, http://doi: 10.1007/s11920-007-0020-z.

Clark, A. L., Sorg, S. F., Schiehser, D. M., Luc, N., Bondi, M. W., Sanderson, M., . . . and Delano-Wood, L. (2016) 'Deep white matter hyperintensities affect verbal memory independent of PTSD symptoms in veterans with mild traumatic brain injury'. *Brain Injury*, *30*(7), pp. 864–871, http://doi : 10.310 9/02 699 052. 2016 1144894.

Copolov, D., Trauer, T., and Mackinnon, A. (2004) 'On the non-significance of internal versus external auditory hallucinations', *Schizophrenia Research*, *69*(1), pp. 1–6, http:// doi: 10.1016/S0920-9964(03)00092-6.

Dekel, S., Solomon, Z., and Ein-Dor, T. (2016) 'PTSD symptoms lead to modification in the memory of the trauma: a prospective study of former prisoners of war', *The Journal of Clinical Psychiatry*, *77*(3), pp. e290–e296, http://doi: 10.10.4088/ JCP.14m. de Leede-Smith, S., and Barkus, E. (2013) 'A comprehensive review of auditory verbal hallucinations: lifetime prevalence, correlates and mechanisms in healthy and clinical individuals;, *Frontiers in Human Neuroscience*, *7*, p. 367, http://doi: 10.3389//fnhum.2013.00367.

Dodgson, G., and Gordon, S. (2009) 'Avoiding false negatives: are some auditory hallucinations an evolved design flaw?', *Behavioural and Cognitive Psychotherapy*, *37*(3), pp. 325–334, http://doi: 10.1017/S1352465809005244.

Edmondson, D., Richardson, S., Fausett, J. K., Falzon, L., Howard, V. J., and Kronish, I. M. (2013) 'Prevalence of PTSD in survivors of stroke and transient ischemic attack: a meta-analytic review', *PLoS One*, *8*(6), p. e66435, http:// doi:10.1371/ journal.pone.0066435.

Freedman, M., Alexander, M. P., and Naeser, M. A. (1984) 'Anatomic basis of transcortical motor aphasia', *Neurology*, *34*(4), pp. 409–409, http://doi: 10.1212/ WNL.34.4.409.

Friederici, A. D., Rueschemeyer, S. A., Hahne, A., and Fiebach, C. J. (2003) 'The role of left inferior frontal and superior temporal cortex in sentence comprehension: localizing syntactic and semantic processes', *Cerebral Cortex*, *13*(2), pp. 170–177, http://doi: 10.1093/cercor/13.2.170.

Haller, M., Angkaw, A. C., Hendricks, B. A., and Norman, S. B. (2016) 'Does reintegration stress contribute to suicidal ideation among returning veterans seeking ptsd treatment?', *Suicide and Life-Threatening Behavior*, *46*(2), pp. 160–171, http://doi: 10.1111/sltb.12181.

Hart Jr, MD, J., Kimbrell, T., Fauver, P., Cherry, B. J., Pitcock, J., Booe, L. Q., . . . and

Freeman, T. W. (2008) 'Cognitive dysfunctions associated with PTSD: evidence from World War II prisoners of war', *The Journal of Neuropsychiatry and Clinical Neurosciences*, *20*(3), pp. 309–316, http://doi: 10.1176/jnp.2008.20.3. 309.

Hart, N. (2015) 'Veterans battling PTSD know the triggers, recognize the symptoms', *North Carolina Medical Journal*, *76*(5), pp. 308–309, http://doi: 10.18043/ncm.76.5.30.

Hickok, G., Erhard, P., Kassubek, J., Helms-Tillery, A. K., Naeve-Velguth, S., Strupp, J. P., . . . and Ugurbil, K. (2000) 'A functional magnetic resonance imaging study of the role of left posterior superior temporal gyrus in speech production: implications for the explanation of conduction aphasia', *Neuroscience Letters*, *287*(2), pp. 156–160, http://doi: 10.1016/ S0304- 3940(00)01143-5.

Hoffer, M. E., Donaldson, C., Gottshall, K. R., Balaban, C., and Balough, B. J. (2009) Blunt and blast head trauma: different entities', *International Tinnitus Journal*, *15*(2), pp. 115–118, http://www.tinnitusjournal.com/ articles/blunt- and-blast-head-trauma-different-entities.pdf.

Homan, P., Kindler, J., Hauf, M., Hubl, D., and Dierks, T. (2012) 'Cerebral blood flow identifies responders to transcranial magnetic stimulation in auditory verbal hallucinations', *Translational Psychiatry*, *2*(11), p. e189, https://www.nature.com/articles/tp2012114.

Hubl, D., Dougoud-Chauvin, V., Zeller, M., Federspiel, A., Boesch, C., Strik, W., . . . and

Koenig, T. (2010) 'Structural analysis of Heschl's gyrus in schizophrenia patients with auditory hallucinations', *Neuropsychobiology*, *61*(1), pp. 1–9, http://doi: 10.1159/000258637.

Kindler, J., Homan, P., Jann, K., Federspiel, A., Flury, R., Hauf, M., . . . and Hubl, D. (2013) 'Reduced neuronal activity in language-related regions after transcranial magnetic stimulation therapy for auditory verbal hallucinations', *Biological psychiatry*, *73*(6), pp. 518–524.

Kandel, E. R., Schwartz, J. H., and Jessell, T. M. (2004) *Principles of Neural Science*, New York: McGraw-Hill, Health Professions Division.

Kuroki, N., Shenton, M. E., Salisbury, D. F., Hirayasu, Y., Onitsuka, T., Ersner, H., . . . and

McCarley, R. W. (2006) 'Middle and inferior temporal gyrus gray matter volume abnormalities in first-episode schizophrenia: an MRI study', *American Journal of Psychiatry*, *163*(12), pp. 2103–2110, http://doi: 10.1176/ajp.2006.163. 12.2103 Leff, A. P., Scholfield, T. M., Crinion, J. T., Seghier, M. L., Grogan, A., Green, D. W.,

Price, C. J. (2009) 'The left superior temoral gyrus is a shared substrate for auditory short-term memory and speech comprehension: evidence from 210 patients with stroke', *Brain (132/12)*, pp. 3398–4116, http://doi: 10.1093/brain /awp273. Lezak, M. D., Howieson, D. B., Loring, D. W., Hannay, H. J., and Fischer, J. S. (2004) *Neuropsychological Assessment* (4th ed.), New York, NY, US: Oxford University Press.

Mahendran, R. (2007) 'The psychopathology of musical hallucinations', *Singapore Medical Journal*, *48*(2), pp. e68–e70.

Manasco, H. (2017) *Introduction to Neurogenic Communication Disorders*, Jones & Bartlett Publishers.

McCarthy-Jones, S. (2012) *Hearing Voices: The Histories, Causes and Meanings of Auditory Verbal Hallucinations*, Cambridge University Press.

Moskowitz, A., and Corstens, D. (2008) 'Auditory hallucinations: Psychotic symptom or dissociative experience?', *Journal of Psychological Trauma*, *6*(2–3), pp. 35–63, doi: 10.1300/J513v06n02_04.

Pedersen, P. M., Vinter, K., and Olsen, T. S. (2004) 'Aphasia after stroke: type, severity and prognosis', *Cerebrovascular Diseases*, *17*(1), pp. 35–43, http://doi: 10.1159/00 0073896.

Steel, C. (2015) 'Hallucinations as a trauma-based memory: implications for psychological interventions', *Frontiers in Psychology*, *6*, p. 1262, http://doi: 10.3389/fpsyg.2015.01262.

Steenkamp, M. M., Litz, B. T., Hoge, C. W., and Marmar, C. R. (2015) 'Psychotherapy for military-related PTSD: a review of randomized clinical trials', *JAMA*, *314* (5), pp. 489– 500, http://doi: 10.1001/jama.2015.8370.

Stewart, C. and Riedel, K. (2016) 'Managing speech and language deficits after stroke', in Gillen, G. (ed.) *Stroke Rehabilitation (fourth edition)* pp. 673–689, http://doi: 10.1016/B978-0-323-17281-3.00029-0.

Swanberg, M. M., Nasreddine, Z. S., Mendez, M. F., and Cummings, J. L. (2007) 'Speech and language', in *Textbook of Clinical Neurology: Third Edition*, Elsevier Inc., http://doi: 10.1016/B978-141603618-0.10006-2.

Taylor, F. K. (1981) 'On pseudo-hallucinations', *Psychological Medicine*, *11*(2), pp. 265–271, http://doi: 10.1017/S0033291700052089. van der Kolk, B. A. (2012) 'Posttraumatic therapy in the age of neuroscience', *Psychoanalytic Dialogues*, *12*(3), pp. 381–392, http://doi: 10.1080/104818812093.

Vermeer, S. E., Kourdstaal, P. J., Oudkerk, M., *et al.* (2002) 'prevalence and risk Factors of silent brain infarcts in the population based Rotterdam Scan Study', *Stroke, 33,* pp. 21–25.

Wade, D. M., Brewin, C. R., Howell, D. C., White, E., Mythen, M. G., and Weinman, J. A. (2015) 'Intrusive memories of hallucinations and delusions in traumatized intensive care patients: an interview study', *British Journal of Health Psychology*, *20*(3), pp. 613–631, http://doi: 10.1111/bjhp.12109.

Yourganov, G., Smith, K. G., Fridriksson, J., and Rorden, C. (2015) Predicting aphasia type from brain damage measured with structural MRI', *Cortex, 73*, pp. 203–215, http://doi: 10.1016/j.cortex.2015.09.005.

Appendix A

Figure from Kuroki *et al.* (2007)

CHAPTER 11

Schizophrenia

*'My good fortune is not that I have recovered
from mental illness. I have not, or will I ever.
My good fortune lies in having found my life.'*

As well as being one of the worst things that can happen to a human being, schizophrenia can also be one of the richest learning and humanising experiences life offers.

Schizophrenia is a severe and chronic mental disorder that impacts how an individual behaves, thinks, feels, relates to other people, and make decisions. According to the World Health Organization, schizophrenia has affected more than twenty million people globally (James *et al.*, 2017). Schizophrenia can occur at any age and to any gender; however, it is more prevalent in males than females. Although psychosocial stress, environment, genetics, and neurobiology can lead to the development of schizophrenia, the specific causes of the disorder remain unknown (Owen and Sawa, 2018).

Some of the likely environmental factors that lead to the development of schizophrenia include substance abuse, situations that are extremely stressful, and viral infections among others. Other environmental factors that increase the risk of developing this mental disorder are the death of a parent, childhood trauma, abuse, or being bullied (Misiak *et al.*, 2017). Schizophrenia is believed to run in families; nonetheless, there is no particular gene that can be attributed to the disorder (Parakh and Basu, 2013). According to *DSM*-5 most individuals diagnosed with schizophrenia often have no history of psychosis in their family (APA, 2013).

An increase in the serotonin levels has been linked to positive symptoms of schizophrenia. Various brain regions such as cortex, thalamus, basal ganglia, hippocampus, and the medial temporal lobe have also been linked to schizophrenia.

The Diagram on the Causes of Schizophrenia

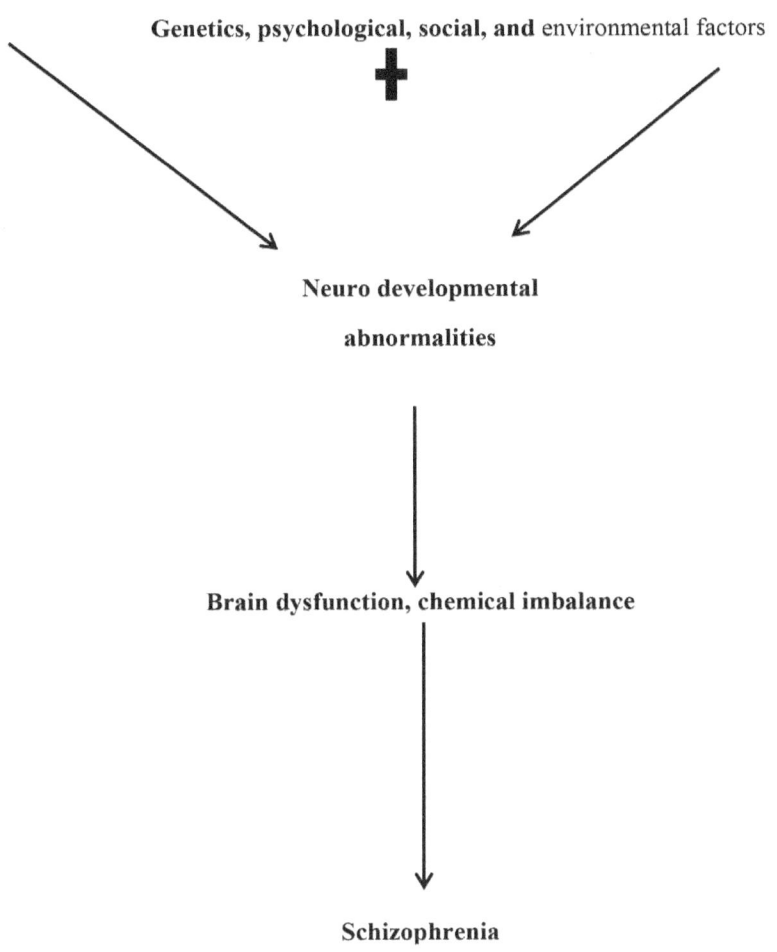

Genetics, psychological, social, and environmental factors

Neuro developmental

abnormalities

Brain dysfunction, chemical imbalance

Schizophrenia

Positive Symptoms of Schizophrenia

Positive symptoms refer to the presence and not the absence of symptoms. In schizophrenia, these symptoms entail ideas, actions, or perceptions that are highly exaggerated. They also refer to features that are added to a person's state of being. Some of these symptoms include disorganised speech and thoughts, hallucinations, and delusions. Hallucinations include hearing, feeling, or seeing things which are not visible or audible to other people (Császár, Kapócs, and Bókkon, 2019). Auditory hallucinations among people diagnosed with schizophrenia involve hearing voices in the head. The person may also become angry, demanding, begin murmuring, or whispering.

There are also auditory hallucinations where the person sees patterns, objects, lights, or people, which mostly include their loved ones who are no longer alive. Visual hallucinations can cause the affected person to experience challenges with distance and depth perception. Hallucinations may also involve the touch, smell, and taste senses. Consequently, the person diagnosed with schizophrenia may start believing that he or she is being poisoned, thereby refusing to eat (Császár, Kapócs, and Bókkon, 2019). Tactile hallucination can also occur when the affected individuals feel things such as insects or hands crawling on their bodies.

Delusions, which also mean false suspicions or beliefs not shared by other people, are common in people diagnosed with schizophrenia. Delusions refer to firmly held views even when there are adequate facts to the contrary. An example of a delusion is when a schizophrenia patient believes that others are trying to control his brain through televisions (Heinz *et al.*, 2016). Those diagnosed with schizophrenia may also believe that they possess superpowers, are the president, or are well-known personalities. There are also persecutory delusions where the patient feels people are hunting, stalking, tricking, or framing them. On the other hand, referential delusion can make the person believe that some public means of communication, such as a particular song, are meant to be a special message for them (Capps, 2010). There are also religious delusions that can lead the person to believe that they possess a unique relationship with a particular deity or that they are demon-possessed. Through grandiose delusions, people with schizophrenia may view themselves as prominent figures such as politicians or entertainers.

Disorganised speech and confused thoughts are other positive symptoms of schizophrenia, causing schizophrenia patients to experience challenges in organising their thoughts (APA, 2013). It becomes difficult for the person to follow a conversation, and when he or she tries to talk, their works are jumbled and rarely make any sense. Disorganised thinking can also involve derailment where the person shifts the topic before completing the initial thought. Circumstantial thinking is another form of disorganised thinking where due to schizophrenia, the person talks in circles and adds details that are unnecessary while not getting to the actual point. Tangential thinking can also occur where the person gives answers that are not related to the question. Disorganised thinking can also manifest through disconnected or illogical thoughts (APA, 2013). Disorganised thinking in people diagnosed with schizophrenia can also be portrayed through incoherence, often referred to as *word salad*. Movement disorders are also common among schizophrenia patients. At times, the person may engage in one movement repeatedly. Other times, schizophrenia can make the person be still for many hours, and this is referred to as catatonia. This condition is often characterised by a significant reduction in the way the person responds to his environment.

Catatonia can involve motor rigidity, stupor, purposeless excitement, or mutism. A person with catatonia may experience stupor or rigidity, become unable to move, respond, or speak. At times, when not treated, these conditions may last for extended periods, such as many hours or days. Catatonia can cause the schizophrenia patient to engage in abnormal movements or stay in uncomfortable positions. Extreme and erratic movement is another common catatonic behaviour.

For instance, the affected individual may repeatedly pace in a particular pattern while making loud exclamations without any specific reason (Capps, 2010). Echoing of words, which is commonly known as echolalia, is another catatonic behaviour. It is necessary to note that hallucinations and delusions often occur together. For instance, an individual affected by schizophrenia may experience delusions about persecution while the evidence may originate from auditory hallucinations. Another example is where the person believes he is an archangel, and this may be arising from *God's voice*. Both delusions and hallucinations can lead to chaos where the affected individual losses touch with reality (Heinz et al., 2016).

Negative Symptoms of Schizophrenia

Negative symptoms in schizophrenia can be described as a reduction in motivation, emotional responses, movement, thought process, speech, and socialisation. Negative symptoms often lead to functional and social decline. When these symptoms are present, they tend to remain, even after positive symptoms have resolved. Negative symptoms are present often for an extended period before the start of positive symptoms, where they are referred to as *prodromal symptoms*. These symptoms are difficult to identify since they are often mistaken for other mental health disorders like depression (Rector, Beck, and Stolar, 2005). Additionally, these symptoms may appear and disappear in the course of schizophrenia.

The five primary domains of negative symptoms include emotional bluntness, alogia, avolition, asociality, and anhedonia (APA, 2013). Emotional bluntness is where the affected person demonstrates little or no emotion. Emotional bluntness is often characterised by facial expressions that are unchanging and apathetic. The lack of expression may be demonstrated in circumstances that generally trigger excitement or sadness. For example, the person diagnosed with schizophrenia on receiving good news may not laugh, become joyful, or even smile. Emotional bluntness is more prevalent in men than women and is often seen in the initial stages of schizophrenia (Li *et al.*, 2016).

Some of the signs of emotional bluntness include an apparent disinterest in the subject at hand.

Flat voice or monotone with no expression or modulation can be another indicator of emotional bluntness. Nonverbal responses or body language that cannot be linked to the current situation, conversation, or experience can also be signs of emotional bluntness. Flat affect or emotional bluntness can adversely affect a person's social functioning (Evensen *et al.*, 2012).

Alogia also referred to as poverty of speech is a symptom of different conditions but mostly linked to schizophrenia. This condition, which involves decreased verbal fluency, is another negative symptom of schizophrenia. Often, it becomes impossible for schizophrenia patients to communicate their thoughts or engage in conversations (Mitra *et al.*, 2016). People who due to schizophrenia have alogia often answer questions with monosyllables. It is necessary to understand that the delays in speech resulting from alogia are not similar to those caused by positive symptoms such as visual or auditory hallucinations of disorganised thoughts. Some of the signs indicating the presence of alogia include pausing for an extended period between words.

Another sign of alogia is when the person answers only what they are asked. Those affected can also have dull facial expressions and a flat tone in their voice. Moreover, schizophrenia patients struggling with alogia have unclear pronunciations of consonants. Their few words usually become a whisper. At times alogia can cause an individual to have the right amount of speech, but the words generally make no sense (Marder and Galderisi, 2017). Poverty in speech originates from the brain's incapacity, making such patients experience challenges in having a mental understanding of the right words.

Alogia can be a secondary impact caused by primary symptoms

like anxiety or psychosis. For instance, the affected individual may decide not to speak due to threats he or she receives from their head. Additionally, these people may not talk since they are anxious, nervous, or paranoid around other people. For those diagnosed with schizophrenia, alogia involves the interruption of the thought pattern leading to challenges in verbal fluency and a lack of speech. Studies have reported that alogia that is caused by schizophrenia may arise from having a disorganised semantic memory (Kuperberg, 2010).

It is believed that alogia can be caused by brain dysfunction; this causes degradation of the semantic store. The semantic store is the brain region that is responsible for processing language and meaning of words. This can explain why individuals with alogia experience challenges in getting the right words to express what they mean. Studies have demonstrated that alogia is associated with finding words and their meanings from long-term memory stores (Kuperberg, 2010). When the different brain regions experience challenges in communicating with one another, it can lead to symptoms related to alogia. This condition can adversely affect the social functioning of the affected individual. The person may become socially withdrawn due to the incapacity to communicate or organise his/her thoughts.

The other negative symptom linked to schizophrenia is asociality or the lack of desire to engage in any kind of relationship. Other words that can be used to refer to asociality include social disinterest, lack of social drive, unsocial, or non-social. Asociality makes the affected individual have an enhanced desire to stay alone (Marder and Galderisi, 2017). The lack of interest in social activities can be secondary to other schizophrenia symptoms such as hallucinations and delusions. These symptoms can damage interpersonal relationships and other social links. Delusions and hallucinations can lead to social withdrawal, depressed mood, or suspicion.

Another negative symptom of schizophrenia is avolition, which refers to a lack of motivation or initiative in completing activities that are goal-directed (Norton et al., 2013). Avolition can be mistaken for procrastination. Avolition causes people diagnosed with schizophrenia to be willing to complete a particular task but has no physical or mental energies to execute their responsibility. Some examples of avolition include the inability to begin or complete payment of bills even when it is urgent. Another example of avolition is the failure to turn up for a scheduled meeting. Not tending to one's appearance or physical hygiene can also be linked to avolition.

One character of avolition is emotional blunting (Norton *et al.*, 2013). As a result, people may label the person lazy or apathetic. Avolition can lead to social withdrawal and make the affected individual not to complete their daily responsibilities or meet their goals. Due to avolition, family and work relationships may be adversely affected. This condition makes it difficult for the person to participate in psychotherapy actively. Avolition can also be mistaken for aboulia, which means a lack of will instead of motivation. It is also necessary to differentiate avolition from anhedonia or asociality.

Anhedonia is another negative emotion commonly associated with schizophrenia. Anhedonia refers to a reduced capacity to experience pleasurable feelings. For schizophrenia patients, anhedonia can mean lacking enthusiasm for passions, activities, pleasures, and hobbies previously enjoyed (Strauss, 2013). Some of the symptoms of anhedonia include experiencing difficulties in adapting to social situations, adverse feelings towards oneself and others, and social withdrawal. Other symptoms of anhedonia include withdrawing from previous relationships, faking emotions such as pretending to be happy when one is sad, and a decrease in emotional capacities, which may involve less verbal or nonverbal expressions.

Cognitive Symptoms of Schizophrenia

Apart from the conventionally recognised positive and negative symptoms, there are also cognitive symptoms of schizophrenia. In schizophrenia, cognitive symptoms affect the way an individual thinks (Targum and Keefe, 2008). The cognitive symptoms include impairment in information procession, executive functioning, and the working memory of the affected individual. These symptoms occur before the onset of schizophrenia and to a considerable extent, influence the morbidity related to this mental disorder (Greene, Horan, and Lee, 2019).

These symptoms are similar to the negative symptoms and often become evident after several psychotic episodes.

Like negative schizophrenia symptoms, cognitive symptoms become noticeable after positive symptoms have been reduced due to age or medication. The impact of cognitive impairments can be subtle and decline (Greene, Horan, and Lee, 2019). For instance, the patient's capacity to participate in intellectual activities previously enjoyed, such as watching drama on television or reading fictional stories, may decline. There have been cases where affected individuals unbeknownst to them, gazing blankly at the pages of a book. The person may also sit in front of the television with a blank stare.

Dopamine and Glutamate in Schizophrenia

Dopamine and glutamate have different neural signalling; however, both significantly contribute to the pathophysiology of schizophrenia (McCutcheon, Krystal, and Howes, 2020). Studies have reported that environmental and genetic causes of schizophrenia are associated with the disruption of dopamine and glutamate functions. Genetic factors can be linked directly to glutamate dysfunction. On the contrary, only a few genetic factors can be directly associated with the dysfunction of the dopamine system. Therefore, abnormal dopamine signalling can be linked to other factors.

Dopamine

Initially, dopamine was believed to be an intermediary compound that was biologically inactive on the synthetic pathway between noradrenaline and tyrosine. However, studies have demonstrated that a reduction in dopamine led to restricted movement. It was possible to reverse this effect through the administration of the dopamine precursor. As a result, dopamine has been viewed to have a significant biological impact. Dysfunction of the dopamine has been associated with the development of various psychotic symptoms and has been linked to the pathophysiology of schizophrenia (McCutcheon, Abi-Dargham, and Howes, 2019).

Several theories have been proposed regarding how disruption of the normal function of dopamine can be linked to positive symptoms of schizophrenia such as hallucinations and delusions (McCutcheon, Abi-Dargham, and Howes, 2019). When the firing of the dopamine neuron is dysregulated, it abnormally signals the significance of irrelevant stimuli. As a result, thoughts and perceptions are instilled with abnormal salience, which further leads to causal attributions and incorrect associations (Sterzer *et al.*, 2018). When dopamine is uncoordinated, it can lead to delusional ideas (McCutcheon, Abi-Dargham, and Howes, 2019).

Various studies have endeavoured to determine more accurately the mechanism through which the dysfunction of dopamine can lead to psychotic symptoms. The stimulus experience relies not just on the sensory inputs coming from the stimulus, but also on previous anticipations concerning the likelihood of a particular perception. Auditory hallucinations seem to be a result of a substantial impact of prior expectations on sensory perception (Powers, Mathys, and Corlett, 2017). The previous expectations have been linked to a release of increased levels of amphetamine-induced dopamine in the striatum (Cassidy *et al.*, 2018).

Studies have reported that dopamine signalling plays a critical role in reorganising the brain (Braun *et al.*, 2019). The primary function of dopamine in coding prediction errors and in the cortical representation of environmental states has been used by various studies to evaluate the behavioural impact of an interrupted dopamine signalling (Maia and Frank, 2011). Cortical D1 receptors have a significant role in accurately shaping the environmental states' neural representations by accurately inhibiting neural activity (Krystal *et al.*, 2017). When the cortical dopamine signalling decreases, stimuli connected to reward cannot be correctly encoded, which inhibits their capacity to guide behaviour.

Additionally, decreased signalling of the cortical dopamine can mean the reward-linked representations last for only a short period (Krystal *et al.*, 2017). Previously, the firing of the dopamine neurons in response to stimuli has been linked to reward and control behaviour towards actions connected to previous rewards. This mechanism can decrease the appetitive characteristics of a particular reward. Consequently, the impact of this reward in shaping future behaviour may be reduced, leading to negative symptoms of schizophrenia, such as lack of motivation and anhedonia (Strauss *et al.*, 2011).

Cognitive Symptoms and Cortical Dopamine

The dorsolateral prefrontal cortex plays a significant role in most cognitive processes.

Dysfunction of the dorsolateral prefrontal cortex has been associated with impairments that are witnessed in schizophrenia (Kelly *et al.*, 2019). Based on the significance of the signalling of the D1 receptor in cognition, a decrease in the cortical dopamine signalling is believed to be a contributing factor in the development of cognitive symptoms in schizophrenia. Studies have demonstrated that excessive signalling of the striatal dopamine signalling can lead to decreased cortical dopamine and the associated cognitive symptoms. Hence, both excessive and reduced dopamine signalling can adversely affect cognition. As a result, success in developing dopamine regulating therapies for cognitive symptoms has been limited (Greene, Horan, and Lee, 2019).

Glutamate

The dopamine model regarding schizophrenia remains significant; however, many features of the disorder cannot be clarified based entirely on dopaminergic dysfunction. Furthermore, most people diagnosed with schizophrenia have not experienced any changes in their symptoms despite receiving treatment with diverse dopaminergic compounds. Significant evidence has implicated the glutamate system in the development of schizophrenia (McCutcheon, Krystal, and Howes, 2020). Glutamatergic models of schizophrenia account for positive, negative, and cognitive symptoms of schizophrenia. These models can lead to new approaches in treating schizophrenia patients.

In the central nervous system, glutamate is the primary excitatory neurotransmitter. This chemical assists in activating neurons among other cells in the brain. When the glutamate-mediated neurotransmission is disturbed, it can lead to neuropsychiatric disorders like mood disorders, schizophrenia, autism spectrum disorders, and substance abuse (McCutcheon, Krystal, and Howes, 2020). Theories that implicate glutamate in the development of schizophrenia are founded on the capacity of the N-methyl-D-aspartate receptor antagonists to trigger schizophrenic symptoms.

Contrary to the cell bodies of the dopamine neurons that are anatomically localised, glutamate neurons are extensively spread in the brain. Glutamate is involved in brain regions that develop memories and helps an individual to learn new things. This chemical also gives instructions to various brain regions regarding what they are expected to do. Some studies have reported that excess glutamate activity in some brain regions enhances the risk of developing schizophrenia.

The different brain regions associated with schizophrenia are linked to a brain cell circuit that depends on glutamate for communication (McCutcheon, Krystal, and Howes, 2020).

There are diverse glutamate receptors that are categorised as either metabotropic or ionotropic.

The ionotropic receptors comprise the NMDA and non-NMDA receptors, commonly localised on neurons (Wang *et al.*, 2013). The NMDA receptors due to slower kinetics often increase depolarisation, which the non-NMDA receptors initiate. The dopamine neurons are restricted to particular anatomical pathways. In contrast, glutamate signalling takes place in every part of the brain. Consequently, a dysfunctional glutamate system can lead to diverse impairments.

NMDA receptors have a significant role in coordinating various cognitive processes that entail working memory (Wang *et al.*, 2013). One of the techniques involved in representing information efficiently through the cortical requires sparse coding. Encoding of information is performed based on the diverse cell classes. As a result, only a small cell area within a particular region spike leading to the spatial encoding of information. Sparse coding entails high spatial exactness concerning the excitation area. The administration of NMDA antagonists to healthy controls and those with schizophrenia leads to symptoms that can be linked to impaired sparse coding.

This phenomenon can also be associated with false alarms in the working memory, reduced mnemonic precision, and a smaller working memory buffer (Buzsák and Watson, 2012). In situations where NMDA receptor antagonists like ketamine and phencyclidine have repeatedly been administered to healthy controls, they have induced behaviours similar to the negative and positive symptoms of schizophrenia. Studies have shown that blocking the NMDA receptors with such compounds can have a psychotic effect (Moghaddam and Javitt, 2020). Evidence has shown that these drugs can aggravate various symptoms in people with schizophrenia.

A reduction in the activity of the NMDAR on the inhibitory neurons can disinhibit glutamate neurons and as a result, increase the synaptic glutamate activity, particularly in the prefrontal cortex. NMDA dysfunction can be caused by a decrease in the glutamate tone in the brain, thereby leading to an overall deficit in glutamatergic neurotransmission. The NMDAR model may be viewed revolutionary since it recommends a diverse set of regions than those predicted by traditional monoaminergic models. Additionally, the NMDAR model proposes what brain areas to target in the treatment of schizophrenia.

Contrary to the dopamine neurotransmission, a large number of the cortical connectional and afferent is glutamatergic. Based on the glutamatergic model, impairments are spread throughout the subcortical and cortical regions (Javitt, 2009). For instance, event-associated potential indexing the functioning of the brain that is referred to as mismatch negativity has been reported to be abnormal in schizophrenia patients (Näätänen, R., and Kähkönen, 2009).

The Striatum and Schizophrenia

The striatum comprises the putamen and caudate and is the basal ganglia input element, a group of subcortical nuclei that conventionally was linked to the motor movement control. The striatum gets its inputs from the hippocampus, thalamus, amygdala, and cortex. The primary basal ganglia output includes the subthalamic nucleus, globus pallidus, the ventral tegmental region, and the substantia nigra. These outputs primarily project to the thalamus, which is the main target of the basal ganglia. Consequently, the thalamus projects back to the cortex, which completes a circle involving the thalamus, striatum, and cortex.

Striatal dysfunction is believed to be a primary factor in the development of schizophrenia. For instance, most patients with schizophrenia demonstrate deficits in their reward system, which has been linked to dysfunctional striatum. The prefrontal cortex and striatum function are to mediate both the executive functions and the working memory. Cognitive symptoms in schizophrenia can occur not only from the impairment of the prefrontal cortex but also from dysfunctional striatum (Strauss *et al.*, 2011). It is necessary to note that enhanced production of the amphetamine-induced dopamine in people affected by schizophrenia is more evident in the associative striatum.

In the striatum, the level of dopamine abnormalities for people affected by schizophrenia differs.

However, it is in the associative striatum where this dysfunction is primarily witnessed. The associative striatum moderates communication between the limbic and the motor regions. The prefrontal cortex sends inputs directly to the associative striatum. Enhanced dopamine production in the caudate can modulate the efficiency of the corticostriatal synapse in the associative striatum. As a result, cognitive processes, which include the working memory, could be adversely affected. Disrupting the striatum's integrative function can lead to associative deficits, which are common in schizophrenia (Strauss *et al.*, 2011).

Various preclinical models have suggested that the fundamental pathophysiology in schizophrenia is caused by enhanced dopamine release and a decrease in adaptive phasic release in responding to relevant stimuli (Maia and Frank). As a result, the noise in dopamine signalling in the associative striatum is increased; this may explain the decreased functional connection between the cortex and associative striatum (Fornito *et al.*, 2013). Dopamine signalling that targets a particular region assists in the accurate selection of some behaviours over others and mediates the correct integration of various signals (Burke, Rostein, and Alavrez, 2017).

On the contrary, when the dopamine transmission is undirected, this mechanism becomes impaired, thereby causing disorganised behaviour. Pharmacology can inhibit the over-activity of the dopamine system; thus, impairing the implementation of the preferred behaviour. Dopamine transmission to the striatum is often enhanced during the psychotic and prodromal states. These high levels of dopamine have been associated with the positive symptoms of schizophrenia.

Studies of perfusion, metabolic rate, and brain structure have linked the dysfunction of the dorsal striatum to auditory hallucinations (Zhuo *et al.*, 2017). Striatal dopamine signalling is also related to the development of negative and cognitive symptoms of schizophrenia. Recent studies have shown that enhanced dopamine signalling in the dorsal striatum can decrease the release of mesocortical dopamine and generate cognitive impairments (Krabbe *et al.*, 2015).

Striatal hyperdopaminergia can lead to cognitive impairments by dysregulating cortical dopamine or interrupting the signalling between the associative striatum and the frontal cortex (Simpson,

Kellendobk, and Kandel, 2010). An animal model intended to mimic the enhanced dopamine signalling common in schizophrenia showed that overexpression of the striatal D2 reduced the turnover of the cortical dopamine and caused cognitive impairments. These deficits remained even after the transmission of the dopamine signalling was normalised.

These findings may suggest that although an increase in the striatal dopamine signalling causes cognitive deficits, succeeding adaptive changes can explain persistence. The model can also explain the results showing that a reduction in the transmission of striatal dopamine through antipsychotics has minimal success in treating cognitive symptoms. Studies have also shown that less connection between the associative striatum and the substantia nigra is associated with the severity of the cognitive symptoms in schizophrenia (Yoon *et al.*, 2014). Evidence also shows that striatal dysfunction can directly lead to negative symptoms, which often develop as a result of reward-based learning that is impaired (Strauss *et al.*, 2011).

Several studies have proven that striatum plays a significant role in the development of this kind of behaviour. Additionally, studies have demonstrated that excess irregular release of the dopamine can conceal the production of adaptive striatal dopamine (Maia and Frank, 2017).

Consequently, this may lead to the behavioural impairments witnessed in schizophrenia.

The Gut and Schizophrenia

The gut microbiome, which comprises various microbes, has been associated with multiple mental health disorders (Bastiaanssen *et al.*, 2019). Studies have reported that the number of microbial cells is more than the human cells in a ratio of 1:3 (Sender, Fuchs and Milo, 2016).

Additionally, the study has shown that 99% of the human bodies' genes contain more than ten million microbial genes (Flint *et al.*, 2012). These microbes have a significant role in immune, satiety, and metabolism regulation. Recent evidence has shown that microbes influence both behaviour and mood. Consequently, their impact on human disease and health cannot be underestimated.

During the birth process, the gastrointestinal tracts are filled with good bacteria that move to the baby through the mother's birth canal. Furthermore, during the birth process, the gastrointestinal tract contacts and maintains regular communication with the microbes in the gut.

This contact and communication can be as a result of direct contact or the discharge of secreted compounds. Studies have reported that lifestyle factors such as stress, sleep, and diet influence the gut microbiome (Benedict *et al.*, 2016). As a result, the overall health and brain development of an individual is affected.

The bacteria composition that inhabits the gastrointestinal in an adult is developed early on in life. The primary microbiota occurs parallel with the sprouting, development, and maturation of neurons in the brain of a young child (Borre *et al.*, 2014). On the contrary, a decrease in microbiota diversity and complexity occurs in old age. As a result, the onset or progression of various mood disorders such as mania, suicidal ideations, anxiety, anhedonia, and depressive symptoms may occur. Gut bacteria help control proteins and other chemicals that affect the brain's capacity in developing new neurons and neuroplasticity. The gut environment affects brain receptors. Brain chemicals can be compared to keys that are designed to fit in a particular receptor. An example of this kind of receptor is the NMDA, a type of glutamate receptor involved in the plasticity of neurons linked to the memory (Wang *et al.*, 2013). When the gut microbiome is not balanced, it can lead to malfunctioning of the NMDA receptors and cause changes to the BDNF, further triggering schizophrenia symptoms.

Microbial maladaptation or imbalance of the population of microorganisms, commonly referred to as microbial dysbiosis, is strongly linked to various health conditions. Some of these health conditions include metabolic disorders, such as obesity and diabetes mellitus. Others include coeliac disease, inflammatory bowel syndrome, irritable bowel syndrome, and psychiatric disorders like schizophrenia (Morris *et al.*, 2017).

The functions carried out by the microbiota are aimed at enhancing organic health and stability.

The brain-gut relationship strongly correlates with psychiatric disorders, and disrupting this connection increases the risk of developing this disorder. The gut microbiome helps in nutrients digestion, generation of short-chain fatty acids, production of metabolites like kynurenine, and modulating gene expression (Moos *et al.*, 2016). In the past few years, the gut-brain axis has gained significance due to evidence-based on the new association between the immune, nervous, and endocrine systems.

Various mechanisms regulate the link between the brain and the gut microbiota. These mechanisms focus on pro-inflammatory mediators produced by the immune system. Alterations in the microorganisms change the bi-directional communication between the gut microbiota and the brain through the vagus nerve. Gut colonisation begins during birth when the baby comes into contact with the maternal microflora (Yang *et al.*, 2016). The first microbiome of neonates differs based on the perinatal period and the kind of delivery, whether through a caesarean section or vaginal birth.

During a caesarean section of birth, the child is not exposed to microbes that are residents in the birth canal; this limits the baby's contact with the typical microbial fauna. In its place, the baby is exposed to other bacteria from the environment. Babies born through caesarean section are at a higher risk of developing autoimmune disorders such as celiac disease, asthma, eczema, and diabetes (Dinan, Stanton, and Cryan, 2013). Furthermore, babies that are not breastfed but instead bottle-fed are also limited in their exposure to the mother's original organisms.

Insufficient interaction with symbiotic bacteria in babies can reduce the number of normal organisms and increase the population of pathogenic microorganisms like Clostridium difficile (Molloy,

2015). The significance of early exposure of a baby to normal microbes has led to diverse researches where the baby's skin, eyes, and mouth are inoculated with swabs from the vagina of the mother instantly after a caesarean section. The purpose of this procedure is to activate the healthy microbiome development in the newborn. The cleaning of pacifiers has also been linked to a reduction in allergies. Mothers who clean baby's pacifiers through sucking have shown that it reduces the rate of eczema and asthma.

Evidence has also shown that a parent can transfer her oral microbiota to the child through saliva by sucking the pacifier when cleaning. Helicobacter pylori, which resides in the host's stomach, is acquired in early childhood and resides in 50% of the human population (Haley and Gaddy, 2016). Helicobacter pylori infection is linked to the malabsorption of nutrients, which often leads to childhood malnutrition. As a result, biochemical abnormalities such as dopamine system dysfunction is induced. These factors play a significant role in the development of schizophrenia (Vitale et al., 2011). Evidence has shown that a dysfunctional immune system is one of the primary causes of schizophrenia.

The gut microbiota, through its communication with the immune system, influences the brain-gut immune responses (Ergün, Urhan, and Ayer, 2018). Immune response dysregulation leads to autoimmune and neuropsychiatric diseases like schizophrenia. Changes in the gut barrier properties can lead to a dysbiotic status, which increases the risk of various diseases (Konig et al., 2016). T helper cells are in control of the IL-17 production, whose levels are often high in schizophrenia (Li et al., 2017). There is a positive correlation between this cytokine and the severity and symptoms of schizophrenia.

The dysfunction of the gut barrier leads to behavioural and neurological changes (Severance et al., 2016). Various factors can alter the composition of the microorganisms in the gut microbiota.

Some of these factors include microbiota modulators like the probiotics and prebiotics and drugs such as vaccines and antibiotics. Mental health conditions like stress or schizophrenia can also alter the microbiota population (Evrensel and Ceylan, 2015). Studies have shown that antibiotics that change the gut microbiota composition can enhance antipsychotics action (Ardakani *et al.*, 2014).

Improper functioning of neurotransmitters such as dopamine and noradrenaline have been associated with the development of mental health disorders like schizophrenia. The gut microbiota can increase the levels of these neurotransmitters in the brain. The gut microbiota can also cause disturbances to the neuroendocrine system, the immune system, and the HPA axis due to the interruption of the brain chemistry. The brain-gut axis functions are connected to the cognitive and emotional centres, such as the enteric, autonomic, enteroendocrine, and central nervous systems. Dysregulation in these systems, particularly the enteroendocrine system, can lead to mental disorders like schizophrenia (Rogers *et al.*, 2016). The gut microbiota is also responsible for metabolising some non-digestible dietary carbohydrates into short-chain fatty acids (SCFAs) (Louis and Flint, 2017). The primary short- chain fatty acids produced by the gut bacteria include the butyric acid, propionic acid, and acetic acid. These metabolites impact various psychological functions such as immune cells and gene expression regulation, suppressing inflammation, which influences brain physiology and behaviour. For instance, acetate can lead to physiological changes in the hypothalamus. Acetate, which is produced by the gut microbiota, can also cause feelings of satisfaction. SCFAs, on the other hand, can lead to anxiety, behavioural changes such as becoming antisocial, which are common in many psychiatric disorders.

Microbiome's Role in Brain Development

Brain development starts from the prenatal stage and spans to post-adolescence. Brain development involves the interplay of environmental and genetic factors (O'Mahony *et al.*, 2015). When these interactions are disrupted, the normal developmental trajectories can be altered, leading to neuropsychiatric conditions. Neural development starts early in embryonic life with several significant stages that happen before birth. During this time, maternal metabolism and immunity exemplify a relationship between neurodevelopmental in the womb and the external environment.

Problems to maternal homeostasis, which may include prenatal stress, poor nutrition, and infections have been linked to neurodevelopmental disorders such as autism, anxiety, schizophrenia, and depression. Disrupting the maternal microbiome often relates foetal development to externals stressors. The maternal gut microbiota can impact foetal neurodevelopment by influencing the circulating 5-hydroxytryptamine levels. Maternal dysbiosis can also affect the formation of the blood-brain barrier, which is vital in developing the central nervous system. Neurodevelopment continues after the baby is born, and it involves cell differentiation and morphological changes (O'Mahony et al., 2015).

The Microbe-Gut Interactions

Despite the various beneficial roles of the gut microbes, the host is required to ensure a physical barrier between the microbiota and host to prevent infections (Pott and Hornef, 2012). The gut epithelial lining is comprised of the secretory cells, gut-related lymphoid tissues, the chemosensory cells, and the enterocytes. The gut's single-cell epithelial layer's primary role is to restrict the direct contact of the visceral tissue with the intestinal microbiota. The single-celled epithelial regulates this kind of connection by producing a protective viscous mucus layer. Host- microbe communication occurs in the mucosal layer.

Antibiotics and the Gut Microbiota

Antibiotics are drugs used to treat bacterial infections by targeting pathogenic bacteria.

Medicines can adversely affect the gut microbiota since the reduction in bacterial diversity can last for more than three months after discontinuing these drugs. Antibiotics treatment enhances a reduction in gut microbiota's bacterial diversity. The bacterial diversity alongside the immunological disturbances and metabolic abnormalities has been linked to unusual behaviours in adults. Some of the abnormal behaviours include cognitive disorders and anxiety (Sherwin *et al.*, 2016).

The use of antibiotics should be controlled since they have the potential to be abused. The use of antibiotics in adulthood or childhood modifies the gut microbiota, leading to bacterial resistance and could also cause neoplastic and metabolic diseases (Blaser, 2016). Ampicillin, which is one type of antibiotics due to its impact in changing, can explain schizophrenia's cognitive symptoms in schizophrenia (Dinah and Cyran, 2017).

Prebiotics

Prebiotics are a kind of dietary ingredient that leads to particular changes in the activity and composition of the gastrointestinal microflora. Intestines through bifidobacterium and lactobacillus help in metabolising prebiotics. Prebiotics are fibres that repel enzymatic hydrolysis, absorption and gastric acidity in the upper gastrointestinal tract. The microflora in the intestines ferment the prebiotics, thereby enhancing the activity of particular intestinal bacteria (Slavin, 2013). The concentration of *bifidobacterium* in the gut reduces with age. Nevertheless, a healthy microbiota among the elderly can be attained through prebiotic supplementation.

Consequently, this can decrease the risk of age-related neurogastrointestinal diseases (Scott *et al.*, 2015).

Probiotics

Probiotics are live bacteria that have health benefits. At times, the natural balance of the gut homeostasis, which includes the intestine and stomach, can be interrupted. In such situations, probiotics can assist in restoring the balance. Probiotics can modulate and reconstruct the gastrointestinal barrier, thereby enhancing the production of mucin and decreasing the intestinal permeability (Shermin *et al.*, 2016). Some probiotics can activate the gut barrier development, changing the expression of the tight junction protein, and enhancing the gut barrier's role (Saulnier *et al.*, 2013). Probiotics can interact with the immune system.

As a result, the inflammatory response is modulated through the stimulation of regulatory cells (Mangiola *et al.*, 2016). The primary benefit of probiotics in mental health disorders is managing symptoms such as depression and anxiety. Furthermore, probiotics help reduce the corticosterone levels generated by depression, anxiety, and stress, all of which are symptoms linked to schizophrenia (Mangolia *et al.*, 2016). Therefore, probiotics are gradually becoming a promising therapy in the treatment of psychiatric disorders and gut dysbiosis.

Brain-Derived Neurotrophic Factor and Schizophrenia

Brain-derived neurotrophic factor is the most predominant growth factors in the central nervous system. BDNF is vital for neuronal plasticity and the development of the central nervous system. Since the brain-derived neurotrophic factor plays a crucial role in plasticity and development of the brain, it has been extensively linked to psychiatric disorders. Neurotrophins belong to the family of proteins and assist in the development and survival of neurons.

Neurotrophins enhance the growth, differentiation, and survival of neurons during brain development. The long-term impact of neurotrophins, including neuroplasticity, dendrite, axonal growth, synaptic connections, and structure, depends on gene regulation (Favalli *et al.*, 2012).

The short-term cytoplasmic effects of neurotrophins influence the neuronal differentiation, synaptic transmission, and modulation of the excitability of neurons. Reduced synaptic connectivity has been linked to a lack of neurotrophins. The correct synaptic function that if often linked to schizophrenia symptoms is influenced by neurotrophins. One of the most extensively studied neurotrophins is the brain-derived neurotrophic factor. BDNF is expressed in the central and periphery nervous systems. The brain-derived neurotrophic factor is involved in brain development, including maturation, differentiation, and maturation of neurons (Nieto, Kukuljan, and Silva, 2013).

In the brain, BDNF is active in the basal forebrain, cortex, and hippocampus. These brain regions are essential in higher thinking, memory, and learning. The prostate, kidney, skeletal muscle, saliva, motor neurons, and the retina are also involved in BDNF expression (Delezie and Handschin, 2018). Studies have demonstrated that BDNF mRNA and TrkB levels are often reduced in the hippocampus and prefrontal cortex of schizophrenia patients. This brain region is involved with working memory (Ray, Weickert, and Webster, 2014). Most schizophrenia patients struggle with impaired working memories; this shows that BDNF plays a significant role in the aetiology of schizophrenia. Schizophrenia also leads to the reduced hippocampus. BDNF is one of the most active neurotrophins involved in stimulating and controlling neurogenesis.

The brain-derived neurotrophic factor can enhance protective pathways and obstruct damaging pathways that influence the brain's neurogenic response by supporting cell survival. BDNF is crucial in neuronal plasticity of an adult's brain, neurotransmitters modulation, and the survival of serotonergic, cholinergic, and dopaminergic neurons. These neurons have been implicated in cognitive and memory changes in schizophrenia patients. BDNF has been linked to various mental health disorders. Brain-derived neurotrophic factor is vital in the development of the central nervous system and regulating the neuronal links that may be associated with the pathophysiology of schizophrenia (Nieto, Kukuljan, and Silva, 2013).

BDNF can enhance the quantity of inhibitory and excitatory synapses, regulate axonal morphology, or promote synapse. Furthermore, BDNF enhances the development and stabilisation of the molecular and cellular components of the production of the neurotransmitter.

Consequently, more functional synapses are developed. Brain-derived neurotrophic factors play a vital role in learning and synaptic plasticity (Lee and Silva, 2009). Primary changes in the neurotrophins activity can incorrectly change the synaptic transmission and cortical circuitry in the brain. Consequently, this could lead to neural dysfunction, which has been linked to mental health disorders like schizophrenia (Favalli *et al.*, 2013). Based on schizophrenia's neurodevelopmental hypothesis, BDNF has been a possible factor in the pathogenesis of this disorder. Insufficient neurotrophic support in brain development can disorganise the network structure, where neural connections are developed sub-optimally. Therefore, changes in BDNF can alter brain development, cause neuroplasticity failures, and disconnect the synapses. Additionally, changes in BDNF can explain some of the cytoarchitectonic, neurochemical, and morphological abnormalities, which are common in schizophrenia patients' brains. Studies have shown that low serum brain-derived neurotrophic factor quantities in the initial stages of schizophrenia have been linked to long periods of untreated psychosis (Rizos *et al.*, 2010).

Deregulation of Synapse in Schizophrenia

Various studies have suggested that changes in neuronal connectivity and synaptic transmission could be among the primary features of schizophrenia. Evidence has shown changes in the dopaminergic, glutamatergic, cholinergic, GABAergic and serotonergic synapses neurotransmission in schizophrenia. These pathways are often involved in schizophrenia pathophysiology. Glutamatergic neurons are responsible for the BDNF expression. The release of BDNF is at the synapse, where it impacts synaptic plasticity generating necessary changes in memory and learning and cognitive functions (Nieto *et al.*, 2013). Susceptibility genes which have a primary role in synaptic plasticity and neural development can influence pathogenic schizophrenia mechanisms in these synaptic pathways (Yin *et al.*, 2012).

Abnormal signalling of the brain-derived neurotrophic factor can influence synaptic function and neuronal differentiation. As a result, the brain function in the synaptic systems may be altered, which can lead to schizophrenia. Although dopamine dysregulation does not lead to schizophrenia, it can trigger positive, negative, and cognitive symptoms of this disorder.

Antipsychotic drugs at the dopamine D2-receptors block the dopamine transmission. Brain- derived neurotrophic factor regulates the expression of the D2 or D3-receptors. Previous approaches regarding schizophrenia aetiology focused on dopamine's neurotransmission due to its strong antipsychotic effect on dopamine antagonists.

However, current evidence supports the glutamate dysfunction in schizophrenia, where dopamine imbalance is viewed as secondary. Insufficient BDNF signalling mediated by the TrkB receptor in schizophrenia patients can decrease the GABA synthesis in the dorsolateral prefrontal cortex. Consequently, changes can occur in perisomatic pyramidal neurons inhibition; this may reduce the ability for frequency in the activity of synchronized gamma neuronal, which is essential for the working memory.

Schizophrenia and BDNF Polymorphisms

Some polymorphism variants have been associated with memory impairment and susceptibility to psychiatric disorders. For instance, changes in the brain volume that occur in schizophrenia patients have been linked to Val66Met polymorphism of the BDNF gene. Several pathophysiological and clinical characteristics of schizophrenia, such as brain pathology and symptoms and age of onset, have been associated with Val66Met polymorphism (Notaras *et al.*, 2015). Studies have reported a significant relationship between the severity of negative symptoms in the first schizophrenia episode and Val66Met polymorphism.

Structural Damage of GI Tract and Antibodies Development in Schizophrenia

The gastrointestinal tract is the largest immune organ in the body. Studies have shown that gut microbiota can control the brain's behaviours and functions through the microbiota-gut-brain axis.

For instance, based on research, the gut microbiota has been linked to locomotor activity, cognition, memory, and anxiety (Huttenhower *et al.*, 2012). The GI system comprises molecular and cellular mechanisms designed to help digestion, assist nutrient absorption, and protect the body from infections, toxins, and harmful antigens. Imbalances in the gut microbiome can be linked to structural damage in the gut.

Furthermore, when the gut microbiome is not balanced, it can lead to autoimmune disorders and inflammation. Structural damage to the gastrointestinal tract in individuals diagnosed with schizophrenia has been associated with the development of antibodies to the brain cells in the frontal cortex, amygdala, and hippocampus. These brain regions impaired in people with schizophrenia are involved in logical thinking, decision-making, motivation, emotion, and working memory (Ray, Weickert, and Webster, 2014). Imbalances in the gut flora can lead to enhanced sensitivity to gluten.

Additionally, imbalances in gut flora have been linked to insulin resistance and obesity, common in schizophrenia. Many studies have linked the GI in the aetiology and pathophysiology of various psychiatric disorders. The relationship between digestive issues with mental disorders spans centuries. Before the last half of the twentieth century, there were minimal distinctions between schizophrenia, psychosis, and bipolar disorder. These psychiatric disorders were commonly referred to as *insanity*.

An ancient famous Greek physician named Galen observed the link between mental problems and gastrointestinal tract symptoms such as constipation, flatulence, and indigestion. Galen prescribed fasting, emetics, diets containing laxatives, moderate wine, and purgatives to improve his patients' mental health. Galen emphasised that early intervention with the above approaches could eliminate or reduce mental problems. By the mid-nineteenth century, many scientists and healthcare professionals had accepted that various psychiatric illnesses were a result of diseases in the stomach, liver, and other organs. Physicians began to adopt Galen's techniques in treating mental illnesses.

An understanding of the gastrointestinal tract conditions linked to schizophrenia helps develop accurate, tailor-made treatment approaches to enhance the quality of life of those diagnosed with mental illnesses. Consideration for the GI system role in the development of schizophrenia should entail mechanisms that affect the brain. The view that bio-active and toxic products leave the GI tract, generate an immune response, and go into the brain requires these products to penetrate the endothelial and epithelial barriers in the blood central nervous system and the GI tract interfaces (Daneman and Rescigno, 2009).

The bi-directional communication between the central nervous system and the gut has been confirmed through the high comorbidity between mental and gastrointestinal illnesses (Kennedy *et al.*, 2014). For instance, more than half of the patients affected by mood disorders have irritable bowel syndrome. The gut-brain axis comprises bi-directional communication networks that integrate and regulate the gut's functions and connect them to emotional and cognitive brain centres. The gut-brain axis, which has been linked to the aetiology of several psychiatric disorders, comprises the enteric, autonomic, neuroimmune, and central nervous systems. This axis mediates the impact of environmental and genetic factors on brain function and development.

Stress, infection, inflammation, diet, disrupted sleep patterns, and exposure to antibiotics are environmental factors that can alter the microbiome (Lambert, 2009). For instance, the relationship between exposure to antibiotics and altered function of the brain are common in the antibiotics' side effects such as panic, anxiety, delirium, and psychosis. A recent study has shown that multiple exposures to antibiotics increase the risk of developing anxiety and depression (Lurie *et al.*, 2015). Further studies have reported that administering non-absorbable antimicrobials orally alter the gut microbiota composition. Therefore, changes to the brain function should be one of the reasons the wrong use of antibiotics should be avoided.

The composition and function of the gut microbiota associated with psychological results are also determined by diet. For instance, consuming a high-fat diet can alter microbial diversity and decrease synaptic plasticity (Liu *et al.*, 2015). Microbiota modulates various proteins and neurotrophins involved in plasticity and brain development. Research has shown that these alterations are significant in the pathophysiology of schizophrenia. For instance, the expression of BDNF is believed to have a primary role in the molecular mechanism leading to altered cognition.

Antipsychotics and Gastrointestinal Tract Motility

The function of the gastrointestinal tract motility is a process that is controlled by the parasympathetic cholinergic nervous system. Studies have shown that clozapine, an atypical antipsychotic due to its strong anticholinergic effect, decreases intestinal motility. As a result, this can lead to colitis, constipation, paralytic ileus, bowel obstruction, and death (De Hert *et al.*, 2011). Other antipsychotics having cholinergic effects can generate various side effects such as vomiting, anorexia, abdominal pain, and nausea. Adverse effects of medication on the GI tract are not restricted to the cholinergic system since the gut contains other neurotransmitters receptors such as noradrenergic, serotonin, and dopamine receptors. For instance, the capacity of clozapine to antagonise serotonin receptors can also disrupt the gut function.

Dopaminergic blocking agents, which include sulpiride and haloperidol, can influence various activities on distal colon motility. Monoamine oxidase inhibitors and lithium, on the other hand, could influence the functions of the gastrointestinal tract functions and appetite. Based on our current knowledge, medications used to fight the brain effects of mental disorders have some benefits. However, regulating the gastrointestinal tract nutritional status and discomfort are often not addressed in the treatment and care of people diagnosed with schizophrenia.

Inflammation of the Gastrointestinal Tract

Gastrointestinal tract dysfunction that is has been caused by medication is common in mental illnesses. This kind of dysfunction can lead to nutritional deficiency in schizophrenia patients. Studies have shown that people diagnosed with schizophrenia struggle with colitis, enteritis, and gastritis. Research has also reported that increased anti-*Saccharomyces cerevisiae* antibodies response, which indicated inflammation of the GI, was considerably linked to schizophrenia.

These results show the gastrointestinal tract's relevance to psychiatric disorders (Severance *et al.*, 2012).

The Immune System, Microbiome, and the Brain

Research has shown that disruption of the bacteria balance in the microbiome can cause an overreaction of the immune system, leading to inflammation of the gastrointestinal tract. As a result, diseases may occur in the body and also the brain. The communication and connection between the brain and the gastrointestinal tract are referred to as the gut-brain axis. Studies have shown that infections that occur early in life can adversely impact the mucosal membrane in the gastrointestinal tract. When the gut-brain axis is disrupted, it can interfere with the healthy development of the brain. Alteration of the mucosal membrane can occur due to various factors such as the use of antibiotics, radiation treatment, chemotherapy, and poor diet.

Understanding that the peripheral immune system components such as major histocompatibility complex and complement CIq influence the synaptic pruning and brain synaptogenesis strengthens the hypotheses on how brain disorders such as autism and schizophrenia develop (Boulangr, 2009). Numerous complement pathway components are biologically and genetically associated with schizophrenia (Severance et al., 2014). For instance, studies have documented evidence of the increased volume of CIq comprising gluten and immune complexes in people diagnosed with schizophrenia (Severance et al., 2012).

Additionally, evidence shows noted that during birth, CIq-related antibodies are higher in mothers whose babies later as adults developed psychoses compared to controls (Severance, 2014). The study raises the likelihood that maternal autoantibodies to CIq can interact with foetal CIq during significant brain development stages such as during synapse formation and pruning.

The gut-brain-immune interactome assumes that any product, including those that are bacterially derived, can activate innate and adaptive immune processes such as the CIq activation. Aerobic bacteria attached to the intestinal lumen can produce numerous poorly characterised toxic metabolites and bio-active toxins.

The absorption of these tiny molecules over a long period can damage enzymatic, immunological, biochemical, epigenetic, hormonal, and nutritional sequelae. The gut microbiota has various functions in the regulation of the development and maturation of the immune system.

Processes attributed to the gut microbiota include the control of lymphocyte diversity and the manipulation of some T-cell responses. Other processes include control of anti-inflammatory responses

Faecal Transplantation as a New Therapy of Schizophrenia

Faecal microbiota transplantation refers to the administration of faecal matter solution from a healthy donor to the gastrointestinal tract of a patient. The goal of FMT is to restore or introduce healthy microbes to the patient. Faecal microbiota transplantation has a history of over 1700 years. In the last fifty years, faecal microbiota transplantation has gradually started to be accepted as a treatment approach for mental disorders. The first known use of faeces material for treatment was performed by a Chinese physician Ge Hong in the fourth century (Zhang *et al.*, 2012). The treatment has been used since then in patients having severe diarrhoea.

No medical records are available regarding faecal microbiota transplantation over the centuries.

However, from the seventeenth century, the treatment was used in veterinary both rectally and orally. During the Second World War, German soldiers with bacterial dysentery were treated with warm camel stool (Smits *et al.*, 2013). In 1958, faecal microbiota transplantation for the first time was implemented in modern medicine. Although there is no standard application of faecal microbiota transplantation, Amsterdam protocol is recommended (Smits *et al.*, 2013).

Faecal Microbiota Transplantation Donor Selection

Minimising the risk of disease transmission or risk of infection requires potential donors to go through intensive screening. The stool donor is needed to be healthy and living close to the patient. The faeces donor could either be a close relative or spouse of the patient.

People who have used antibiotics within the last three months have a history of piercing or tattoo, abuse drugs, have metabolic, infectious autoimmune, or allergic diseases are excluded from being faeces donors (Smits *et al.*, 2013). Donor stool is usually from two sources: universal donors through stool banks or patient-directed donors from family members and friends.

Donors that have been selected by a patient are rarely used unless preferred since the patient knows their diet. The patient may also prefer a specific donor to avoid infectious agents that occur in universal donors. Using the stool of patient-directed donors can delay the treatment due to sourcing, testing, and screening the donor (Kim, Schwartz, and Gluck, 2018). Moreover, a donor selected by the patient can also feel coerced to reveal confidential information (Kassam et al., 2013).

It is recommended that faeces be taken from a stool bank since it contains healthy and reliable donors. Additionally, these stool banks undergo regular health screening (Di Bella *et al.*, 2013).

Using universal donors has enhanced various advances in faecal microbiota transplantation. The use of faecal material from several healthy donors can increase the treatment efficacy of ingestion or infusion. Additionally, using thawed or frozen stool in FMT as compared to fresh stool ensures the microbes' viability after freezing. Frozen faeces from stool banks also decreases the recipient's costs and time (Kim, Schwartz, and Gluck, 2018).

The convenience and cost-effectiveness of faecal materials from universal donors has led to the emergence of stool banks like the OpenBiome. This stool bank has strict guidelines on recruiting healthy volunteers. In OpenBiome stool bank, the volunteers are first screened, then the faecal materials produced and stored after freezing. Stool banks also can be used for research and tracking registries from several sites conducting faecal microbiota transplantations (Kazerouni *et al.*, 2015). However, stool banks pose a risk to multiple recipients due to the transmission process or undetectable infections.

Processing of the Faecal Matter

Although slight variations are there depending on specific circumstances, most institutions use the same procedure to prepare the faecal material. One month after the screening, the donor gives fresh stool (Bakken *et al.*, 2011). The stool is collected by the potential donor into a fresh plastic bag and taken to the microbiology laboratory. The faecal material is then diluted with milk, saline, or water. A household hand mixer is used to obtain the faeces suspension. Afterwards, the faeces are passed through a coffee filter or gauze to filter it from solid particles. The subsequent suspension is then put in syringes (Evrensel and Ceylan, 2015).

There are various opinions on whether the faeces material should be mixed with an electric or hand mixer. Additionally, there are diverse views on whether the content should be combined with saline, milk, or water. Faecal microbiota transplantation containing saline has a double recurrence rate compared to one mixed with water. Moreover, the use of an electric mixer reduces the quantity of anaerobic bacteria because of the air mixed in the suspension (Smits et al., 2013). Studies have demonstrated that egg, buttermilk, and yoghurt can dilute the faeces material (Demirci and Uygun, 2014).

The healthy stool solution can be inserted through a tube to the nose, stomach, stomach, and oesophagus into the patient's intestines. Since this is not a pleasant therapy, other options have been developed over time. One alternative option includes faecal transplant through an enema, which means injecting the stool into the lower bowel via the rectum. The faecal material can also be transferred through a capsule comprising freeze-dried bacteria. Most patients prefer the latter treatment. Currently, in humans, faecal microbiota transplantation is used to treat gastrointestinal diseases such as clostridium difficile infections (Wilcox, McGovern, and Hecht, 2020).

These infections are difficult to treat, severe, and frequent. Generally, antibiotics are used to treat bacterial infections. Although antibiotics eliminate pathogens, they also destroy healthy bacteria in the gut, causing an imbalance in the microbiome. Furthermore, antibiotics increase the incidences of bacteria that are resistant to antibiotics. Introducing a healthy microbiome through faecal transplantation can restore the microbiome's imbalance and reduce the number of bacteria that are resistant to antibiotics (Woodworth *et al.*, 2019).

The Impact of Faecal Microbiota Transplantation on Schizophrenia

There is a high rate of comorbidity between schizophrenia and gastrointestinal disturbances. The gut microbiota can influence brain function, development, and behaviour. Faecal microbiota transplantation is a plausible treatment technique for various mental disorders, including schizophrenia (Cryan and Dianh, 2012). Microbiota regulates the hypothalamic-pituitary-glands, which monitor responses to stress, emotions, mood, and immune system. The human gut microbiota also directly influences the functions of the central nervous system. Studies have reported that the gut bacteria through the vagus nerve can trigger a stress response.

Evidence has shown that microbiome composition influences behaviour and stress response (Foster and Neufeld, 2013). Research on faecal microbiota transplantation has demonstrated that the administration of stool from a donor to a recipient causes the patient to mimic the donor's, noticeable characteristics, and phenotype. For instance, an obese donor in an experiment with mice led the recipient to take on the obese phenotype (Million *et al.*, 2013). This mechanism can be used to explain why faecal microbiota transplantation can be an effective therapy for schizophrenia.

Side Effects of Faecal Microbiota Transplantation

Faecal microbiota transplantation is a safe procedure when done in a clinical setting with pre- screened and healthy donors. In such cases, there are few and mild side effects of FMT. However, significant faecal microbiota transplantation risks can occur when there is no care or proper screening during the procedure. Some of the common and mild side effects of FMT include changes in stool where the faecal matter may look and smell different. Another side effect associated with the procedure consists of diarrhoea, which may last for a short period (Smits *et al.*, 2013).

Constipation can also occur after faecal microbiota transplantation; however, if the discomfort progresses to pain, the patient should seek medical intervention (Smits *et al.*, 2013). Cramping and bloating are also normal in the days or hours following the FMT procedure. These side effects are safe and common. Nevertheless, if the symptoms persist for more than a few days, it can be dangerous and could indicate severe complications. There are also significant risks associated with the faecal microbiota transplantation, which can be avoided through adequate preparation and screening.

Some of the significant risks of FMT include perforation of the intestines, although this is rare.

Physical injuries can also occur through nasoenteric tube, colonoscopy, or enema. Additionally, there is a possibility of cutting or scrapping interior walls. Pathogens or parasites can also be transferred through faecal microbiota transplantation. The risk of dysbiosis or imbalance in the gut microbiota is also increased, which may exacerbate the recipient's dysbiosis. Although not common, donors can also transfer some of their characteristics, such as obesity to the recipient (Million *et al.*, 2013).

The above are some of the known side effects of faecal microbiota transplantation. More studies are required to identify other risks that are associated with the procedure. It is not advisable to perform the FMT procedure in a do-it-yourself fashion since the lack of screening and adequate care can increase the risks.

Dietary Balance of the Gut to Reduce Inflammations in Schizophrenia

Over the last two decades, various studies have demonstrated the correlation between high inflammation biomarkers for patients diagnosed with bipolar disorder, schizophrenia, and major depressive disorder (Pariante, 2015). The high levels of these inflammatory cytokines referred to as cytokines show a connection between inflammation and psychiatric symptoms. Inflammation can be caused by various factors such as infections, pollution, toxins, obesity, and a poor diet.

Between 15%–20% of people will struggle with psychiatric disorders, which include anxiety, disorders, depressive disorders, and schizophrenia in their lifetime (Lépine and Briley, 2011). Unfortunately, many mental health disorders have not been adequately treated since most do not sufficiently respond to psychological or pharmacological therapies. As a result, there has been a call for more research on effective treatment for mental health disorders. Studies over the past few years have investigated the connection between diet and mood (Oriach *et al.*, 2016).

Additionally, the impact of the gut microbiota on behaviour and neurobiology has been extensively studied.

Evidence is emerging, showing the strong impact of the gut and diet on neurological processes and emotional behaviour. Since diet has a strong influence on the gut microbiota, the two factors are interlinked (Oriach *et al.*, 2016). Understanding the association between the gut microbiome and diet and its effect on mental health disorders can help prevent or manage the symptoms of these disorders. Studies in the past few years have reported the significant impact of the gut microbiota on human health.

Changes in the gut microbiota affect the immune system, gut microbiome, metabolic pathways, and intestinal homeostasis of the host. Diet influences the population of the gut microbial.

Studies have shown that diet can affect gut microbiota composition. The symbiotic connection between diverse gut microbial communities modulates the immune system. Hence any dysbiosis can lead to the dysregulation of the immune system (Rajoka *et al.*, 2017). Dysbiosis of the function of the gut microbiota has been linked to various neurophysical and behavioural deficits.

As a result, studies have been dedicated to developing treatment approaches for psychiatric disorder by focusing on the gut microbiota.

Several factors can impact the composition and health of the gut microbiota. Some of these factors include genetics and birth delivery method. For instance, shortly after birth, the human gut is colonised by microbiota. Natural delivery ensures that the babies have a higher count of gut bacteria than those delivered through caesarean section (Huurre *et al.*, 2008). However, the diet has been one of the most vital factors affecting the human gut microbiota from childhood to old age. Therefore, dietary interventions can regulate the psychiatric symptoms linked to the brain-gut axis dysfunction.

Studies have also focused on the connection between gut microbiota and food and their impact on health. A disruption of the microbiome, metabolism, and nutrition are some of the factors associated with deregulating the host's normal homeostasis. Such interruption in the microbiome's function and structure has been linked to the development of diverse illnesses. The human gut comprises thousands of types of microorganisms. This taxonomic variety needs different energy and nutrients sources for microbial development and function.

In the past few years, there have been studies on the relationship between mental health and diet.

For instance, a high-quality diet has been linked to reduced suicidal risk (Lai *et al.*, 2014).

Nutrition has a significant effect on mental health. Severe nutritional deficits can lead to psychotic and depressive disorders (O'Neil *et al.*, 2014). Furthermore, people diagnosed with schizophrenia when in asymptomatic episodes frequently display an unhealthy diet. Over the years, there have been changes in dietary patterns. There has been a gradual increase in the consumption of refined sugars, high-fat foods, and red meat.

Westernised diet combined with a sedentary lifestyle often changes the composition of the gut microbiota. As a result, higher incidences of inflammatory disorders, including diabetes, autoimmune diseases, allergies, depression, and obesity, have been reported (Maslowski and Mackay, 2011). Therefore, it is evident that there is a need to enhance the nutritional value of food and hence human health. Additionally, it is necessary to comprehend the biological connection between microbiota and diet. The consumption of a diet saturated with refined sugar and saturated fat accompanied by little fibre is common in people diagnosed with schizophrenia (Andrade, 2016).

A study was conducted, which showed that a high intake of refined sugars leads to a poor state of mind in schizophrenia patients experiencing poor social functioning. The role of diet in regulating the human gut microbiota metabolic activity and composition is growing in recognition. Diet, especially one with high-fibre content, is considered the best way to enhance the health of the gut microbiota. Healthy gut microbiota is necessary for the immune system's development (O'Neil et al., 2014).

Western vs. Rural Diet

Most studies comparing Western and rural communities have reported that gut microbiota adapts to their environments. Western diet has been linked to the loss of bacterial species leading to a subsequent decrease in microbial stability and diversity. Studies have presented a reduction in microbiota diversity, comparing it to a hunter-gatherer community (Schnorr et al., 2014). Other studies have demonstrated the effect of diet on microbial biodiversity in diverse human populations (De Filippo et al., 2010). African children who have a high intake of fibre and a low-fat diet have demonstrated a higher degree of microbial richness and diversity.

On the contrary, based on the study, European children's high intake of Western diet showed reduced microbial richness and diversity (Ou *et al.*, 2013). African children had less firmicutes and more phylum bacteroidetes. In contrast, European children demonstrated a high level of firmicutes and enterobacteriaceae (De Filippo *et al.*, 2010). Unhealthy foods such as fast foods, trans-fatty acids, processed meat, and refined grains can increase inflammation by influencing gut health. The gut, as earlier discussed, is a significant link between our biological systems and diet.

Junk food can weaken the lining of the gut barrier that protects the food particles from entering the bloodstream. When food articles are in the wrong region in the blood, an inflammatory response is activated. When a person's diet primarily consists of poor-quality foods, the inflammatory response is unlikely to be triggered; this increases the risk of mental health disorders like schizophrenia.

Mediterranean Diet

A Mediterranean diet consists of grains, vegetables, fruits, polyunsaturated, or monounsaturated fats (Mörkl *et al.*, 2020). Therefore, it is often regarded as a diet that enhances physical and mental health. A study has reported that a Mediterranean diet can decrease inflammation in Crohn's disease. A Mediterranean diet rich in nutrients is critical for regulating mood as it provides necessary probiotics and fibre essential for proper digestion. A poor diet that interacts with the gut microbiota and immune system can affect the brain function. Processed food lacks enzymes and nutrients that are essential for mental health.

A diet that lacks foods that contain nutrients such as fish, whole grains, vegetables, and fruits can adversely affect the immune system and the gene expression. Additionally, such a diet can damage the gut microbiota and mental health. The human gut microbiota depends on the adequate consumption of food rich in fibre (Mörkl *et al.*, 2020). On the contrary, a diet with high refined sugars and saturated fats adversely affects neurotrophins whose role is to shield the brain from oxidative stress and enhance the development of new cells.

Studies have shown that there is a connection between diet and the volume of the hippocampus.

Additionally, based on studies, saturated fats impact the stress response system. A high-fat diet and processed foods are particularly harmful to the gut (Mörkl *et al.*, 2020). Processed foods should be avoided since they contain refined carbohydrates and unhealthy fats, which, according to studies, adversely affect the gut microbiota.

Vegetarian Diet

Over the past few years, a vegetarian diet has gained recognition as a therapeutic and healthy diet for various chronic diseases. Studies have shown that a diet comprising whole grains, unprocessed fruits, and whole vegetables can reduce inflammation (Glick-Bauer and Yeh, 2014).

A vegan diet can protect against inflammatory and metabolic diseases. Studies have reported fewer symptoms of mood disturbance, stress, anxiety, and depression among vegetarians. High antioxidant levels in the blood from fruits and vegetables have been linked to low risk of depression and suicide. Studies have also shown that a diet that has high-fibre content enhances stable and healthy gut bacteria.

A high-fibre intake alongside other plant-based diet enhances the growth of bacteria that are beneficial and reduces inflammation. Fibre is known to increase short-chain fatty acids associated with better immunity and intestinal function. The gastrointestinal tract microbiota is responsible for producing short-chain fatty acids (Macfarlane and Macfarlane, 2012). A plant- based or vegetarian diet is an effective way of making sure the gut health is optimal. A vegetarian diet enhances the growth of a highly diverse gut microbial system.

Research has demonstrated that large food particles such as those found in plants can lead to more nutrients reaching the gastrointestinal system. As a result, the nutrient transmission to the gut microbiota is enhanced. Therefore, a plant-based diet is believed to support the development of fibre-degrading bacteria beneficial in the colon.

Gluten-Free Diet

Gluten is a protein that is found in barley, rye, wheat, and milk among other foods. Intriguing studies have reported that individuals who are genetically intolerant to gluten are at a high risk of developing schizophrenia (Ergün, Urhan, and Ayer, 2018). During the gluten metabolism, casomorphin and gliadorphin can adversely affect the brain function. Casomorphin and gliadorphin are neuropeptides that have a structural resemblance to the dairy items' by-products.

These neuropeptides interrupt the brain's neurotransmitter's communication, leading to psychological symptoms. Some of the symptoms include aggression, fatigue, and hallucinations.

People diagnosed with celiac disease, a genetic digestive disorder is three times more likely to develop schizophrenia. Evidence has shown that a gluten-free diet can enhance the symptoms of schizophrenia in some patients. Evidence has also demonstrated that schizophrenia patients with high antibodies, especially antigliadin antibodies who adhere to a gluten-free diet, experienced a greater decrease in negative symptoms than those who did not follow a similar diet (Porcelli et al., 2014).

Most schizophrenia patients have a high intolerance to gluten. High levels of antigliadin antibodies (AGA IgG) in schizophrenia patients have been linked to having fewer positive symptoms of schizophrenia (Porcelli *et al.*, 2014). An example of an immune response to gluten is the generation of antibodies like the anti-gliadin. An increase in the levels of such antibodies has been witnessed in people diagnosed with schizophrenia. Abnormal breakdown of gliadorphin by dipeptidyl peptidase IV causes an accumulation in the neurotoxic levels, further generating psychoactive effects. A study conducted on schizophrenia patients who had high levels of AGA IgG on a gluten-free diet showed that after a short period, their intestinal and psychiatric symptoms were enhanced.

However, the treatment did not reduce the positive symptoms of schizophrenia but significantly enhanced negative symptoms such as the inability to experience pleasure, a lack of emotions, and motivation. Nevertheless, more research is required in the future regarding a gluten-free diet as an alternative treatment for schizophrenia (Brietzke *et al.*, 2018).

Omega 3

The common treatment for people diagnosed with schizophrenia includes antipsychotic drugs.

However, these medications are not effective for every patient and have various side effects.

Additionally, these medications have to be used for a lifetime. Several alternatives exist to antipsychotic drugs in treating the onset of psychiatric drugs such as schizophrenia. Omega- 3 fatty acids are one such treatment and are often linked to fewer side effects and risks (Watson, 2014).

Fatty acids from Omega-3 are normally found in walnuts, eggs, and fatty fish. Several studies have suggested that Omega-3 fatty acids may reduce inflammation and enhance symptoms of different psychiatric disorders. Schizophrenia patients frequently have elevated inflammatory chemicals and reduced levels of Omega-3 fatty acids. Evidence has shown that Omega-3 fatty acids can impede the development of schizophrenia in individuals who are at a high risk of developing this mental disorder (Watson, 2014).

Omega-3 fatty acids can have a positive impact on schizophrenia symptoms. Additionally, these fatty acids can increase the antipsychotic medication efficacy. Studies have also reported that adding two or three grams of Omega-3 fatty acids to antipsychotic drugs can reduce schizophrenia symptoms (Watson, 2014). These treatments can also hinder psychosis development in a population that is at high risk (Amminger *et al.*, 2010).

Probiotics for Schizophrenia

From historical times, probiotics have been used for psychological enhancement, treatment, and health supplements. In the past few decades, research has found the role of the gut microbiota in the brain-gut axis that can change the human mind and behaviour through the central nervous system. Knowledge of the gut microbiome has led to the development of probiotics. When administered, probiotics refer to living microorganisms that confer health benefits to the host (Butel, 2014). *Bifidobacterium* and l*actobacillus* genera are commonly used probiotics in both humans and animals.

Bifidobacterium longum, according to studies, has a positive impact on cognition (Dickerson eta l., 2018). *Lactobacillus rhamnosus* enhances the GABA metabolism and receptor stimulation in the amygdala, hippocampus, and prefrontal cortex. A probiotic supplementation randomised trial has shown that exposure to *Bifidobacterium animalis* and *Lactobacillus rhamnosus* probiotics is linked to reduced re-hospitalisation rates and decreases inpatient admissions (Dickerson *et al.*, 2018). Currently, probiotics are available as capsules, fermented drinks or milk, wafers, tablets, chocolates, cheese, sachets, and yoghurts.

Probiotics can be obtained from drugstores, health food stores, pharmacies, webshops, or grocery stores (McFarland, 2015). Schizophrenia patients who often struggle with stress, lactose sensitivity, low nutrition, and inflammatory stress can benefit from probiotic supplementation. Administration of probiotics for schizophrenia can also be considered since it helps address the gastrointestinal tract upset, particularly constipation, which is common in these patients. Studies have shown that over 50% of schizophrenia patients struggle with constipation (Dinan, T. Borre, and Cryan, 2014).

In the recent past, probiotics have gained recognition for diverse clinical applications such as the treatment for mood and gastrointestinal disorders. Studies have also shown that in some schizophrenia patients, probiotics can reduce hallucinations and delusions. Probiotics are also useful in reversing inflammation that is common in schizophrenia. Probiotics bacteria can generate neurotransmitters and monoamines, such as serotonin and GABA. These bacteria can activate an anti-inflammatory effect on the immune system. Additionally, the microbes can reduce the hypothalamic-pituitary-adrenal axis activation.

Probiotics supplementation is also useful in managing the negative symptoms of schizophrenia.

Probiotic supplementation is beneficial to gut microbiota as it contains immune-modulatory and anti-inflammatory properties (Frei, Akdis, and O'Mahony, 2015). Probiotics have been used to alter the functions of the central nervous system. Probiotics can change the composition of gut microbiota, thereby enhancing mental health. The functions of the central nervous system that have been changed by probiotics include memory abilities and psychiatric disorders. Probiotics can directly change the central nervous system's biochemistry by affecting the levels of dopamine, serotonin, and BDNF. As a result, the human mind and behaviour are influenced (Liu *et al.*, 2016).

The enteric and vagus nerve is involved in the brain-gut interaction and can be influenced by some probiotics (Bravo *et al.*, 2011). Probiotics communicate with the brain through the endocrine system, spinal cord, and the vagus nerve. Studies have reported that the hypothalamic pituitary adrenal axis stress response involved in regulating the emotion and mood can be reduced by probiotics, thereby lessening the corticosteroid levels. Probiotics could also influence the immune system; this limits inflammation and the production of the pro-inflammatory cytokine. Consequently, the nervous and endocrine systems are affected (Desbonnet *et al.*, 2010).

Furthermore, probiotics can manipulate the gut microbiota by enhancing the microbiota composition and diversity. Better gut microbiota alters metabolites, including tryptophan and short-chain fatty acids; this may indirectly enhance the function of the central nervous system (Desbonnet *et al.*, 2010). Probiotics are also useful in reducing the high levels of cortisol in most mood disorders. Most psychiatric and neurodegenerative disorders such as schizophrenia, bipolar disorder, major depressive disorder, and epilepsy activate a dysregulated BDNF expression with low plasma and serum levels (Martinez-Levy *et al.*, 2018). BDNF alterations have been associated with cognitive deficits that are common in schizophrenia. Studies have reported an enhancement in the brain-derived neurotrophic factor (BDNF) levels through the use of probiotic supplementation. Probiotics enhance the differentiation of brain development, brain plasticity, and memory (Hwang, Castelli, and Gonzalez-Lima, 2017). Negative metabolic effects, weight gain, and constipation are also common in schizophrenia due to the use of antipsychotics; all this can be alleviated through the use of probiotics (Tomasik *et al.*, 2015).

Probiotics stimulate positive immunomodulatory impact by regulating the host's immune system responses against non-pathogenic and pathogenic organisms. Probiotics achieve this effect by stimulating receptors that recognise patterns and mediate the identification of bacterial antigens.

The signalling cascades are then activated, further regulating the immune response (Reid *et al.*, 2011). A recent study has demonstrated the potential impact of *Bifidobacterium breve strain A1in*, enhancing depressive and anxiety symptoms in twenty-nine schizophrenia patients (Okubo *et al.*, 2019). The study reported that administering probiotics in people diagnosed with schizophrenia helped normalise the levels of *Candida albicans* antibody. *Candida albicans* was linked to gut problems in twenty-two schizophrenia male patients. In another study, fifty-seven chronic schizophrenia patients had their immune-related serum proteins measured after probiotic supplementation. The result showed that after this procedure, the von Willebrand factor levels reduced (Tomasik *et al.*, 2015).

On the other hand, BDNF and monocyte chemotactic protein-1 levels increased. These results may be an indication of decreased intestinal permeability (Tomasik *et al.*, 2015). The results also reported that schizophrenia patients under probiotic supplementation had less risk of developing severe bowel issues. According to the studies, probiotics can eliminate bowel problems, which are common in schizophrenia. The immunomodulatory effect, which is activated by probiotics on schizophrenia patients, affects molecules that are not responsive to antipsychotic treatment.

The quality of the gut flora can be enhanced by regular consumption of foods rich in probiotics.

Evidence has shown that probiotics play a significant role in improving the gut-brain and brain homeostasis. Therefore, it is recommended and beneficial to consume foods that have high probiotic content. It is necessary to note that not every individual who has inflammation is diagnosed with mental health disorders. Additionally, not every person who has a psychiatric disorder has high levels of inflammatory biomarkers. Consequently, not all people with mental health disorders will benefit from anti-inflammatory therapy. Studies have reported that people diagnosed with mental health disorders and have increased immune markers are the most responsive to anti-inflammatory treatment (Papakostas *et al.*, 2013). As a result, there is a need to recognise inflammatory biomarkers through a diagnostic blood test.

This test can be used to identify the kind of therapy that is necessary for a particular patient.

Research suggests that there is a psychiatric patient who can benefit most from inflammatory augmentation. Some patients who struggle with mental health issues are resistant to conventional therapies and can benefit from inflammatory agent augmentation (Kiecolt-Glaser, Derry, and Fagundes, 2015)

References

Aaronson, S. T., Sears, P., Ruvuna, F., Bunker, M., Conway, C. R., Dougherty, D. D., . . . and Zajecka, J. M. (2017) 'A 5-year observational study of patients with treatment-resistant depression treated with vagus nerve stimulation or treatment as usual: comparison of response, remission, and suicidality', *American Journal of Psychiatry*, *174*(7), pp. 640–648.

Abraham, P. F., and Calabrese, J. R. (2008) 'Evidenced-based pharmacologic treatment of borderline personality disorder: A shift from SSRIs to anticonvulsants and atypical antipsychotics?', *Journal of Affective Disorders*, *111*(1), pp. 21–30.

American Psychiatric Association, and American Psychiatric Association (2013) *Diagnostic And Statistical Manual of Mental Disorders*: *DSM-5*.

American Psychiatric Association (2013) 'Diagnostic and statistical manual of mental Disorders', *BMC Med*, *17*, pp. 133–137.

American Psychiatric Association (2013) *Diagnostic and statistical manual of mental disorders (DSM-5)*, American Psychiatric Pub.

Andrade, C. (2016) *Cardiometabolic Risks in Schizophrenia and Directions for Intervention, 2: Nonpharmacological Interventions*.

Andrews, L. W. (2010) *Encyclopedia of Depression (2 volumes)*, ABC-CLIO.

Arntz, A., and Van Genderen, H. (2011) *Schema Therapy for Borderline Personality Disorder*, John Wiley & Sons.

Bakken, J. S., Borody, T., Brandt, L. J., Brill, J. V., Demarco, D. C., Franzos, M. A., . . . and Moore, T. A. (2011) 'Treating Clostridium difficile infection with fecal microbiota Transplantation', *Clinical Gastroenterology and Hepatology*, *9*(12), pp. 1044–1049.

Bastiaanssen, T. F., Cowan, C. S., Claesson, M. J., Dinan, T. G., and Cryan, J. F. (2019) 'Making sense of . . . the microbiome in psychiatry', *International Journal of Neuropsychopharmacology*, *22*(1), pp. 37–52.

Bateman, A. W. (2012) 'Treating borderline personality disorder in clinical practice'.

Bateman, A. W., and Fonagy, P. E. (2012) *Handbook of Mentalizing in Mental Health Practice*, American Psychiatric Publishing, Inc.

Bateman, A. W., and Krawitz, R. (2013) *Borderline Personality Disorder: An Evidence-Based Guide for Generalist Mental Health Professionals*, Oxford University Press.

Bateman, A., and Fonagy, P. (2010) 'Mentalization based treatment for borderline personality Disorder', *World Psychiatry*, *9*(1), p. 11.

Bateman, A., and Fonagy, P. (2016) *Mentalization-Based Treatment for Personality Disorders: A Practical Guide*, Oxford University Press.

Beatson, J. A., and Rao, S. (2013) 'Depression and borderline personality disorder', *Medical Journal of Australia*, *199*, pp. S24–S27.

Bechter, K. (2013) 'Updating the mild encephalitis hypothesis of schizophrenia', *Progress in Neuro-Psychopharmacology and Biological Psychiatry*, *42*, pp. 71–91.

Bellino, S., Paradiso, E., and Bogetto, F. (2008) 'Efficacy and tolerability of pharmacotherapies for borderline personality disorder', *CNS Drugs*, *22*(8), pp. 671–692.

Benedict, C., Vogel, H., Jonas, W., Woting, A., Blaut, M., Schürmann, A., and Cedernaes, J. (2016) 'Gut microbiota and glucometabolic alterations in response to recurrent partial sleep deprivation in normal-weight young individuals', *Molecular Metabolism*, *5*(12), pp. 1175–1186.

Bergfeld, I. O., Mantione, M., Figee, M., Schuurman, P. R., Lok, A., and Denys, D. (2018) 'Treatment-resistant depression and suicidality', *Journal of Affective Disorders*, *235*, pp. 362–367.

Bertsch, K., Schmidinger, I., Neumann, I. D., and Herpertz, S. C. (2013) 'Reduced plasma oxytocin levels in female patients with a borderline personality disorder', *Hormones and Behavior*, *63*(3), pp. 424–429.

Bewernick, B. H., Hurlemann, R., Matusch, A., Kayser, S., Grubert, C., Hadrysiewicz, B., . . . and Brockmann, H. (2010) 'Nucleus accumbens deep brain stimulation decreases ratings of depression and anxiety in treatment-resistant depression', *Biological Psychiatry*, *67*(2), pp. 110–116.

Blaser, M. J. (2016) 'Antibiotic use and its consequences for the normal microbiome', *Science*, *352*(6285), pp. 544–545.

Blum, N., St. John, D., Pfohl, B., Stuart, S., McCormick, B., Allen, J., . . . and Black, D. W. (2008) 'Systems Training for Emotional Predictability and Problem Solving (STEPPS) for outpatients with borderline personality disorder: a randomized controlled trial and 1-year follow-up', *American Journal of Psychiatry*, *165*(4), pp. 468–478.

Boisseau, C. L., Yen, S., Markowitz, J. C., Grilo, C. M., Sanislow, C. A., Shea, M. T., . . . and McGlashan, T. H. (2013) 'Individuals with single versus multiple suicide attempts over 10 years of prospective follow-up', *Comprehensive Psychiatry*, *54*(3), pp. 238–242. *Borderline Personality Disorder*, Oxford University Press.

Bornovalova, M. A., Hicks, B. M., Iacono, W. G., and McGue, M. (2009) 'Stability, change, and heritability of borderline personality disorder traits from adolescence to adulthood: A longitudinal twin study', *Development and Psychopathology*, *21*(4), pp. 1335–1353.

Borre, Y. E., O'Keeffe, G. W., Clarke, G., Stanton, C., Dinan, T. G., and Cryan, J. F. (2014) 'Microbiota and neurodevelopmental windows: implications for brain disorders, *Trends in Molecular Medicine*, *20*(9), pp. 509–518.

Boulanger, L. M. (2009) 'Immune proteins in brain development and synaptic plasticity.' *Neuron*, *64*(1), pp. 93–109.

Braun, U., Harneit, A., Pergola, G., Menara, T., Schaefer, A., Betzel, R. F., . . . and Blasi, G. (2019) 'Brain state stability during working memory is explained by network control theory, modulated by dopamine D1/D2 receptor function, and diminished in schizophrenia', *arXiv preprint arXiv:1906.09290*.

Bravo, J. A., Forsythe, P., Chew, M. V., Escaravage, E., Savignac, H. M., Dinan, T. G., . . . and Cryan, J. F. (2011) 'Ingestion of Lactobacillus strain regulates emotional behavior and central GABA receptor expression in a mouse via the vagus nerve', *Proceedings of the National Academy of Sciences*, *108*(38), pp. 16050–16055.

Bresin, K. (2014) 'Five indices of emotion regulation in participants with a history of nonsuicidal self-injury: A daily diary study', *Behavior Therapy*, *45*(1), pp. 56–66.

Bridler, R., Häberle, A., Müller, S. T., Cattapan, K., Grohmann, R., Toto, S., . . . and Greil, W. (2015) 'Psychopharmacological treatment of 2195 in-patients with borderline personality disorder: a comparison with other psychiatric disorders', *European Neuropsychopharmacology*, *25*(6), pp. 763–772.

Brietzke, E., Cerqueira, R. O., Mansur, R. B., and McIntyre, R. S. (2018) 'Gluten related illnesses and severe mental disorders: a comprehensive review', *Neuroscience and Biobehavioral Reviews*, *84*, pp. 368–375.

Brown, J., Blum, N., and Black, D. W. (2013) 'Systems Training for Emotional Predictability and Problem Solving: An Advanced Understanding', *Journal of Law Enforcement*, *3*(4).

Brüne, M., Dimaggio, G., and Edel, M. A. (2013) 'Mentalization-Based Group Therapy for Inpatients with Borderline Personality Disorder: Preliminary Findings', *Clinical Neuropsychiatry*, *10*(5).

Brunner, R., Henze, R., Richter, J., and Kaess, M. (2015) 'Neurobiological findings in youth with a borderline personality disorder', *Scandinavian Journal of Child and Adolescent Psychiatry and Psychology*, *3*(1), pp. 22–30.

Burke, D. A., Rotstein, H. G., and Alvarez, V. A. (2017) 'Striatal local circuitry: a new framework for lateral inhibition', *Neuron*, *96*(2), pp. 267–284.

Butel, M. J. (2014) 'Probiotics, gut microbiota and health', *Médecine et Maladies Infectieuses*, *44*(1), pp. 1–8.

Buzsáki, G., and Watson, B. O. (2012) 'Brain rhythms and neural syntax: implications for efficient coding of cognitive content and neuropsychiatric disease', *Dialogues in Clinical Neuroscience*, *14*(4), p. 345.

Cailhol, L., Roussignol, B., Klein, R., Bousquet, B., Simonetta-Moreau, M., Schmitt, L., . . . and Birmes, P. (2014) 'Borderline personality disorder and rTMS: a pilot trial', *Psychiatry Research*, *216*(1), pp. 155–157.

Caine, E. D. (2012) 'Suicide prevention is a winnable battle', *American Journal of Public Health*, *102*(S1), pp. S1–S6.

Capps, D. (2010) *Understanding Psychosis: Issues, Treatments, and Challenges for Sufferers and Their Families*, Rowman & Littlefield Publishers.

Carlstedt, R. A. (2009) *Handbook of Integrative Clinical Psychology, Psychiatry, and Behavioral Medicine: Perspectives, Practices, and Research*, Springer Publishing Company.

Carrion, V. G., Weems, C. F., Watson, C., Eliez, S., Menon, V., and Reiss, A. L. (2009) 'Converging evidence for abnormalities of the prefrontal cortex and evaluation of midsagittal structures in pediatric posttraumatic stress disorder: an MRI study', *Psychiatry Research: Neuroimaging*, *172*(3), pp. 226–234.

Cassidy, C. M., Balsam, P. D., Weinstein, J. J., Rosengard, R. J., Slifstein, M., Daw, N. D., . . . and Horga, G. (2018) 'A perceptual inference mechanism for hallucinations linked to striatal dopamine', *Current Biology*, *28*(4), pp. 503–514.

Castro-Nallar, E., Bendall, M. L., Pérez-Losada, M., Sabuncyan, S., Severance, E. G., Dickerson, F. B., . . . and Crandall, K. A. (2015) 'Composition, taxonomy and functional diversity of the oropharynx microbiome in individuals with schizophrenia and controls', *PeerJ*, *3*, e1140.

Chalker, S. A., Carmel, A., Atkins, D. C., Landes, S. J., Kerbrat, A. H., and Comtois, K. A. (2015) 'Examining challenging behaviors of clients with a borderline personality Disorder', *Behavior Research and Therapy*, *75*, pp. 11–19.

Chanen, A. M., and McCutcheon, L. (2013) 'Prevention and early intervention for borderline personality disorder: current status and recent evidence', *The British Journal of Psychiatry*, *202*(s54), pp. s24–s29.

Chanen, A. M., Jackson, H. J., McCutcheon, L. K., Jovev, M., Dudgeon, P., Yuen, H. P., . . . and

Clarkson, V. (2009) 'Early intervention for adolescents with borderline personality disorder: quasi-experimental comparison with treatment as usual', *Australian and New Zealand Journal of Psychiatry*, *43*(5), pp. 397–408.

Chanen, A. M., Jovev, M., Djaja, D., McDougall, E., Yuen, H. P., Rawlings, D., and Jackson, H. J. (2008) 'Screening for borderline personality disorder in outpatient youth', *Journal of Personality Disorders*, *22*(4), pp. 353–364.

Chanen, A. M., Jovev, M., McCutcheon, L. K., Jackson, H. J., and McGorry, P. D. (2008) 'Borderline personality disorder in young people and the prospects for prevention and early intervention', *Current Psychiatry Reviews*, *4*(1), pp. 48–57.

Chanen, A. M., Mccutcheon, L. K., Germano, D., Nistico, H., Jackson, H. J., and Mcgorry, P. D. (2009) 'The HYPE Clinic: an early intervention service for borderline personality Disorder', *Journal of Psychiatric Practice*, *15*(3), pp. 163–172.

Chapman, A., and Gratz, K. (2007) *The Borderline Personality Disorder Survival Guide: Everything You Need to Know About Living with BPD*, New Harbinger Publications.

Choi-Kain, L. W., and Gunderson, J. G. (eds.) (2019) *Applications of Good Psychiatric Management for Borderline Personality Disorder: A Practical Guide*, American Psychiatric Pub.

Choi-Kain, L. W., Albert, E. B., and Gunderson, J. G. (2016) 'Evidence-based treatments for borderline personality disorder: implementation, integration, and stepped care', *Harvard Review of Psychiatry*, *24*(5), pp. 342–356.

Clarkin, J. F., Levy, K. N., Lenzenweger, M. F., and Kernberg, O. F. (2013) 'Evaluating three treatments for borderline personality disorder: A multiwave study', *Focus*, *11*(2), pp. 269–276.

Cloitre, M., Garvert, D. W., Weiss, B., Carlson, E. B., and Bryant, R. A. (2014) 'Distinguishing PTSD, complex PTSD, and borderline personality disorder: A latent class analysis', *European Journal of Psychotraumatology, 5*(1), p. 25097.

Coyle, T. N., Shaver, J. A., and Linehan, M. M. (2018) 'On the potential for iatrogenic effects of psychiatric crisis services: the example of dialectical behavioral therapy for adult women with a borderline personality disorder', *Journal of Consulting and Clinical Psychology, 86*(2), p. 116.

Cristea, I. A., Gentili, C., Cotet, C. D., Palomba, D., Barbui, C., and Cuijpers, P. (2017) 'Efficacy of psychotherapies for borderline personality disorder: a systematic review and meta-analysis', *JAMA Psychiatry, 74*(4), pp. 319–328.

Crowell, S. E., and Kaufman, E. A. (2016) 'Development of self-inflicted injury: Comorbidities and continuities with borderline and antisocial personality traits', *Development and Psychopathology, 28*(4pt1), pp. 1071–1088.

Cryan, J. F., and Dinan, T. G. (2012) 'Mind-altering microorganisms: the impact of the gut microbiota on brain and behaviour', *Nature Reviews Neuroscience, 13*(10), pp. 701–712.

Császár, N., Kapócs, G., and Bókkon, I. (2019) 'A possible key role of vision in the development of schizophrenia', *Reviews in the Neurosciences, 30*(4), pp. 359–379.

Cyprien, F., Courtet, P., Malafosse, A., Maller, J., Meslin, C., Bonafé, A., . . . and Artero, S. (2011) 'Suicidal behavior is associated with reduced corpus callosum area', *Biological Psychiatry, 70*(4), pp. 320–326.

Daneman, R., and Rescigno, M. (2009) 'The gut immune barrier and the blood-brain barrier: are they so different?', *Immunity, 31*(5), pp. 722–735.

Das, P., Calhoun, V., and Malhi, G. S. (2014) 'Bipolar and borderline patients display differential patterns of functional connectivity among resting state networks. *Neuroimage, 98*, pp. 73–81.

De Filippo, C., Cavalieri, D., Di Paola, M., Ramazzotti, M., Poullet, J. B., Massart, S., . . . and Lionetti, P. (2010) 'Impact of diet in shaping gut microbiota revealed by a comparative study in children from Europe and rural Africa', *Proceedings of the National Academy of Sciences*, *107*(33), pp. 14691–14696.

de Leon, V. C., Drysdale, A. T., Conway, C. R., and Aaronson, S. T. (2019) 'Predictors of response for vagus nerve stimulation in treatment-resistant depression', *Personalized Medicine in Psychiatry*.

Delaloye, S., and Holtzheimer, P. E. (2014) 'Deep brain stimulation in the treatment of Depression', *Dialogues in Clinical Neuroscience*, *16*(1), p. 83.

Delezie, J., and Handschin, C. (2018) 'Endocrine crosstalk between skeletal muscle and the Brain', *Frontiers in Neurology*, *9*, p. 698.

Demirci, H., and Uygun, A. (2014) 'Fekal Transplantasyon Nasıl ve Kime Uygulanmalı?', *Güncel Gastroenteroloji*, *18*, pp. 444–447.

Desbonnet, L., Garrett, L., Clarke, G., Kiely, B., Cryan, J. F., and Dinan, T. G. (2010) 'Effects of the probiotic Bifidobacterium infantis in the maternal separation model of depression', *Neuroscience*, *170*(4), pp. 1179–1188.

Desmyter, S., Duprat, R., Baeken, C., Van Autreve, S., Audenaert, K., and van Heeringen, K. (2016) 'Accelerated intermittent theta burst stimulation for suicide risk in therapy- resistant depressed patients: a randomized, sham-controlled trial', *Frontiers in Human Neuroscience*, *10*, p. 480.

Di Bella, S., Drapeau, C., García-Almodóvar, E., and Petrosillo, N. (2013) 'Fecal microbiota transplantation: the state of the art', *Infectious Disease Reports*, *5*(2).

Dickerson, F., Adamos, M., Katsafanas, E., Khushalani, S., Origoni, A., Savage, C., . . . and Yolken, R. H. (2018) 'Adjunctive probiotic microorganisms to prevent rehospitalization in patients with acute mania: a randomized controlled trial', *Bipolar Disorders*, *20*(7), pp. 614–621.

Dimeff, L. A., and Koerner, K. E. (2007) *Dialectical Behavior Therapy in Clinical Practice: Applications Across Disorders and Settings*, Guilford Press.

Dinan, T. G., Borre, Y. E., and Cryan, J. F. (2014) 'Genomics of

schizophrenia: time to consider the gut microbiome?',
Molecular Psychiatry, *19*(12), pp. 1252–1257.

Dinan, T. G., Stanton, C., and Cryan, J. F. (2013) 'Psychobiotics: a
novel class of psychotropics', *Biological Psychiatry*, *74*(10), pp.
720–726.

Donse, L., Padberg, F., Sack, A. T., Rush, A. J., and Arns, M. (2018)
'Simultaneous rTMS and psychotherapy in major depressive
disorder: clinical outcomes and predictors from a large
naturalistic study', *Brain Stimulation*, *11*(2), pp. 337–345.

Dougherty, D. D., and Widge, A. S. (2017) 'Neurotherapeutic
interventions for psychiatric Illness', *Harvard Review of
Psychiatry*, *25*(6), p. 253.

Dougherty, D. D., Rezai, A. R., Carpenter, L. L., Howland, R. H.,
Bhati, M. T., O'Reardon, J. P., . . . and Cusin, C. (2015) 'A
randomized sham-controlled trial of deep brain stimulation
of the ventral capsule/ventral striatum for chronic treatment-
resistant depression', *Biological Psychiatry*, *78*(4), pp. 240–248.

Douglas, B., and James, P. (2013) *Common Presenting Issues in
Psychotherapeutic Practice*, Sage.

Ducasse, D., Lopez-Castroman, J., Dassa, D., Brand-Arpon, V.,
Dupuy-Maurin, K., Lacourt, L., . . . and Olié, E. (2019)
'Exploring the boundaries between borderline personality
disorder and suicidal behavior disorder', *European Archives of
Psychiatry and Clinical Neuroscience*, pp. 1–9.

Durand, V. M., and Barlow, D. H. (2012) *Essentials of Abnormal
Psychology*, Cengage Learning.

Edelstein, B. A., Hersen, M., and Thase, M. E. (eds.) (2013) *Handbook
of Outpatient Treatment of Adults: Nonpsychotic Mental Disorders*,
Springer Science+Business Media.

Emsell, L., Leemans, A., Langan, C., Van Hecke, W., Barker, G.
J., McCarthy, P., . . . and McDonald, C. (2013) 'Limbic
and callosal white matter changes in euthymic bipolar I
disorder: an advanced diffusion magnetic resonance imaging
tractography study', *Biological Psychiatry*, *73*(2), pp. 194–201.

Epstein, J., Pan, H., Kocsis, J. H., Yang, Y., Butler, T., Chusid,

J., . . . and Silbersweig, D. A. (2006) 'Lack of ventral striatal response to positive stimuli in depressed versus normal Subjects', *American Journal of Psychiatry*, *163*(10), pp. 1784–1790.

Ergün, C., Urhan, M., and Ayer, A. (2018) 'A review on the relationship between gluten and schizophrenia: Is gluten the cause?', *Nutritional Neuroscience*, *21*(7), pp. 455–466.

Evensen, J., Røssberg, J. I., Barder, H., Haahr, U., ten Velden Hegelstad, W., Joa, I., . . . and Rund, B. R. (2012) 'Flat affect and social functioning: a 10 year follow-up study of first episode psychosis patients', *Schizophrenia Research*, *139*(1–3), pp. 99–104.

Evrensel, A., and Ceylan, M. E. (2015) 'The gut-brain axis: the missing link in depression', *Clinical Psychopharmacology and Neuroscience*, *13*(3),

Evrensel, A., and Ceylan, M. E. (2015) 'The role of fecal microbiota transplantation in psychiatric treatment/Fekal mikrobiyota nakli ve psikiyatrik tedavideki yeri', *Anadolu Psikiyatri Dergisi*, *16*(5), pp. 380–381.

Favalli, G., Li, J., Belmonte-de-Abreu, P., Wong, A. H., and Daskalakis, Z. J. (2012) 'The role of BDNF in the pathophysiology and treatment of schizophrenia', *Journal of Psychiatric Research*, *46*(1), pp. 1–11.

Flint, H. J., Scott, K. P., Duncan, S. H., Louis, P., and Forano, E. (2012) 'Microbial degradation of complex carbohydrates in the gut', *Gut Microbes*, *3*(4), pp. 289–306.

Fornito, A., Harrison, B. J., Goodby, E., Dean, A., Ooi, C., Nathan, P. J., . . . and Bullmore, E. T. (2013) 'Functional dysconnectivity of corticostriatal circuitry as a risk phenotype for psychosis', *JAMA Psychiatry*, *70*(11), pp. 1143–1151.

Foster, J. A., and Neufeld, K. A. M. (2013) 'Gut-brain axis: how the microbiome influences anxiety and depression', *Trends in Neurosciences*, *36*(5), pp. 305–312.

Frei, R., Akdis, M., and O'Mahony, L. (2015) 'Prebiotics, probiotics, synbiotics, and the immune system: experimental data and clinical evidence', *Current Opinion in Gastroenterology*, *31*(2), pp. 153–158.

Gan, J., Yi, J., Zhong, M., Cao, X., Jin, X., Liu, W., and Zhu, X. (2016) 'Abnormal white matter structural connectivity in treatment-naïve young adults with borderline personality disorder', *Acta Psychiatrica Scandinavica*, *134*(6), pp. 494–503.

Gerull, F., Meares, R., Stevenson, J., Korner, A., and Newman, L. (2008) 'The beneficial effect on family life in treating borderline personality', *Psychiatry*, *71*(1), pp. 59–70.

Gerull, F., Meares, R., Stevenson, J., Korner, A., and Newman, L. (2008) 'The beneficial effect on family life in treating borderline personality', *Psychiatry*, *71*(1), pp. 59–70.

Glick-Bauer, M., and Yeh, M. C. (2014) 'The health advantage of a vegan diet: exploring the gut microbiota connection', *Nutrients*, *6*(11), pp. 4822–4838.

Gold, L. H., and Frierson, R. L. (Eds.). (2017) *The American Psychiatric Publishing Textbook of Forensic Psychiatry*, American Psychiatric Pub.

Goodman, W. K., Foote, K. D., Greenberg, B. D., Ricciuti, N., Bauer, R., Ward, H., . . . and Okun, M. S. (2010) 'Deep brain stimulation for intractable obsessive compulsive disorder: pilot study using a blinded, staggered-onset design', *Biological Psychiatry*, *67*(6), pp. 535–542.

Green, M. F., Horan, W. P., and Lee, J. (2019) 'Nonsocial and social cognition in schizophrenia: current evidence and future directions', *World Psychiatry*, *18*(2), pp. 146–161.

Greenberg, B. D., Gabriels, L. A., Malone, D. A., Rezai, A. R., Friehs, G. M., Okun, M. S., . . . and Malloy, P. F. (2010) 'Deep brain stimulation of the ventral internal capsule/ventral striatum for obsessive-compulsive disorder: worldwide experience', *Molecular Psychiatry*, *15*(1), pp. 64–79.

Guilé, J. M., Boissel, L., Alaux-Cantin, S., and de La Rivière, S. G. (2018) 'Borderline personality disorder in adolescents: prevalence, diagnosis, and treatment strategies', *Adolescent Health, Medicine, and Therapeutics*, *9*, p. 199.

Gunderson, J. G. (2009) 'Borderline personality disorder: ontogeny of a diagnosis', *American Journal of Psychiatry*, *166*(5), pp. 530–539.

Gunderson, J. G. (2011) 'Borderline personality disorder', *New England Journal of Medicine*, *364*(21), pp. 2037–2042.

Gunderson, J. G. (2016) 'The emergence of a generalist model to meet public health needs for patients with borderline personality disorder', *American Journal of Psychiatry*, *173*(5), pp. 452–458.

Gunderson, J. G., Stout, R. L., McGlashan, T. H., Shea, M. T., Morey, L. C., Grilo, C. M., . . . and Ansell, E. (2011) 'The ten-year course of borderline personality disorder: psychopathology and function from the Collaborative Longitudinal Personality Disorders Study', *Archives of General Psychiatry*, *68*(8), pp. 827–837.

Gunderson, J. G., Stout, R. L., Shea, M. T., Grilo, C. M., Markowitz, J. C., Morey, L. C., . . . and McGlashan, T. H. (2014) 'Interactions of borderline personality disorder and mood disorders over ten years', *Journal of Clinical Psychiatry*, *75*(8), p. 829.

Gunderson, J. G., Weinberg, I., and Choi-Kain, L. (2013) 'Borderline personality disorder', *Focus*, *11*(2), pp. 129–145.

Gunderson, John G. (2009) 'Borderline personality disorder: ontogeny of a diagnosis', *American Journal of Psychiatry* 166.5, pp. 530–539.

Haesebaert, F., Moirand, R., Schott-Pethelaz, A. M., Brunelin, J., and Poulet, E. (2018) 'Usefulness of repetitive transcranial magnetic stimulation as a maintenance treatment in patients with major depression', *The World Journal of Biological Psychiatry*, *19*(1), pp. 74–78.

Haley, K. P., and Gaddy, J. A. (2016) 'Nutrition and Helicobacter pylori: host diet and nutritional immunity influence bacterial virulence and disease outcome', *Gastroenterology Research and Practice*.

Hallett, M. (2007) 'Transcranial magnetic stimulation: a primer', *Neuron*, *55*(2), pp. 187–199.

Hancock-Johnson, E., Griffiths, C., and Picchioni, M. (2017) 'A focused systematic review of pharmacological treatment for borderline personality disorder', *CNS Drugs*, *31*(5), pp. 345–356.

HarIz, M. I., Blomstedt, P., and Zrinzo, L. (2010) 'Deep brain stimulation between 1947 and 1987: the untold story', *Neurosurgical Focus*, *29*(2), E1.

Harned, M. S., Rizvi, S. L., and Linehan, M. M. (2010) 'Impact of co-occurring posttraumatic stress disorder on suicidal women with a borderline personality disorder', *American Journal of Psychiatry*, *167*(10), pp. 1210–1217.

Heinz, A., Voss, M., Lawrie, S. M., Mishara, A., Bauer, M., Gallinat, J., . . . and Strik, W. (2016) 'Shall we really say goodbye to first rank symptoms?', *European Psychiatry*, *37*, pp. 8–13.

Herpertz, S. C., Zanarini, M., Schulz, C. S., Siever, L., Lieb, K., and Möller, H. J. (2007) 'Treatment of personality disorders: World Federation of Societies of Biological Psychiatry (WFSBP) Guidelines for Biological Treatment of Personality Disorders', *World J Biol Psychiatry*, *8*(4), pp. 212–244.

Higgins, E. S., and George, M. S. (2019) *Brain Stimulation Therapies for Clinicians*, American Psychiatric Pub.

Hirsh, J. B., Quilty, L. C., Bagby, R. M., and McMain, S. F. (2012) 'The relationship between agreeableness and the development of the working alliance in patients with a borderline personality disorder', *Journal of Personality Disorders*, *26*(4), pp. 616–627.

Holtzheimer, P. E., and Mayberg, H. S. (2011), 'Deep brain stimulation for psychiatric disorders', *Annual Review of Neuroscience*, *34*, pp. 289–307.

Hopwood, C. J., Swenson, C., Bateman, A., Yeomans, F. E., and Gunderson, J. G. (2014) 'Approaches to psychotherapy for borderline personality: Demonstrations by four master Clinicians', *Personality Disorders: Theory, Research, and Treatment*, *5*(1), p. 108.

Horvath, A. O., Del Re, A. C., Flückiger, C., and Symonds, D. (2011) 'Alliance in individual Psychotherapy', *Psychotherapy*, *48*(1), p. 9.

Huttenhower, C., Gevers, D., Knight, R., Abubucker, S., Badger, J. H., Chinwalla, A. T., . . . and Giglio, M. G. (2012) 'Structure, function and diversity of the healthy human Microbiome', *Nature*, *486*(7402), p. 207.

Huurre, A., Kalliomäki, M., Rautava, S., Rinne, M., Salminen, S., and Isolauri, E. (2008) 'Mode of delivery–effects on gut microbiota and humoral immunity', *Neonatology*, *93*(4), pp. 236–240.

Hwang, J. W., Xin, S. C., Ou, Y. M., Zhang, W. Y., Liang, Y. L., Chen, J., . . . and Ma, W. H. (2016) 'Enhanced default mode network connectivity with ventral striatum in subthreshold depression individuals', *Journal of psychiatric research*, *76*, pp. 111–120.

Hwang, J., Castelli, D. M., and Gonzalez-Lima, F. (2017) 'The positive cognitive impact of aerobic fitness is associated with peripheral inflammatory and brain-derived neurotrophic biomarkers in young adults', *Physiology and Behavior*, *179*, pp. 75–89.

James, S. L., Abate, D., Abate, K. H., Abay, S. M., Abbafati, C., Abbasi, N., . . . and Abdollahpour, I. (2018) 'Global, regional, and national incidence, prevalence, and years lived with disability for 354 diseases and injuries for 195 countries and territories, 1990–2017: a systematic analysis for the Global Burden of Disease Study 2017', *The Lancet*, *392*(10159), pp. 1789–1858.

Kaess, M., von Ceumern-Lindenstjerna, I. A., Parzer, P., Chanen, A., Mundt, C., Resch, F., and Brunner, R. (2013) 'Axis I and II comorbidity and psychosocial functioning in female adolescents with a borderline personality disorder', *Psychopathology*, *46*(1), pp. 55–62.

Kaiser, R. H., Andrews-Hanna, J. R., Wager, T. D., and Pizzagalli, D. A. (2015) 'Large-scale network dysfunction in major depressive disorder: a meta-analysis of resting-state functional connectivity', *JAMA Psychiatry*, *72*(6), pp. 603–611.

Kaplan, C., Tarlow, N., Stewart, J. G., Aguirre, B., Galen, G., and

Auerbach, R. P. (2016) 'Borderline personality disorder in youth: The prospective impact of child abuse on non- suicidal self-injury and suicidality', *Comprehensive Psychiatry*, *71*, pp. 86–94.

Kassam, Z., Lee, C. H., Yuan, Y., and Hunt, R. H. (2013) 'Fecal Microbiota Transplantation For Clostridium difficile infection: Systematic Review and Meta-Analysis', *American Journal of Gastroenterology*, *108*(4), pp. 500–508.

Kazerouni, A., Burgess, J., Burns, L. J., and Wein, L. M. (2015) 'Optimal screening and donor management in a public stool bank', *Microbiome*, *3*(1), pp. 75.

Kelly, S., Guimond, S., Lyall, A., Stone, W. S., Shenton, M. E., Keshavan, M., and Seidman, L. J. (2019) 'Neural correlates of cognitive deficits across developmental phases of Schizophrenia', *Neurobiology of Disease*, *131*, p. 104353.

Kennedy, P. J., Cryan, J. F., Dinan, T. G., Clarke, G. (2014) 'Irritable bowel syndrome: a microbiome-gut-brain axis disorder?', *World Journal Gastroenterol*, 20, pp. 14105–14125.

Kennedy, S. H., and Giacobbe, P. (2007) 'Treatment resistant depression—advances in somatic Therapies', *Annals of Clinical Psychiatry*, *19*(4), pp. 279–287.

Kibleur, A., Polosan, M., Favre, P., Rudrauf, D., Bougerol, T., Chabardès, S., and David, O. (2017) 'Stimulation of subgenual cingulate area decreases limbic top-down effect on ventral visual stream: A DBS-EEG pilot study', *NeuroImage*, *146*, pp. 544–553.

Kiecolt-Glaser, J. K., Derry, H. M., and Fagundes, C. P. (2015) 'Inflammation: depression fans the flames and feasts on the heat', *American Journal of Psychiatry*, *172*(11), pp. 1075–1091.

Kim, K. O., Schwartz, M., and Gluck, M. (2018) '1011-Reducing Cost and Scheduling Complexity of Fecal Microbiota Transplantation by Using Universal Donor over Patients-Directed Donors in Patients with Recurrent Clostrodium Difficile Infections', *Gastroenterology*, *154*(6), S-191.

Kimmel, C. L., Alhassoon, O. M., Wollman, S. C., Stern, M. J.,

Perez-Figueroa, A., Hall, M. G., . . . and Radua, J. (2016) 'Age-related parieto-occipital and other gray matter changes in borderline personality disorder: a meta-analysis of cortical and subcortical structures', *Psychiatry Research: Neuroimaging*, *251*, pp. 15–25.

Koenigs, M., and Grafman, J. (2009) 'The functional neuroanatomy of depression: distinct roles for ventromedial and dorsolateral prefrontal cortex', *Behavioural Brain Research*, *201*(2), pp. 239–243.

Krabbe, S., Duda, J., Schiemann, J., Poetschke, C., Schneider, G., Kandel, E. R., . . . and Simpson, E. H. (2015) 'Increased dopamine D2 receptor activity in the striatum alters the firing pattern of dopamine neurons in the ventral tegmental area', *Proceedings of the National Academy of Sciences*, *112*(12), E1498–E1506.

Krawitz, R., and Jackson, W. (2008) *Borderline Personality Disorder*, Oxford University Press. Krystal, J. H., Anticevic, A., Yang, G. J., Dragoi, G., Driesen, N. R., Wang, X. J., and Murray, J. D. (2017) 'Impaired tuning of neural ensembles and the pathophysiology of schizophrenia: a translational and computational neuroscience perspective', *Biological Psychiatry*, *81*(10), pp. 874–885.

Kulacaoglu, F., and Kose, S. (2018) 'Borderline Personality Disorder (BPD): In the Midst of Vulnerability, Chaos, and Awe', *Brain Sciences*, *8*(11), p. 201.

Kuperberg, G. R. (2010) 'Language in schizophrenia part 1: an introduction', *Language and Linguistics Compass*, *4*(8), pp. 576–589.

Lai, J. S., Hiles, S., Bisquera, A., Hure, A. J., McEvoy, M., and Attia, J. (2014) 'A systematic review and meta-analysis of dietary patterns and depression in community-dwelling adults', *The American Journal of Clinical Nutrition*, *99*(1), pp. 181–197.

Lambert, G. P. (2009) 'Stress-induced gastrointestinal barrier dysfunction and its inflammatory Effects', *Journal of Animal Science*, *87*(suppl_14), E101–E108.

Laurenssen, E. M., Hutsebaut, J., Feenstra, D. J., Bales, D. L., Noom, M. J., Busschbach, J. J., . . . and Luyten, P. (2014) 'Feasibility of mentalization-based treatment for adolescents with borderline symptoms: A pilot study', *Psychotherapy*, *51*(1), p. 159.

Leander, N. P., Moore, S. G., and Chartrand, T. L. (2009) *Mystery Moods: Their Origins and Consequences*, Na.

Lee, Y. S., and Silva, A. J. (2009) 'The molecular and cellular biology of enhanced cognition, *Nature Reviews Neuroscience*, *10*(2), pp. 126–140.

Leiberich, P., Nickel, M. K., Tritt, K., and Gil, F. P. (2008) 'Lamotrigine treatment of aggression in female borderline patients, Part II: an 18-month follow-up', *Journal of Psychopharmacology*, *22*(7), pp. 805–808.

Lépine, J. P., and Briley, M. (2011) 'The increasing burden of depression', *Neuropsychiatric Disease and Treatment*, *7*(Suppl. 1), p. 3.

Levkovitz, Y., Isserles, M., Padberg, F., Lisanby, S. H., Bystritsky, A., Xia, G., . . . and Hafez, H. M. (2015) 'Efficacy and safety of deep transcranial magnetic stimulation for major depression: a prospective multicenter randomized controlled trial', *World Psychiatry*, *14*(1), pp. 64–73.

Li, B., Piriz, J., Mirrione, M., Chung, C., Proulx, C. D., Schulz, D., . . . and Malinow, R. (2011) 'Synaptic potentiation onto habenula neurons in the learned helplessness model of Depression', *Nature*, *470*(7335), pp. 535–539.

Li, H., Zhang, Q., Li, N., Wang, F., Xiang, H., Zhang, Z., . . . and Zhou, R. (2016) 'Plasma levels of Th17-related cytokines and complement C3 correlated with aggressive behavior in patients with schizophrenia', *Psychiatry Research*, *246*, pp. 700–706.

Li, R., Ma, X., Wang, G., Yang, J., and Wang, C. (2016) 'Why sex differences in schizophrenia?', *Journal of Translational Neuroscience*, *1*(1), p.37.

Lieb, K., Völlm, B., Rücker, G., Timmer, A., and Stoffers, J. M.

(2010) 'Pharmacotherapy for borderline personality disorder: Cochrane systematic review of randomised trials', *The British Journal of Psychiatry*, *196*(1), pp. 4–12.

Linehan, M. M. (2018) *Cognitive-Behavioral Treatment of Borderline Personality Disorder*, Guilford Publications.

Linehan, M. M., Korslund, K. E., Harned, M. S., Gallop, R. J., Lungu, A., Neacsiu, A. D., . . . and Murray-Gregory, A. M. (2015) 'Dialectical behavior therapy for high suicide risk in individuals with borderline personality disorder: a randomized clinical trial and component analysis', *JAMA Psychiatry*, *72*(5), pp. 475–482.

Liu, Y. W., Liu, W. H., Wu, C. C., Juan, Y. C., Wu, Y. C., Tsai, H. P., . . . and Tsai, Y. C. (2016) 'Psychotropic effects of Lactobacillus plantarum PS128 in early life-stressed and naïve adult mice' *Brain Research*, *1631*, pp. 1–12.

Liu, Z., Patil, I. Y., Jiang, T., Sancheti, H., Walsh, J. P., Stiles, B. L., . . . and Cadenas, E. (2015) 'High-fat diet induces hepatic insulin resistance and impairment of synaptic plasticity', *PloS one*, *10*(5), e0128274.

Livesley, J. (2008) 'Toward a genetically-informed model of borderline personality disorder', *Journal of Personality Disorders*, *22*(1), pp. 42–71.

Loonen, A. J., and Ivanova, S. A. (2016) 'Circuits regulating pleasure and happiness mechanisms of depression', *Frontiers in Human Neuroscience*, *10*, p. 571.

Lopez-Castroman, J., Galfalvy, H., Currier, D., Stanley, B., Blasco-Fontecilla, H., Baca-Garcia, E., . . . and Oquendo, M. A. (2012) 'Personality disorder assessments in acute depressive episodes: stability at follow-up', *The Journal of Nervous and Mental Disease*, *200*(6), p. 526.

Louis, P., and Flint, H. J. (2017) 'Formation of propionate and butyrate by the human colonic Microbiota', *Environmental Microbiology*, *19*(1), pp. 29–41.

Lozano, A. M., Giacobbe, P., Hamani, C., Rizvi, S. J., Kennedy, S. H., Kolivakis, T. T., . . . and Ilcewicz-Klimek, M. (2012)

'A multicenter pilot study of subcallosal cingulate area deep brain stimulation for treatment-resistant depression', *Journal of Neurosurgery*, *116*(2), pp. 315–322.

Lurie, I., Yang, Y. X., Haynes, K., Mamtani, R., and Boursi, B. (2015) 'Antibiotic exposure and the risk for depression, anxiety, or psychosis: a nested case-control study', *The Journal of Clinical Psychiatry*, *76*(11), pp. 1522–1528.

Macfarlane, G. T., and Macfarlane, S. (2012) 'Bacteria, colonic fermentation, and gastrointestinal health', *Journal of AOAC International*, *95*(1), pp. 50–60.

Maia, T. V., and Frank, M. J. (2011) 'From reinforcement learning models to psychiatric and neurological disorders', *Nature Neuroscience*, *14*(2), p. 154.

Maltsberger, J. T., Schechter, M., Herbstman, B., Ronningstam, E., and Goldblatt, M. J. (2015) 'Suicide studies today'.

Mangiola, F., Ianiro, G., Franceschi, F., Fagiuoli, S., Gasbarrini, G., and Gasbarrini, A. (2016) 'Gut microbiota in autism and mood disorders', *World Journal of Gastroenterology*, *22*(1), p. 361.

Marder, S. R., and Galderisi, S. (2017) 'The current conceptualization of negative symptoms in Schizophrenia', *World Psychiatry*, *16*(1), pp. 14–24.

Marks Jr, W. J. (ed.) (2015) *Deep Brain Stimulation Management*, Cambridge University Press.

Martin, Donel M., Shawn M. McClintock, Jane J. Forster, Tin Yan Lo, and Colleen K. Loo. (2017) 'Cognitive enhancing effects of rTMS administered to the prefrontal cortex in patients with depression: A systematic review and meta-analysis of individual task effects', *Depression and Anxiety* 34, no. 11, pp. 1029–1039.

Martinez-Levy, G. A., Rocha, L., Rodriguez-Pineda, F., Alonso-Vanegas, M. A., Nani, A., Buentello-García, R. M., . . . and Cruz-Fuentes, C. S. (2018) 'Increased expression of brain-derived neurotrophic factor transcripts I and VI, cAMP response element binding, and glucocorticoid receptor in the cortex of patients with temporal lobe epilepsy', *Molecular Neurobiology*, *55*(5), pp. 3698–3708.

Maslowski, K. M., and Mackay, C. R. (2011) 'Diet, gut microbiota and immune responses', *Nature Immunology*, *12*(1), pp. 5–9.

May, J. M., Richardi, T. M., and Barth, K. S. (2016) 'Dialectical behavior therapy as treatment for borderline personality disorder', *Mental Health Clinician*, *6*(2), pp. 62–67. 'Borderline personality disorder in adolescents', *Clinical Psychology Review*, *28*(6), pp. 969–981.

McCutcheon, R. A., Abi-Dargham, A., and Howes, O. D. (2019) 'Schizophrenia, dopamine and the striatum: from biology to symptoms', *Trends in Neurosciences*, *42*(3), pp. 205–220.

McCutcheon, R. A., Krystal, J. H., and Howes, O. D. (2020), 'Dopamine and glutamate in schizophrenia: biology, symptoms and treatment', *World Psychiatry*, *19*(1), pp. 15–33.

McFarland, L. V. (2015) 'From yaks to yogurt: the history, development, and current use of Probiotics', *Clinical Infectious Diseases*, *60*(suppl_2), S85–S90.

McMain, S. F., Links, P. S., Gnam, W. H., Guimond, T., Cardish, R. J., Korman, L., and Streiner, D. L. (2009) 'A randomized trial of dialectical behavior therapy versus general psychiatric management for borderline personality disorder', *American Journal of Psychiatry*, *166*(12), pp. 1365–1374.

Meguins, L. C. (2012) 'Deep brain stimulation for treatment-resistant depression: a state-of-the- art review', *Juruena MF. Clinical, Research and Treatment Approaches to Affective Disorders*, pp. 357–64.

Mercer, D., Douglass, A. B., and Links, P. S. (2009) 'Meta-analyses of mood stabilizers, antidepressants and antipsychotics in the treatment of borderline personality disorder: effectiveness for depression and anger symptoms', *Journal of Personality Disorders*, *23*(2), pp. 156–174.

Mertens, A., Raedt, R., Gadeyne, S., Carrette, E., Boon, P., and Vonck, K. (2018) 'Recent advances in devices for vagus nerve stimulation', *Expert Review of Medical Devices*, *15*(8), pp. 527–539.

Miller, A. L., Muehlenkamp, J. J., and Jacobson, C. M. (2008) 'Fact or fiction: Diagnosing'.

Million, M., Lagier, J. C., Yahav, D., and Paul, M. (2013) 'Gut bacterial microbiota and obesity', *Clinical Microbiology and Infection*, *19*(4), pp. 305–313.

Minichino, A., Bersani, F. S., Capra, E., Pannese, R., Bonanno, C., Salviati, M., . . . and Biondi, M. (2012) 'ECT, rTMS, and deepTMS in pharmacoresistant drug-free patients with unipolar depression: a comparative review', *Neuropsychiatric Disease and Treatment*, *8*, pp. 55.

Mitra, S., Mahintamani, T., Kavoor, A. R., and Nizamie, S. H. (2016) 'Negative symptoms in Schizophrenia', *Industrial Psychiatry Journal*, *25*(2), p. 135.

Modirrousta, M., Meek, B. P., and Wikstrom, S. L. (2018) 'Efficacy of twice-daily vs once-daily sessions of repetitive transcranial magnetic stimulation in the treatment of major depressive disorder: a retrospective study', *Neuropsychiatric Disease and Treatment*, *14*, p. 309.

Moffitt, T. E., in alphabetical order, Arseneault, L., Jaffee, S. R., Kim-Cohen, J., Koenen, K. C., . . . and Viding, E. (2008) 'Research review: DSM-V conduct disorder: Research needs for an evidence base', *Journal of Child Psychology and Psychiatry*, *49*(1), pp. 3–33.

Moghaddam, B., and Javitt, D. (2012) 'From revolution to evolution: the glutamate hypothesis of schizophrenia and its implication for treatment', *Neuropsychopharmacology*, *37*(1), pp. 4–15.

Molloy, A. 'Mothers facing C-sections look to vaginal "seeding" to boost their babies' health', *Guardian* (accessed on 17 August 2015).

Moos, W. H., Faller, D. V., Harpp, D. N., Kanara, I., Pernokas, J., Powers, W. R., and Steliou, K. (2016) 'Microbiota and neurological disorders: a gut feeling', *BioResearch Open Access*, *5*(1), pp. 137–145.

Morishita, T., Fayad, S. M., Higuchi, M. A., Nestor, K. A., and Foote, K. D. (2014) 'Deep brain stimulation for treatment-resistant depression: systematic review of clinical outcomes', *Neurotherapeutics*, *11*(3), pp. 475–484.

Mörkl, S., Wagner-Skacel, J., Lahousen, T., Lackner, S., Holasek, S. J., Bengesser, S. A., . . . and Reininghaus, E. (2020) 'The role of nutrition and the gut-brain axis in psychiatry: a review of the literature', *Neuropsychobiology*, *79*(1–2), pp. 80–88.

Morris, G., Berk, M., Carvalho, A., Caso, J. R., Sanz, Y., Walder, K., and Maes, M. (2017) 'The role of the microbial metabolites including tryptophan catabolites and short chain fatty acids in the pathophysiology of immune-inflammatory and neuroimmune diseases', *Molecular Neurobiology*, *54*(6), pp. 4432–4451.

Motter, J. N., Pimontel, M. A., Rindskopf, D., Devanand, D. P., Doraiswamy, P. M., and Sneed, J. R. (2016) 'Computerized cognitive training and functional recovery in major depressive disorder: a meta-analysis', *Journal of Affective Disorders*, *189*, pp. 184–191.

Näätänen, R., and Kähkönen, S. (2009) 'Central auditory dysfunction in schizophrenia as revealed by the mismatch negativity (MMN) and its magnetic equivalent MMNm: a review', *International Journal of Neuropsychopharmacology*, *12*(1), pp. 125–135.

Naidich, T. P., Castillo, M., Cha, S., and Smirniotopoulos, J. G. (2012) *Imaging of the Brain: Expert Radiology Series*, Elsevier Health Sciences.

Neacsiu, A. D., Rizvi, S. L., and Linehan, M. M. (2010) 'Dialectical behavior therapy skills use as a mediator and outcome of treatment for borderline personality disorder', *Behavior Research and Therapy*, *48*(9), pp. 832–839.

Niedtfeld, I., Schulze, L., Krause-Utz, A., Demirakca, T., Bohus, M., and Schmahl, C. (2013) 'Voxel-based morphometry in women with borderline personality disorder with and without comorbid posttraumatic stress disorder', *PloS One*, *8*(6).

Nieto, R., Kukuljan, M., and Silva, H. (2013) 'BDNF and

schizophrenia: from neurodevelopment to neuronal plasticity, learning, and memory', *Frontiers in Psychiatry, 4*, p. 45.

Norton, S., Cosco, T., Doyle, F., Done, J., and Sacker, A. (2013) 'The Hospital Anxiety and Depression Scale: a meta confirmatory factor analysis', *Journal of Psychosomatic Research, 74*(1), pp. 74–81.

O'Mahony, S. M., Clarke, G., Borre, Y. E., Dinan, T. G., and Cryan, J. F. (2015) 'Serotonin, tryptophan metabolism and the brain-gut-microbiome axis', *Behavioural Brain Research, 277*, pp. 32–48.

O'neil, A., Quirk, S. E., Housden, S., Brennan, S. L., Williams, L. J., Pasco, J. A., . . . and Jacka, F. N. (2014) 'Relationship between diet and mental health in children and adolescents: a systematic review', *American Journal of Public Health, 104*(10), e31–e42.

Okubo, R., Koga, M., Katsumata, N., Odamaki, T., Matsuyama, S., Oka, M., . . . and Matsuoka, Y. J. (2019) 'Effect of bifidobacterium breve A-1 on anxiety and depressive symptoms in schizophrenia: a proof-of-concept study', *Journal of Affective Disorders, 245*, pp. 377–385.

O'Reardon, J. P., Cristancho, P., and Peshek, A. D. (2006) 'Vagus nerve stimulation (VNS) and treatment of depression: to the brainstem and beyond', *Psychiatry (Edgmont), 3*(5), p. 54

Oriach, C. S., Robertson, R. C., Stanton, C., Cryan, J. F., and Dinan, T. G. (2016) 'Food for thought: The role of nutrition in the microbiota-gut–brain axis', *Clinical Nutrition Experimental, 6*, pp. 25–38.

Ou, J., Carbonero, F., Zoetendal, E. G., DeLany, J. P., Wang, M., Newton, K., . . . and O'Keefe, S. J. (2013) 'Diet, microbiota, and microbial metabolites in colon cancer risk in rural Africans and African Americans', *The American Journal of Clinical Nutrition, 98*(1), pp. 111–120.

Oumaya, M., Friedman, S., Pham, A., Abou, T. A., Guelfi, J. D., and Rouillon, F. (2008) 'Borderline personality disorder, self-mutilation, and suicide: a literature review', *L'Encephale*, *34*(5), pp. 452–458.

Owen, M. J., and Sawa, A. (2016) 'Mortensen PB', *Schizophrenia Lancet*, *388*, pp. 86–97.

Papakostas, G. I., Shelton, R. C., Kinrys, G., Henry, M. E., Bakow, B. R., Lipkin, S. H., . . . and Bilello, J. A. (2013) 'Assessment of a multi-assay, serum-based biological diagnostic test for major depressive disorder: a pilot and replication study', *Molecular Psychiatry*, *18*(3), pp. 332–339.

Parakh, P., and Basu, D. (2013) 'Cannabis and psychosis: Have we found the missing links?', *Asian Journal of Psychiatry*, *6*(4), pp. 281–287.

Pariante, C. M. (2015) 'Psychoneuroimmunology or immunopsychiatry?', *The Lancet Psychiatry* 2(3), pp. 197–199.

Paris, J. (2008) 'Clinical trials of treatment for personality disorders', *Psychiatric Clinics of North America*, *31*(3), pp. 517–526.

Paris, J. (2009) 'The treatment of borderline personality disorder: implications of research on diagnosis, etiology, and outcome', *Annual Review of Clinical Psychology*, *5*, pp. 277–290.

Paris, J. (2010) 'Estimating the prevalence of personality disorders in the community', *Journal of Personality Disorders*, *24*(4), pp. 405–411.

Paris, J. (2019) *Treatment of Borderline Personality Disorder: A Guide to Evidence-Based Practice*, Guilford Publications.

Parker, G. (2011) 'Clinical differentiation of bipolar II disorder from personality-based "emotional dysregulation" conditions', *Journal of Affective Disorders*, *133*(1–2), pp. 16–21.

Parry, G. D., Crawford, M. J., and Duggan, C. (2016) 'Iatrogenic harm from psychological therapies–time to move on', *The British Journal of Psychiatry*, *208*(3), pp. 210–212.

Paton, C., Crawford, M. J., Bhatti, S. F., Patel, M. X., and Barnes, T. R. (2015) 'The use of psychotropic medication in patients with emotionally unstable personality disorder under the care of UK mental health services', *The Journal of Clinical Psychiatry*, *76*(4), pp. 512–518. Patten, C. A., Goggin, K., Harris, K. J.,

Richter, K. P., Williams, K., Decker, P. A., . . . and Catley, D. (2016) 'Relationship of autonomy social support to quitting motivation in diverse smokers', *Addiction Research and Theory*, *24*(6), pp. 477–482.

Perera, T., George, M. S., Grammer, G., Janicak, P. G., Pascual-Leone, A., and Wirecki, T. S. (2016) 'The clinical TMS society consensus review and treatment recommendations for TMS therapy for major depressive disorder', *Brain Stimulation*, *9*(3), pp. 336–34

Philip, N. S., Barredo, J., van't Wout-Frank, M., Tyrka, A. R., Price, L. H., and Carpenter, L. L. (2018) 'Network mechanisms of clinical response to transcranial magnetic stimulation in posttraumatic stress disorder and major depressive disorder', *Biological psychiatry*, *83*(3), pp. 263–272.

Porcelli, B., Verdino, V., Bossini, L., Terzuoli, L., and Fagiolini, A. (2014) 'Celiac and non-celiac gluten sensitivity: a review on the association with schizophrenia and mood disorders', *Autoimmunity Highlights*, *5*(2), pp. 55–61.

Porr, V. (2010) *Overcoming Borderline Personality Disorder: A Family Guide for Healing and Change*, Oxford University Press.

Pott, J., and Hornef, M. (2012) 'Innate immune signalling at the intestinal epithelium in homeostasis and disease', *EMBO Reports*, *13*(8), pp. 684–698.

Powers, A. R., Mathys, C., and Corlett, P. R. (2017) 'Pavlovian conditioning–induced hallucinations result from overweighting of perceptual priors', *Science*, *357*(6351), pp. 596–600.

Quevedo, K., Ng, R., Scott, H., Kodavaganti, S., Smyda, G., Diwadkar, V., and Phillips, M. (2017) 'Ventral striatum functional connectivity during rewards and losses and symptomatology in depressed patients', *Biological Psychology*, *123*, pp. 62–73.

Rajoka, M. S. R., Shi, J., Mehwish, H. M., Zhu, J., Li, Q., Shao, D., . . . and Yang, H. (2017) 'Interaction between diet composition and gut microbiota and its impact on gastrointestinal tract health', *Food Science and Human Wellness*, *6*(3), pp. 121–130.

Ranft, K., Dobrowolny, H., Krell, D., Bielau, H., Bogerts, B., and Bernstein, H. G. (2010) 'Evidence for structural abnormalities of the human habenular complex in affective disorders but not in schizophrenia', *Psychological Medicine*, *40*(4), pp. 557–567.

Rasmussen, K. G. (2011) 'Some considerations in choosing electroconvulsive therapy versus transcranial magnetic stimulation for depression', *The Journal of ECT*, *27*(1), pp. 51–54.

Rausch, J., Gäbel, A., Nagy, K., Kleindienst, N., Herpertz, S. C., and Bertsch, K. (2015) 'Increased testosterone levels and cortisol awakening responses in patients with borderline personality disorder: gender and trait aggressiveness matter', *Psychoneuroendocrinology*, *55*, pp. 116–127.

Ray, M. T., Weickert, C. S., and Webster, M. J. (2014) 'Decreased BDNF and TrkB mRNA expression in multiple cortical areas of patients with schizophrenia and mood disorders', *Translational Psychiatry*, *4*(5), e389–e389.

Rector, N. A., Beck, A. T., and Stolar, N. (2005) 'The negative symptoms of schizophrenia: a cognitive perspective', *The Canadian Journal of Psychiatry*, *50*(5), pp. 247–257.

Reddy, L. F., Green, M. F., Rizzo, S., Sugar, C. A., Blanchard, J. J., Gur, R. E., . . . and Horan, W. P. (2014) 'Behavioral approach and avoidance in schizophrenia: an evaluation of motivational profiles', *Schizophrenia Research*, *159*(1), pp. 164–170.

Reddy, M. S., and Vijay, M. S. (2017) 'Empirical reality of dialectical behavioral therapy in borderline personality', *Indian journal of Psychological Medicine*, *39*(2), pp. 105.

Reid, G., Younes, J. A., Van der Mei, H. C., Gloor, G. B., Knight, R., and Busscher, H. J. (2011) 'Microbiota restoration: natural and supplemented recovery of human microbial Communities', *Nature Reviews Microbiology*, *9*(1), pp. 27–38.

Ripke, S., Neale, B. M., Corvin, A., Walters, J. T., Farh, K. H., Holmans, P. A., . . . and Pers, T. H. (2014) 'Biological insights from 108 schizophrenia-associated genetic loci', *Nature*, 511(7510), pp. 421–427.

Ripoll, L. H. (2012) 'Clinical psychopharmacology of borderline personality disorder: an update on the available evidence in light of the Diagnostic and Statistical Manual of Mental Disorders–5', *Current Opinion in Psychiatry*, *25*(1), pp. 52–58.

Ripoll, L. H. (2013) 'Psychopharmacologic treatment of borderline personality disorder', *Dialogues in Clinical Neuroscience*, *15*(2), p. 213.

Rizos, E. N., Michalopoulou, P. G., Siafakas, N., Stefanis, N., Douzenis, A., Rontos, I., . . . and Lykouras, L. (2010) 'Association of serum brain-derived neurotrophic factor and duration of untreated psychosis in first-episode patients with schizophrenia', *Neuropsychobiology*, *62*(2), pp. 87–90.

Rogers, B., and Acton, T. (2012) '"I think we're all guinea pigs really": a qualitative study of medication and borderline personality disorder', *Journal of Psychiatric and Mental Health Nursing*, *19*(4), pp. 341–347.

Rogers, G. B., Keating, D. J., Young, R. L., Wong, M. L., Licinio, J., and Wesselingh, S. (2016) 'From gut dysbiosis to altered brain function and mental illness: mechanisms and pathways', *Molecular psychiatry*, *21*(6), pp. 738–748.

Ruocco, A. C., Amirthavasagam, S., Choi-Kain, L. W., and McMain, S. F. (2013) 'Neural correlates of negative emotionality in borderline personality disorder: an activation- likelihood-estimation meta-analysis', *Biological Psychiatry*, *73*(2), pp. 153–160.

Sack, A. T., Cohen Kadosh, R., Schuhmann, T., Moerel, M., Walsh, V., and Goebel, R. (2009) 'Optimizing functional accuracy of TMS in cognitive studies: a comparison of Methods', *Journal of Cognitive Neuroscience*, *21*(2), pp. 207–221.

Sadock, B. J., Sadock, V. A., and Levin, Z. E. (eds.) (2007) *Kaplan and Sadock's Study Guide and Self-Examination Review in Psychiatry*, Lippincott Williams and Wilkins.

Sartorius, A., Kiening, K. L., Kirsch, P., von Gall, C. C., Haberkorn,

U., Unterberg, A. W., . . . and Meyer-Lindenberg, A. (2010) 'Remission of major depression under deep brain stimulation of the lateral habenula in a therapy-refractory patient', *Biological Psychiatry*, *67*(2), e9–e11.

Saulnier, D. M., Ringel, Y., Heyman, M. B., Foster, J. A., Bercik, P., Shulman, R. J., . . . and Guarner, F. (2013) 'The intestinal microbiome, probiotics and prebiotics in neurogastroenterology', *Gut Microbes*, *4*(1), pp. 17–27.

Schlaepfer, T. E., Bewernick, B. H., Kayser, S., Mädler, B., and Coenen, V. A. (2013) 'Rapid effects of deep brain stimulation for treatment-resistant major depression', *Biological Psychiatry*, *73*(12), pp. 1204–1212.

Schlaepfer, T. E., Cohen, M. X., Frick, C., Kosel, M., Brodesser, D., Axmacher, N., . . . and Sturm, V. (2008) 'Deep brain stimulation to reward circuitry alleviates anhedonia in refractory major depression', *Neuropsychopharmacology*, *33*(2), pp. 368–377.

Schnorr, S. L., Candela, M., Rampelli, S., Centanni, M., Consolandi, C., Basaglia, G., . . . and Fiori, J. (2014) 'Gut microbiome of the Hadza hunter-gatherers', *Nature Communications*, *5*(1), pp. 1–12.

Schulze, L., Schmahl, C., and Niedtfeld, I. (2016) 'Neural correlates of disturbed emotion processing in borderline personality disorder: a multimodal meta-analysis', *Biological Psychiatry*, *79*(2), pp. 97–106.

Scott, K. P., Jean-Michel, A., Midtvedt, T., and van Hemert, S. (2015) 'Manipulating the gut microbiota to maintain health and treat disease', *Microbial Ecology in Health and Disease*, *26*(1), p. 25877.

Sender, R., Fuchs, S., and Milo, R. (2016) 'Are we really vastly outnumbered? Revisiting the ratio of bacterial to host cells in humans', *Cell*, *164*(3), pp. 337–340.

Severance, E. G., Alaedini, A., Yang, S., Halling, M., Gressitt, K. L., Stallings, C. R., . . . and Dickerson, F. B. (2012) 'Gastrointestinal inflammation and associated immune activation in schizophrenia', *Schizophrenia Research, 138*(1), pp. 48–53.

Severance, E. G., Gressitt, K. L., Buka, S. L., Cannon, T. D., and Yolken, R. H. (2014) 'Maternal complement C1q and increased odds for psychosis in adult offspring', *Schizophrenia Research, 159*(1), pp. 14–19.

Severance, E. G., Prandovszky, E., Castiglione, J., and Yolken, R. H. (2015) 'Gastroenterology issues in schizophrenia: why the gut matters', *Current Psychiatry Reports, 17*(5), p. 27.

Shaffer, D., and Jacobson, C. (2009) 'Proposal to the DSM-V childhood disorder and mood disorder work groups to include non-suicidal self-injury (NSSI) as a DSM-V disorder', *American Psychiatric Association*, pp. 1–21.

Sher, L., Mindes, J., and Novakovic, V. (2010) 'Transcranial magnetic stimulation and the treatment of suicidality', *Expert Review of Neurotherapeutics, 10*(12), pp. 1781–1784.

Sherwin, E., Sandhu, K. V., Dinan, T. G., and Cryan, J. F. (2016) 'May the force be with you: the light and dark sides of the microbiota-gut-brain axis in neuropsychiatry', *CNS Drugs, 30*(11), pp. 1019–1041.

Siever, L. J. (2008) 'Neurobiology of aggression and violence', *American Journal of Psychiatry, 165*(4), pp. 429–442.

Silk, K. R. (2008) 'Personality disorder in adolescence: The diagnosis that dare not speak its name'.

Silvers, J. A., Hubbard, A. D., Biggs, E., Shu, J., Fertuck, E., Chaudhury, S., . . . and Brodsky, B. S. (2016) 'Affective lability and difficulties with regulation are differentially associated with the amygdala and prefrontal response in women with Borderline Personality Disorder', *Psychiatry Research: Neuroimaging, 254*, pp. 74–82.

Simpson, E. H., Kellendonk, C., and Kandel, E. (2010) 'A possible role for the striatum in the pathogenesis of the cognitive symptoms of schizophrenia', *Neuron, 65*(5), pp. 585–596.

Skodol, A. E., Gunderson, J. G., Shea, M. T., McGlashan, T. H., Morey, L. C., Sanislow, C. A., . . . and Pagano, M. E. (2005)

'The collaborative longitudinal personality disorders study (CLPS): Overview and implications', *Journal of Personality Disorders*, *19*(5), pp. 487–504.

Smits, L. P., Bouter, K. E., de Vos, W. M., Borody, T. J., and Nieuwdorp, M. (2013) 'Therapeutic potential of fecal microbiota transplantation', *Gastroenterology*, *145*(5), pp. 946–953.

Smoski, M. J., Salsman, N., Wang, L., Smith, V., Lynch, T. R., Dager, S. R., . . . and Linehan, M. M. (2011) 'Functional imaging of emotion reactivity in opiate-dependent borderline personality disorder', *Personality Disorders: Theory, Research, and Treatment*, *2*(3), p. 230.

Soloff, P., Nutche, J., Goradia, D., and Diwadkar, V. (2008) 'Structural brain abnormalities in borderline personality disorder: a voxel-based morphometry study', *Psychiatry Research: Neuroimaging*, *164*(3), pp. 223–236.

Stanley, B., and New, A. (eds.) (2017) *'Borderline Personality Disorder*, Oxford University Press.

Stanley, B., and Siever, L. J. (2009) 'The interpersonal dimension of borderline personality disorder: toward a neuropeptide model', *American Journal of Psychiatry*, *167*(1), pp. 24–39.

Starcevic, V., and Janca, A. (2018) 'Pharmacotherapy of borderline personality disorder: replacing confusion with prudent pragmatism', *Current Opinion in Psychiatry*, *31*(1), pp. 69–73.

Steele, H., and Siever, L. (2010) 'An attachment perspective on borderline personality disorder: Advances in gene–environment considerations', *Current Psychiatry Reports*, *12*(1), pp. 61–67.

Sterzer, P., Adams, R. A., Fletcher, P., Frith, C., Lawrie, S. M., Muckli, L., . . . and Corlett, P. R. (2018) 'The predictive coding account of psychosis', *Biological Psychiatry*, *84*(9), pp. 634–643.

Stoffers-Winterling, J. M., Völlm, B. A., Rücker, G., Timmer, A., Huband, N., and Lieb, K. (2012) 'Psychological therapies for people with borderline personality disorder', *Cochrane Database of Systematic Reviews*, (8).

Strauss, G. P. (2013) 'The emotion paradox of anhedonia in schizophrenia: or is it?', *Schizophrenia bulletin*, *39*(2), pp. 247–250.

Strauss, G. P., Frank, M. J., Waltz, J. A., Kasanova, Z., Herbener, E. S., and Gold, J. M. (2011) 'Deficits in positive reinforcement learning and uncertainty-driven exploration are associated with distinct aspects of negative symptoms in schizophrenia', *Biological Psychiatry*, *69*(5), pp. 424–431.

Targum, S. D., and Keefe, R. S. (2008) 'Cognition and schizophrenia: is there a role for cognitive assessments in diagnosis and treatment?', *Psychiatry (Edgmont)*, *5*(12), p. 55.

Tomasik, J., Yolken, R. H., Bahn, S., and Dickerson, F. B. (2015) 'Immunomodulatory effects of probiotic supplementation in schizophrenia patients: a randomized, placebo-controlled trial', *Biomarker Insights*, *10*, BMI-S22007.

Torgersen, S., Myers, J., Reichborn-Kjennerud, T., Røysamb, E., Kubarych, T. S., and Kendler, K. S. (2012) 'The heritability of Cluster B personality disorders assessed both by personal interview and questionnaire', *Journal of Personality Disorders*, *26*(6), pp. 848–866.

Torrey, E. F., Bartko, J. J., and Yolken, R. H. (2012) 'Toxoplasma gondii and other risk factors for schizophrenia: an update', *Schizophrenia Bulletin*, *38*(3), pp. 642–647.

Tottenham, N., Hare, T. A., Quinn, B. T., McCarry, T. W., Nurse, M., Gilhooly, T., . . . and Thomas, K. M. (2010) 'Prolonged institutional rearing is associated with atypically large amygdala volume and difficulties in emotion regulation', *Developmental Science*, *13*(1), pp. 46–61.

Trull, T. J., Jahng, S., Tomko, R. L., Wood, P. K., and Sher, K. J. (2010) 'Revised NESARC personality disorder diagnoses: gender, prevalence, and comorbidity with substance dependence disorders', *Journal of Personality Disorders*, *24*(4), pp. 412–426.

Ustohal, L. (ed.) (2018) *Transcranial Magnetic Stimulation in Neuropsychiatry*, BoD–Books on Demand.

Voigt, J., Carpenter, L., and Leuchter, A. (2017) 'Cost effectiveness analysis comparing repetitive transcranial magnetic stimulation to antidepressant medications after a first treatment failure for major depressive disorder in newly diagnosed patients–A lifetime analysis', *PLoS One*, *12*(10).

Völlm, B. A., Chadwick, K., Abdelrazek, T., and Smith, J. (2012) 'Prescribing of psychotropic medication for personality disordered patients in secure forensic settings', *The Journal of Forensic Psychiatry and Psychology*, *23*(2), pp. 200–216.

Wacker, J., Dillon, D. G., and Pizzagalli, D. A. (2009) 'The role of the nucleus accumbens and rostral anterior cingulate cortex in anhedonia: integration of resting EEG, fMRI, and volumetric techniques', *Neuroimage*, *46*(1), pp. 327–337.

Walsh, C., Ryan, P., and Flynn, D. (2018) 'Exploring dialectical behaviour therapy clinicians' experiences of team consultation meetings', *Borderline Personality Disorder and Emotion Dysregulation*, *5*(1), p. 3.

Wang, L., Ross, C. A., Zhang, T., Dai, Y., Zhang, H., Tao, M., . . . and Xiao, Z. (2012) 'Frequency of borderline personality disorder among psychiatric outpatients in Shanghai', *Journal of Personality Disorders*, *26*(3), pp. 393–401.

Wang, M., Yang, Y., Wang, C. J., Gamo, N. J., Jin, L. E., Mazer, J. A., . . . and Arnsten, A. F. (2013) 'NMDA receptors subserve persistent neuronal firing during working memory in dorsolateral prefrontal cortex', *Neuron*, *77*(4), pp. 736–749.

Watson, R. R. (ed.) (2014) *Omega-3 Fatty Acids in Brain and Neurological Health*, Elsevier.

Wedig, M. M., Frankenburg, F. R., Reich, D. B., Fitzmaurice, G., and Zanarini, M. C. (2013) 'Predictors of suicide threats in patients with borderline personality disorder over 16 years of prospective follow-up', *Psychiatry Research*, *208*(3), pp. 252–256.

Weniger, G., Lange, C., Sachsse, U., and Irle, E. (2009) 'Reduced amygdala and hippocampus size in trauma-exposed women with borderline personality disorder and without posttraumatic stress disorder', *Journal of Psychiatry and Neuroscience*, 34, pp. 383–388

Widiger, T. A. (ed.) (2012) *The Oxford Handbook of Personality Disorders*. Oxford University Press.

Wilcox, M. H., McGovern, B. H., and Hecht, G. A. (2020) 'The Efficacy and Safety of Fecal Microbiota Transplant for Recurrent Clostridium difficile infection: Current Understanding and Gap Analysis', in *Open Forum Infectious Diseases*, Vol. 7, No. 5, p. ofaa114. US: Oxford University Press.

Williams, L. M. (2016) 'Precision psychiatry: a neural circuit taxonomy for depression and anxiety', *The Lancet Psychiatry*, *3*(5), pp. 472–480.

Wingenfeld, K., Spitzer, C., Rullkötter, N., and Löwe, B. (2010) 'Borderline personality disorder: hypothalamus pituitary adrenal axis and findings from neuroimaging studies', *Psychoneuroendocrinology*, *35*(1), pp. 154–170.

Winograd, G., Cohen, P., and Chen, H. (2008) 'Adolescent borderline symptoms in the community: prognosis for functioning over 20 years', *Journal of Child Psychology and Psychiatry*, *49*(9), pp. 933–941.

Woodworth, M. H., Hayden, M. K., Young, V. B., and Kwon, J. H. (2019) 'The role of fecal microbiota transplantation in reducing intestinal colonization with antibiotic-resistant organisms: the current landscape and future directions', in *Open Forum Infectious Diseases*, Vol. 6, No. 7, p. ofz288. US: Oxford University Press.

Yang, I., Corwin, E. J., Brennan, P. A., Jordan, S., Murphy, J. R., and Dunlop, A. (2016) *Implications for Infant Health and Neurocognitive Development*.

Yin, D. M., Chen, Y. J., Sathyamurthy, A., Xiong, W. C., and Mei, L. (2012) 'Synaptic dysfunction in schizophrenia', in *Synaptic Plasticity*, pp. 493–516. Springer, Vienna.

Yoon, J. H., Westphal, A. J., Minzenberg, M. J., Niendam, T., Ragland, J. D., Lesh, T., . . . and Carter, C. S. (2014)

'Task-evoked substantia nigra hyperactivity associated with prefrontal hypofunction, prefrontonigral disconnectivity and nigrostriatal connectivity predicting psychosis severity in medication naïve first episode schizophrenia', *Schizophrenia Research, 159*(2–3), pp. 521–526.

Yoshimatsu, K., and Palmer, B. (2014) 'Depression in patients with borderline personality Disorder', *Harvard Review of Psychiatry, 22*(5), pp. 266–273.

Zanarini, M. C., Frankenburg, F. R., Reich, D. B., and Fitzmaurice, G. (2010) 'Time to the attainment of recovery from borderline personality disorder and stability of recovery: A 10-year prospective follow-up study', *American Journal of Psychiatry, 167*(6), pp. 663–667.

Zanarini, M. C., Frankenburg, F. R., Reich, D. B., Harned, A. L., and Fitzmaurice, G. M. (2015) 'Rates of psychotropic medication use reported by borderline patients and axis II comparison subjects over 16 years of prospective follow-up', *Journal of Clinical Psychopharmacology, 35*(1), p. 63. 'English 11-year-olds and 34,653 American adults', *Journal of Personality Disorders, 25*(5), pp. 607–619.

Zanarini, M. C., Frankenburg, F. R., Reich, D. B., Harned, A. L., and Fitzmaurice, G. M. (2015) 'Rates of psychotropic medication use reported by borderline patients and axis II comparison subjects over 16 years of prospective follow-up', *Journal of Clinical Psychopharmacology, 35*(1), p. 63.

Zanarini, M. C., Horwood, J., Wolke, D., Waylen, A., Fitzmaurice, G., and Grant, B. F. (2011) 'Prevalence of *DSM*-IV borderline personality disorder in two community samples: 6,330'.

Zhang, F., Luo, W., Shi, Y., Fan, Z., and Ji, G. (2012) 'Should we standardize the 1,700-year-old fecal microbiota transplantation?', *American Journal of Gastroenterology, 107*(11), p. 1755.

Zhou, C., Zhang, H., Qin, Y., Tian, T., Xu, B., Chen, J., . . . and Lian, B. (2018) 'A systematic review and meta-analysis of deep brain stimulation in treatment-resistant depression',

Progress in Neuro-Psychopharmacology and Biological Psychiatry, 82, pp. 224–232.

Zhuo, C., Zhu, J., Qin, W., Qu, H., Ma, X., and Yu, C. (2017) 'Cerebral blood flow alterations specific to auditory verbal hallucinations in schizophrenia], *The British Journal of Psychiatry, 210*(3), pp. 209–215.

Zimmerman, M., Chelminski, I., and Young, D. (2008) 'The frequency of personality disorders in psychiatric patients', *Psychiatric Clinics of North America, 31*(3), pp. 405–420.

INDEX

M

macrophages 84, 91, 94-5, 97, 101, 105, 118-19, 124

magnesium 61-2

MAOIs (monoamine oxidase inhibitors) 341-2, 370

MBCT (mindfulness-based cognitive therapy) 165-7, 208-9, 213

medications
  adjunctive 332
  antidepressant 131, 148, 187, 192, 383, 418, 518
  antipsychotic 12, 210
  opioid 129

melancholia 6-8, 109, 366

melatonin v, 21, 37, 109, 112, 114, 157

melatonin levels 157

melatonin production 114, 162

memory cells 85-6, 108

memory loss 67, 384

mental disorders 1, 4, 9, 43-4, 47-8, 71-2, 81, 92, 99-100, 109, 119, 127, 186, 201, 211-12, 223, 231-3, 256, 271, 273, 289, 293, 334, 338-9, 349, 351, 366, 369, 375, 380, 382-3, 400, 440, 448, 459, 467, 469, 471, 482, 487, 490
  severe 339, 380, 383, 490

mental health xi, 2, 23, 31, 70, 87, 159, 173, 176, 178, 193, 198, 202, 204-5, 208, 212-13, 228, 234, 345, 467, 477, 479, 509

mental health disorders 204, 229, 231, 234, 336, 346, 370, 375, 444, 459, 462, 464, 476, 479, 486

mental health practitioners 1, 4, 73, 75, 193, 221, 223, 234, 377, 382

mentalisation 248, 323-4

metabolism 6, 114, 269, 341, 477

metabolites 124, 457, 485

methadone 133-9

microbes 89, 108, 175, 456-8, 472, 484

microbiome vii, 48, 174, 468-9, 474, 477, 488, 501

microbiota 457, 460, 468, 474, 477-8, 485, 489, 507, 509

microorganisms 177, 456, 458, 477

mindfulness 6, 165-7, 201, 208-9, 245, 318

mindset, positive 8, 55, 61

minerals 62, 173-4, 179

misdiagnosis vi, 231, 234, 343

monoamine oxidase inhibitors 182, 341, 370, 469

monocytes 83-4, 97, 103, 105

moodiness 31, 59, 227

morbidity 186, 191, 448

morphine 133, 137-8

morphology 197, 204, 304

MRI (magnetic resonance imaging) 275, 290, 304, 402, 436, 491

mu-opioid receptors 127-8, 130, 133-4, 138, 148

muscles 6, 29, 34, 36, 52, 55-6, 63, 65-6, 94, 173-4, 342

N

naloxone 126-7, 129, 134, 146, 151

naltrexone 127, 148, 202

narcissism vi, xi-xii, 239, 242-3

narcissists 239-44

nausea 129, 150-1, 340, 344, 365, 392, 398, 469

neglect 219-20, 226, 230

nerve cells 12, 39, 81, 112, 133, 138, 156

nerves 39, 69, 80, 393-5

nervous system 48-9, 68-9, 80, 104, 120, 198, 365, 393
  parasympathetic 52, 69, 71
  sympathetic 49, 52, 63, 69

neurobiology 206, 364, 440, 476

pharmacotherapy 183, 202, 280, 315-16, 334-5, 338, 346, 348, 357, 365, 370, 376-7, 384, 410, 504
phencyclidine 452
pituitary gland 30, 32, 49, 268-9
plasma 108
plasma levels 114, 124, 503
plasticity 64, 309, 311, 456, 462, 468
  neuronal 212, 462-3, 509
  synaptic 35, 64, 464-5, 468, 489, 504, 519
pollutants, airborne 197
polypharmacy 336, 347, 349
prebiotics vii, 458, 461, 496, 514
prefrontal cortex 28-9, 34, 37, 39, 128, 163, 198, 264-6, 275, 300, 374, 387, 402, 411, 452-4, 463, 483, 491, 505
  dorsolateral 371, 373, 409, 450, 465, 502, 518
  medial 163, 397
probiotics vii, 174, 458, 462, 483-6, 490, 496, 506, 514
procrastination 57, 446
prostaglandins 78-9
proteins 38-9, 51, 53, 84-5, 103, 112, 114, 116, 173-4, 176, 462, 481
psychiatric disorders 44, 123, 130, 160, 186, 199, 229, 274, 352, 364-6, 368-9, 375, 377, 380-3, 391-3, 398, 402, 408, 457, 459, 462, 465, 467-9, 476-7, 482, 484, 486, 490, 499
psychiatric patients 179, 262, 286, 363, 376-7, 386, 395, 420, 486, 521
psychiatric symptoms 392, 476-7, 482
psychiatrists 218-20, 326, 338, 340, 348, 377, 393
psychoeducation 18, 231, 325, 332
psychological therapies 284, 329, 338, 361, 417, 516
psychologists 171-2, 321, 323

psychopathologists 293
psychosis 11, 125, 293, 311, 424-5, 427, 441, 446, 467-8, 496, 505, 510, 515-16
psychosocial therapies 183-4, 329
psychotherapies 5, 8, 10, 18, 20, 158, 171-2, 184, 195, 279, 315-17, 326-7, 329, 331, 334, 337, 339, 345, 347-8, 356-7, 364-5, 370, 376, 378, 382-4, 394, 404-5, 408-9, 437, 447, 493, 495, 499, 503
  supportive 331, 333-4
PTSD (post-traumatic stress disorder) vii, xi, 221, 231, 234-5, 265-6, 272, 354, 404, 421-2, 424-8, 431-2, 434-5
  symptoms of xii, 422, 426-7, 433-4
pulse generator 381-2, 395-6, 398
pyrazinamide 124

Q

quinolinic acid v, 112, 118-21, 124-5
  high levels of 120
  production of 119, 121
quinolinic acid levels 119-20, 124-5

R

rage 47, 225, 241
receptors 5, 34, 41, 95, 97, 106, 127, 129-31, 133-4, 136-9, 199, 269, 450, 456, 485
  delta-opioid 126-7, 138
  ionotropic 451
  mu 126, 129, 134, 136-8, 148
relapse 22, 141, 145, 160, 162, 165, 168, 182-3, 185, 188, 209, 252, 348, 370, 382-3
relaxation 56, 65, 69, 161, 164, 180
remission 145, 250-1, 348, 370, 372, 378, 385, 387, 400, 487

www.ingramcontent.com/pod-product-compliance
Lightning Source LLC
Chambersburg PA
CBHW021347210526
45463CB00001B/5